Your Aching Back

A Doctor's Guide to Relief

Augustus A. White III, MD, PhD, with Preston J. Phillips, MD, MS

Simon & Schuster Paperbacks

NEW YORK   LONDON   TORONTO   SYDNEY

Simon & Schuster Paperbacks
A Division of Simon & Schuster, Inc.
1230 Avenue of the Americas
New York, NY 10020

This Simon & Schuster trade paperback edition September 2010

SIMON & SCHUSTER PAPERBACKS and colophon are
registered trademarks of Simon & Schuster, Inc.

For information about special discounts for bulk purchases,
please contact Simon & Schuster Special Sales at
1-866-506-1949 or business@simonandschuster.com.

The Simon & Schuster Speakers Bureau can bring authors
to your live event. For more information or to book an event,
contact the Simon & Schuster Speakers Bureau at
1-866-248-3049 or visit our website at www.simonspeakers.com.

Designed by Paul Dippolito

Manufactured in the United States of America

1 3 5 7 9 10 8 6 4 2

Library of Congress Cataloging-in-Publication Data
White, Augustus A.
Your aching back : a doctor's guide to relief / Augustus A. White, III,
with Preston J. Phillips. Updated and rev. ed.
p.   cm.
Includes bibliographical references and index.   1. Backache.   I. Title.
RD771.B217W49   2010
617.5'64—dc22   2009047789

ISBN 978-1-4165-9301-0

Dr. A. A. White wishes to disclose that he is a member of the Board of Directors of
Orthologic Corp. (Capstone, Inc.) and was a member of Zimmer Holdings 2001–2010.

Dedicated with enthusiasm to all our family,
friends, and patients past, present, and future

—A. A. W.
and
—P. J. P.

Contents

Acknowledgments

It is impossible to acknowledge all of those very important individuals who are part of our community, who in a direct and indirect manner have created an environment conducive to the completion of this work. The goal of this body of work is to aid those seeking proper CARE for their special conditions. We believe that in order to CARE for people, one must CARE for each person. Our hope is that this book will serve as a tool that can be used in such a manner. We acknowledge the CARE and support that we have received from the institutions in which we work and the extended family members thereof, the diligence of our agent, and the professionalism of our publisher. We gratefully and humbly extend a warm thank-you.

Dear Reader:

The advice and suggestions presented here represent our best opinion based on updated contemporary scientific and clinical knowledge, as well as the experience gleaned from many years of practice. While we fully believe that the information is useful and the advice is the same as would be given to family, friends, and ourselves, nevertheless, there can be no guarantees about your back condition. It could get better or worse with time. If you choose to follow the advice presented here, *you* must assume full responsibility.

There may be instances where the offered opinion differs from what you have been told by your own physician. He/she has examined you and knows your unique situation. When there is a discrepancy, follow the advice of your own doctor, in whom you have confidence, or, if you are unsure, consult another doctor. The information and advice provided here are accurate and reliable for *most* people, but any individual patient can be an exception.

Sincerely,
A. A. White III, MD, PhD,
and P. J. Phillips, MD, MS

Introduction

Raison d'Être

During many years as a physician, I have found low back pain to be one of the most complex and troubling problems to handle. If that's so for me, it's doubly or triply true for my patients, the backache sufferers themselves. It is for you, my backache sufferers, that this book is written and dedicated.

I'm writing this book to tell those of you with back problems what scientific and clinical research has substantiated to be *true* about backache. Unfortunately, as many of you may have already discovered, there's a tangle of confusion and misunderstanding surrounding low back pain. And sometimes the diagnosis, or the treatment, is just plain wrong. I will try to be clear and simple, but I won't withhold important concepts and facts just because they are technical or complex. I think it's to your benefit to be exposed to all the relevant and current knowledge on this topic.

I'm working on the assumption that, all things being equal, it's better to know the truth. This book has several purposes. It will help you understand the cause and prevention of back pain. The contents are selected so as to inform you as to what you can expect once you get a backache. It will tell you about the diagnosis and treatment of back problems and provide information to help you to decide among treatment options. There are numerous specific tips to help you ease the difficulties associated with a bad back. Knowing the facts is your best ammunition. For many of you, the knowledge and understanding provided here will spell relief from your problems.

This book contains the necessary information to keep you "out of trouble," should you get a backache. Forewarned is forearmed.* Finally, I want

---

* *Checklists* designed to summarize specific key information that you may want or need at a particular time have been provided.

you to get this message and theme: *Things take time.* Please be assured that you won't have backache forever. You will gradually get better. Be patient. You will gradually get better.

How to Read This Book

People should read books however they please. Nevertheless, here are some thoughts that will help you get the most out of this book. I suggest that you skim through the entire book very quickly. You can even limit yourself to the pictures and captions the first time through. This will give you an overview: a perspective of what the book may do for you, and a preview of the various treatment strategies available for dealing with your particular back problem. I would then suggest that you read the book again, this time carefully picking out the parts of special interest to you. These parts should be read in depth and studied. Having done that, you should read the whole thing through once more. This will allow you another opportunity to pick up on points that may be especially meaningful for you. If there are times when you get a bit more information than is absolutely necessary, be patient. I decided that it would be better to overestimate your interest and inquisitiveness than to underestimate it.

The annotated bibliography at the end of the book is almost completely from the medical literature. The most important new references have been included. The articles vary in the amount of technical terminology they use. However, those readers interested in delving deeper into a particular topic presented in this book will be put well on their way by the references listed. Most public libraries can now provide medical literature through interlibrary loan programs. These references are also a way of reminding you that you're not just getting "one man's opinion"; there is a lot of evidence to back up the information that is being offered to help you.

I wish you the best. I *know* that the information here will help you *some*—and I *trust* that it will help you a *great deal!*

Your
Aching
Back

— CHAPTER 1 —

Who Suffers?

TRY LISTING THE NAMES OF TEN ADULT FRIENDS AT RAN-dom. If seven of them are backache victims, and only three are free of the sufferings addressed in this book, they are a typical set of persons. If you are one of the seven unfortunates (and the fact that you are opening this book means you probably are), the problem becomes acutely personal in terms of pain and inconvenience. However, if this is a new backache, there is an 85 percent chance that you will be just fine within the next four to five weeks. Nonetheless, there is the risk of recurrence, if one considers the natural history of back pain.

In any case, you are not alone. In the Western world, epidemiological studies reveal that back pain afflicts a staggering 65 percent to 85 percent of the population. Out of every ten people under forty-five who have chronic medical conditions limiting their activities, four are victims of back or spine pain. Backache takes a backseat only to headache as the most common medical complaint, and is second only to the common cold as a reason for missed work. In fact, absence from the workplace due to disabling back pain has soared.

There was a fourteenfold increase in the prevalence of low back pain in the United States between 1970 and 1981, and even more of an increase in England and Sweden. Unfortunately, 5 percent of the total population will complain of low back pain in a given year, including 15 percent of adults. Furthermore, *sciatica* (pain down the leg) may be associated with back pain. Two in five adults will experience sciatica at some point in their lives.

A sore back becomes even more sobering when you realize how often it can become chronic, debilitating, and life diminishing. Chronic symptoms develop in 5 percent to 10 percent of patients. If you are laboring under a difficult back, you do not need to be reminded. However, consider

1

the following: If you're a worker who is absent from work with a bad back for more than six months, statistics indicate that you have only a 50 percent chance of ever regaining full productivity. Individual, genetic, social, and occupational factors are significant contributors to this fact; nonetheless, after one year, your chances dip to 25 percent. Add the high cost of treatment, and you have a more graphic portrait of the social and financial sufferings involved. In 1998, the average bad-back episode would have cost you $9,000, according to data from the Liberty Mutual Insurance Company. The cost of diagnosing and treating back pain in the United States exceeds $20 billion annually, and when we include lost productivity, disability payments, workmen's compensation insurance, and lawsuits, that figure soars to in excess of $90 billion. A Texas oil company study revealed that new hires with a preemployment history of a back injury were 50 percent more likely to be reinjured. Such data have disturbing implications when one considers the current desire of employers to minimize their workers' compensation exposure.

Here is one more way you can grasp the magnitude of the financial problem. The U.S. Postal Service is one of the largest employers in the country. There was a time when we paid 20 cents for a first-class stamp. Can you guess how much of that 20 cents was applied to cost of providing back pain medical care and related expenses for postal employees? Approximately 5 percent, or 1 cent per stamp! The U.S. Postal Service paid $830 million in workers' compensation in 2004. Nationally, fewer than 25 percent of the cases of low back pain generate 75 percent of the cost.

The purpose of reviewing this statistical data is not to depress you but rather to convince you that back pain is a major social problem. Of equal or greater importance are facts that cannot always be expressed in numbers: the profound human suffering and compromised quality of life that back pain sufferers experience. It is ironic to learn that the great work of Florence Nightingale, the nineteenth-century British nurse, was prematurely halted by illness. She was bedridden for thirty years. Among other ailments, she suffered from back pain and sciatica. The leading spinal specialist of that period, Dr. Charles-Édouard Brown-Séquard, arrived at a diagnosis of "congestion of the spine." Nightingale's writings to her mother reveal that she longed for death or amputation of her left leg due to the unrelenting pain.

Why is the human back such a vulnerable, annoying, and frequently painful part of the anatomy? Has it always been thus? Certainly, the spine has been a preoccupation for centuries—as attested to by sayings such as "He's a spineless person," "She really has her back up about it," "He's got a yellow streak down his back," and "She's carrying the team on her back." William Shakespeare aficionados will recall the insinuating words of Iago, the villain of *Othello*, who whispers to Desdemona's father: "Your daughter and the Moor [her husband, Othello] are now making the beast with two backs"—Elizabethan jargon for sexual intercourse. Perhaps echoing the Elizabethans, Jamaican men complaining of impotence will say that they have "lost the strength of their backs." Treachery, we know, is conveyed as a "stab in the back," and paranoia in the phrase "They're laughing behind my back." We could go on cataloguing spinal metaphors in art and life, but if you are lying on a painful back or "with your back against the wall," you will probably want to get to the treatment/prevention chapter pretty quick.

Some researchers have reflected that we humans have only recently evolved into two-legged creatures, and that staying on all fours might have saved us from backaches. There are several problems with this theory. Reversion to four-legged locomotion would require some radical lifestyle changes— perhaps driving shoemakers out of business or placing undue market demands on glove and knee-pad manufacturers. Besides, animals also have back pain; they just do not complain to us about it. Most important is the fact that the hypothesis does not fit the anatomic and evolutionary facts: Our spines are perfectly suited for an upright stance and do not differ significantly from those of our hominid ancestors. Finally, even though there are sexual problems associated with backache (see chapter 8), back problems could not play a part in the evolutionary process because the genes can readily be passed on well before the age by which the incidence of backache is more prevalent—usually in one's thirties.

If we are to look for reasons for the epidemic of back pain, we would do better to examine the quality of our lives: specifically, what we do with our backs. The increasingly sedentary lifestyle in Western industrialized countries has been hypothesized, on a molecular basis, to contribute to the prevalence of back pain. Frankly, even an extensive analysis of all the data does not provide a simple, clear answer. Nevertheless, you will certainly acquire a better understanding, so read on!

Who's at Risk?

Of course, if you are a backache sufferer, your interest is this book is more apt to be personal than sociological. How do the back pain statistics apply to you? How is your type of backache categorized? What are your risk factors and how can you reduce them? One of the goals of this book is to provide this information, along with specific recommendations for managing your back condition on the job and at home. The next section outlines facts gathered from various studies and can help you calculate your risks, because we now understand that gender, age, occupation, leisure activities, and lifestyle all influence the state of your back.

Organized medicine has utilized the scientific method in conjunction with clinical experience, testing, and outcome analysis to pursue the best course of treatment. You may have heard the phrase *evidence-based medicine*. This refers to a concerted effort to improve our decision-making process through structured review, critique, and stratification of strength of the data. These data/studies are assigned a level (level I to level V) based upon the quality of the methods and study design versus that of case reports and expert opinion. The objective is to minimize and/or recognize bias in the information presented, in an effort to arrive at a reproducible high-quality outcome following a course of treatment. Such an approach allows for a more objective assessment of the associated risks and benefits. Level I evidence is gleaned from highly crafted randomized controlled prospective clinical trials. At the other end of the spectrum is Level V data, yielded from expert opinion. This allows for a judicious use of the best available evidence.

Age

Back pain patients tend to seek out their doctors for the first time between the ages of thirty and fifty-five. Why? Simply put, the discs between the vertebrae (bones) of your lower back (figure 1.1) change during the normal course of aging. The young disc is elastic and the cells have a high water content. However, starting at about age thirty, the disc gradually becomes desiccated and scarred, which changes its mechanical properties. This change makes it more susceptible to fragmentation, rupture, or herniation (shifting out of place), causing pain. The disc is analogous to a jelly doughnut. When it's fresh, the pastry is pliable and resilient, and the center contains jelly. As it ages, the outer portion hardens, becomes more brittle, cracks, and flakes. The jelly in the middle dries out. The puzzle is that while all discs undergo this transformation, not all cause pain, and certainly all do not herniate.

Interestingly, the risk of back pain episodes decreases for men after age fifty, but not for women. This is because of the problem of osteoporosis, which is more prevalent in the aging woman. Osteoporosis affects men as well and increases their risk of back pain. In the next section, gender-related issues and low back pain will be discussed further.

Gender

Epidemiological studies suggest that men are slightly more prone to developing herniated discs. They are also more likely than women to undergo surgery for disc problems of equal severity. A herniated disc is an abnormality whereby the central part of the disc moves out from its normal position between the vertebral bodies, causing severe back and/or leg pain. Perhaps the differences in occupation and athletics and the amount of driving account for these male tendencies, rather than genetics. Another factor to consider is the possibility that men simply tolerate pain poorly and are thus more afflicted, resulting in their being more likely to end up with the most rigorous treatment.

On the female side, elderly women are at greatest risk for developing osteoporosis. This condition results in a loss of bone density, weakens the vertebrae, and sometimes causes them to collapse. The relative risks are even greater for a woman who has had more than two full-term pregnancies. Hormonal changes after menopause have been deemed responsible. There is evidence that estrogen replacement therapy together with adequate vitamin D and sunlight, dietary calcium, vigorous physical activity, and exposure to fluorides can be of help in treating osteoporosis. Treatment of osteoporosis may also include the use of bisphosphonates such as alendronate (Fosamax) or the recombinant parathyroid hormone teriparatide (Forteo).

Full-term pregnancy is notoriously hard on the lower back. For one thing, it brings with it mechanical problems such as increased weight and a protruding abdomen that combine to shift the mother-to-be's center of gravity forward. Such conditions place additional stress on her back. Levels of the hormones relaxin, estrogen, progesterone, and cortisol increase during pregnancy. Relaxin has been implicated in pregnancy-related low back pain due to its effect of increasing ligament and joint laxity in the pelvis and lumbar spine. Such an effect results in greater joint mobility and diminished ligament tensile strength, undermining the back's mechanical strength. Back pain during pregnancy should be evaluated to ensure that the unborn child is stable and to screen for other potential coexisting medical conditions. After her child is born, the mother will have to take repeated trips to an appropriate changing table and so forth. The new mother should learn the proper biomechanics of lifting, outlined in chapter 2.

An abnormal forward displacement of the vertebra can occur due to a variety of reasons. The condition is called *spondylolisthesis* (pronounced: SPON-dil-low-lis-THESIS) and will be discussed in greater detail in chapter 3. This condition can result in worsening back pain during pregnancy. A type of arthritis of the spine can also cause this condition. It is known as degenerative spondylolisthesis. The degenerative form is four times more common in women. I am sorry, folks, but the reason for this finding remains to be discovered.

Heredity

Certain back problems seem to run in families, such as intervertebral disc disease, forms of spondylolisthesis, and scoliosis, to name a few. Data suggest that racial differences may be a factor in certain situations. American whites, for example, are overall more prone to spondylolisthesis than African-Americans. However, a study has indicated that African-American women age sixty-five years or older have a higher incidence of spondylolisthesis than white women in a similar age group. The prevalence was lower in women on estrogen replacement therapy. Eskimos have about a ten times greater tendency to develop the disease than whites. The basis for these "hereditary" differences remains unclear.

There is evidence that herniated disc problems run in families. There may be a hereditary predisposition in the chemical makeup of the disc that makes it more likely to fragment and move out of its normal anatomic position and cause nerve irritation.

Occupation

You cannot do very much about your sex, age, or race, but you can change your job. The other option is to alter some of the tasks that your job requires you to perform, when necessary. This is fortunate, since your job may affect your back more than anything else.

People who spend at least half their time on the job driving a motor vehicle are three times more likely than the average worker to suffer a herniated disc. This fact has some cogent and interesting associated observations. A key issue here is that of road vibrations. Most vehicles vibrate in a range of 4.5 Hz to 5.0 Hz, or cycles per second. The first resonant frequency (that frequency likely to cause perturbation or damage) of our spines is in the same range. Laboratory tests have shown that vibrating the spine at this frequency range can damage the spine and cause disc herniation. Vibration in this range has also been shown experimentally to increase the production of pain-causing substances. To put it simply, most cars, buses, and trucks vibrate at 4.5 to 5.0 cycles per second. This is a range that can damage the spine, potentially leading to back pain and disc herniation. The reader should know that some Swedish and Japanese cars do not vibrate at 4.5 to 5.0 cycles per second.

Sedentary occupations in general are bad news for your back, as sitting puts great pressure on the discs between the vertebrae. The concerns regarding driving and the low back are the prolonged sitting without changing position and, more important, a spine constantly jarred by vibrations. Cabbies, truck drivers, bus drivers, train conductors, beware: Your job could be hazardous to your back. Chapter 6 is full of helpful advice, should you be one of these at-risk individuals.

It takes about five years for sedentary occupations or damaging leisure pursuits to do their evil work on your back. Weekend sitting, for example, has been linked to herniated disc disease in men, a fact that spouses of football sofa warriors may find useful as ammunition. Obviously, most office jobs fall into the sedentary category. Therefore administrative assistants, accountants, lawyers, academicians, computer programmers, and middle managers alike would do well to change position during the day, stand, walk to appointments, and relax from time to time.

However, if you get off your backside to spare your back, do not turn around and lift the big box of files, either. Jobs involving heavy lifting and twisting, pulling, or carrying probably lead to lumbar disc disease. Sudden unexpected bouts of lifting—as when you're helping a friend move his piano, and he lets go—appear to be followed by complaints of acute (new onset) back pain leading to visits to doctors' offices. Certainly, for those engaged in heavy manual labor, the risk factors include the weight lifted, frequency of lifting, as well as improper lifting and body mechanics. These all go hand in hand when considering the onset of low back pain. Is it a coincidence that heavy-industrial workers, farmers, nurses, and nurse's aides are more often afflicted with bad backs than most of us? Based on experience, one would also have to put the following occupations in the high-risk group: firefighters, police officers, and emergency medical technicians. They must perform extensive lifting quickly and often without proper positioning. An additional consideration: Twisting injuries are often associated with back pain and disc damage.

One noteworthy condition that appears to be an occupational hazard is degenerative disc disease of the lumbar spine. The term is unfortunate, as it sounds as though we were moldering away and falling apart inside. Actually, lumbar disc degeneration is probably little more than normal wearing of the spine. The X-rays reveal to the doctor a narrowed disc space and osteophyte (bony outgrowth, or spur) formation. As people age, these changes tend to show up on the X-rays of half of all women and about 70 percent of men. However, mechanical stress does appear to hasten the process. Miners, dockworkers, and outdoor laborers such as farmers and road workers are at higher risk, while that of sedentary workers appears to be significantly less.

A similar problem is arthritis or degenerative changes in the *facet joints.* Facet joint arthritis can result in the onset of low back pain. See figure 1.1 to understand facet joints. Two facets from adjacent vertebrae come together, along with a joint capsule, to form a facet joint. Arthritis of the facet joints can come on with age, although it can occur independently of degenerative disc changes. Degenerative changes in the facet joints have been observed in miners and even more frequently in obese individuals.

In summary, here is how Dr. Gunnar Anderson of Rush Medical College, in Chicago, has mapped out the occupational danger signals for your back:

1. Physically heavy work
2. Static work postures
3. Frequent bending and twisting

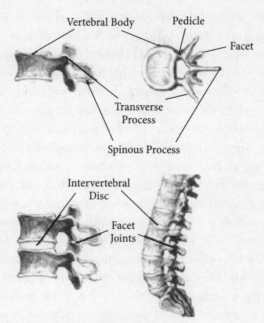

FIGURE 1.1. Basic Anatomy of the Lumbar Vertebrae

4. Lifting and forceful movements
5. Repetitive work (such as assembly-line occupations)
6. Vibrations

In chapter 5, you will learn how to minimize the wear and tear on your back at home and on the job.

Sociological Risks

Back in the 1960s, we doctors cared for a number of patients who complained of back pain associated with a new dance craze called the twist. To the rock-and-roll beat of Chubby Checker and others, the twist dancer held his upper torso relatively fixed while rotating the pelvis as vigorously as possible about the long axis of the body. Nowadays, twist injuries are as rare as smallpox, although one wonders about the effects on the lumbar spine of gyrations, break dancing, hip-hop, step dancing, dirty dancing, modern ballroom, and certain Latin/Afro-Cuban dances, as well as acrobatics and gymnastics.

In a more sober vein, some studies have linked the tendency to take sick leave from work to lower educational level, lower intelligence, and lower socioeconomic status. Workers with a low sense of self-importance, or those who describe their jobs as boring, dissatisfying, and repetitious, are also more apt to stay in bed with backaches. These fellow humans should not be patronized but must be treated with compassion and careful attention to the quality of their work life. Of course, pain can also be a signal of depression. The onset of back pain can also be associated with various life situational stressors: seeking and obtaining a promotion, a vacation, receiving an honor, the loss of a friend and/or loved one, loss of a job, or the necessity to relocate to a new city. Recently, psychiatrists have reported that a sadomasochistic patient may complain of spine pain in the hopes of obtaining a surgical procedure. As in the notorious psychiatric disorder Munchausen syndrome, in which a patient feigns illness and achieves a collection of surgical scars, these patients are usually found to be free of disease when their backs are needlessly opened up.

Cultural factors also play a role in low back pain, or lack thereof. Backache appears to be far less common in cultures in which the squatting position is common. Squatting curves the lumbar spine into a slightly flexed position, in contrast to the Western mode of standing and sitting, where the lumbar spine curves in the opposite, slightly extended direction. One study comparing X-rays of individuals from a squatting culture with those from a sitting culture noted less evidence of disc degeneration in those from the squatting culture. A second theory is that people in developing countries are less prone to back problems because they work harder, walk more, and lead less sedentary lives. Therefore, they are presumed to be in better physical condition. Nevertheless, although the evidence for both theories remains meager, it is thought provoking.

Body Build and Posture

"For heaven's sake, stand up straight, or you'll get a bad back!" your parents may have innocently instructed you. Well, parental dogmas notwithstanding, most studies maintain that there is no real connection between voluntary posture and back pain. A flat back and a slumped back are equal in the eyes of the spine. Mild scoliosis, or sideways curvature of the spine, is probably unrelated to back pain, although severe lumbar *lateral* (sideways) curvature probably is hard on your back.

An interesting study allowed by an outdated tradition helps to prove this point. The postures of students attending certain women's colleges in the eastern United States were carefully evaluated. As part of the study, they were photographed standing nude, to permit an unencumbered evaluation of posture. A careful study of the pictures of the classes of 1957, 1958, and 1959, as well as a review of the department of physical education's written evaluations, led to the following conclusion: Posture, neither good nor bad, was in no way associated with a higher or lower incidence of low back pain over a twenty-five-year period.

Also, contrary to folklore, moderate differences in leg length (as much as three-fourths of an inch) are inconsequential to your back.

As for body build, most studies support the contention that there is not a strong correlation between height, weight, body build, and backache. The importance of exercise therapy in the treatment of chronic low back pain has been shown to be beneficial. Although researchers do not always agree, a few studies have shown a tendency for tall and obese people to develop backache.

Miscellaneous Causes

A Vermont study turned up the unexpected fact that people with chronic coughs and bronchitis frequently suffer from herniated disc disease. In addition, subsequent research has implicated cigarette smoking in disc disease and low back pain. Here is yet another health negative for smokers: There is pretty good evidence that nicotine interferes with the blood flow to the vertebral body and around the disc. This may cause abnormalities in the normal biological function and nutrition of the disc, as well as its ability to recover from injury, thus contributing to back pain.

The size and shape of your spinal canal (the space through which the spinal cord passes) may predispose you to develop sciatica (leg pain and weakness that may or may not be associated with back pain). When the canal is small or triangular in shape, the nerves that can cause sciatica are more easily irritated. This will be outlined in greater detail in chapter 3.

Perhaps after perusing the last few pages, you have concluded that the most likely candidate for back pain is a socially maladjusted male truck driver who is tall and does a lot of loading and unloading during his work-

Relationship of Certain Risk Factors to Lumbar Disc Disease or Low Back Pain

Well-Established Risks

- Age greater than thirty
- Driving motor vehicles more than two hours a day
- Exposure to vibrations
- Cigarette smoking
- Osteoporosis
- Standing, carrying, pushing, pulling, twisting, bending
- Lifting (especially if associated with twisting or with knees straight or arms extended)

Possible Risks

- Use of jackhammers
- Cross-country skiing
- Emotional stress/stressful work
- More than two full-term pregnancies
- Working as a nurse or nurse's aide
- Sedentary occupation
- Leg-length discrepancy greater than one inch.
- Race
- Baseball, golf, bowling, tennis
- Height
- Obesity

day with poor lifting techniques. It would make matters worse for him if he has a family history of low back pain, is divorced, drinks as well as smokes, does not like his job, and belongs to a lower socioeconomic stratum. If he is not particularly proud of his work and spends his weekends vegetating in front of the TV, give him up as a hopeless back pain invalid! Well, this sort of composite portrait is an improper use of statistics, of course, since each individual defies easy categorization. Many a TV-addicted, sedentary, depressed truck driver has never had a backache in his life. This characterization, of course, is presented to emphasize several points. I certainly mean no disrespect to these frequently helpful and lifesaving fellow humans of the highways.

Yet, all of the lifestyle factors that we have mentioned *can* translate into an aching back. It is best to start with a good, hard look at yourself and your life. Do not despair; soon we will tell you what you can do for your back.

CHAPTER 2

Basic Back Mechanics

*The spinal column is a long chain of bones. The head sits at
the top and you sit on the bottom.*

—ANONYMOUS

YOU MAY THINK THAT SPINAL ANATOMY IS TOO COMPLI-
cated, boring, or scary to contemplate in any depth, particularly if your
own back is acting up. Nevertheless, take heart: Many philosophers since
classical times have extolled the beauty of the human anatomy, and I just
happen to agree with them!

On a more practical note, you cannot properly operate your automobile if you do not understand its controls and instrument panel. Therefore,
consider this chapter an abbreviated owner's manual for the spine. Some
of the information may strike you as unduly technical and unsuitable for
bedtime reading. By all means, skim this section if you are in a hurry to get
to the real basics of back care. You can always use this chapter as a reference guide or dictionary. However, if you want the "nuts-and-bolts" basics,
then read on.

Does your doctor ever refer to specific anatomical structures that
sound to your ears like distant galaxies or exotic topographical points?
Well, this chapter can help you interpret your doctor's conversation, although you should always feel free to ask him or her to explain things in
plain English! The goal is to help you better understand this part of your
body and something about your troubling back as well.

The Spinal Column

The human spine is one of the most fascinating and elegant mechanical
structures in the animal kingdom. The segmented bony structures of the

spine are called *vertebrae.* The spine consists of twenty-four vertebrae plus the *sacrum* and the *coccyx,* or tailbone. (The sacrum is the triangular bone between the lowest vertebrae and the tailbone.) The rigid vertebrae are separated by cartilaginous *discs* and elastic *ligaments,* which together form the *spinal column.* The spinal cord and nerve roots are protected by the spinal column. These important structures lie with the *spinal canal* (figure 2.1). The whole structure is balanced and controlled by a complex series of muscles.

What is the function of the spinal column? What makes it so fancy, anyway? Well, first of all, it can move in many different directions with speed and agility. Secondly, it can stiffen yet remain supple enough to withstand and cushion powerful applied mechanical forces. Finally, it performs the crucial job of protecting the vital spinal cord and nerves. You might suppose that the ideal way to shield the spinal cord would be with a straight bony rod, much as the skull protects the brain. However, such a spine would not allow motion or possess the necessary protective energy-absorbing properties.

Therefore, what we have is a mobile curvaceous spine, if you will, that consists of multiple bony segments, each connected via joints, ligaments, and discs. Such a modular structure permits flexibility with strength and stability, plus superior shock-absorbing capacity. Your spine curves forward at the neck (the *cervical spine*) and lower back (*lumbar spine*), while at the midback (*thoracic spine*) and the bottom of the spine (sacrum), it curves slightly backward (figure 2.1). You may not have been aware of it, but you have probably already admired the graceful curvature of the lumbar region in some of your fellow humans.

What we call the "functional spinal unit" consists of two adjacent vertebrae and their intervening soft tissues, ligaments, discs, and muscles. Extensive research has defined the mechanical behavior of the functional spinal units, including their stiffness, flexibility, reaction to various stresses, and so on. Validated data sets are used to generate mathematical formulas that allow a computer to construct a functional model of the entire human spine. Such a model can provide information about the spine's expected mechanical behavior under conditions of normal or threshold pressures, including those that could cause failure or injury.

This futuristic mathematical model will not be like a living spine, nor will it be a replica of a particular patient's back. However, it will be a reliable portrayal of the spine's mechanical properties. As such, this model

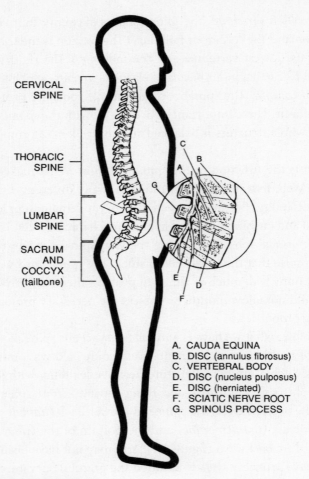

CERVICAL
SPINE

THORACIC
SPINE

LUMBAR
SPINE

SACRUM
AND
COCCYX
(tailbone)

A. CAUDA EQUINA
B. DISC (annulus fibrosus)
C. VERTEBRAL BODY
D. DISC (nucleus pulposus)
E. DISC (herniated)
F. SCIATIC NERVE ROOT
G. SPINOUS PROCESS

FIGURE 2.1. Spinal Anatomy

This anatomic picture is the key to understanding the anatomy of the spine, disc disease, and its associated leg pain. The upper portion of the spine is known as the neck, or the cervical spine; the midportion is the midback, or thoracic spine, to which the ribs are attached; and the lower region of the spine, featured in this book, is the lumbar spine, or the low back. As you can see, the nerves run from the spinal canal down toward the leg. *(COURTESY OF WELL-BEING, THE MEDICAL MAGAZINE OF BOSTON'S BETH ISRAEL HOSPITAL.)*

could provide information more effectively than actual experiments can. This model may provide some breakthrough information to help your aching back in the future. As discussed in chapter 7, current technological advances have sought to preserve, improve, or restore the mechanical properties of the functional spinal unit.

Let us examine exactly what your spine is made of and how nature has designed it.

THE LUMBAR SPINE

Since this book focuses on the lumbar spine, considered to be the major source of low back pain, let us start there.

The lumbar vertebrae have several anatomic features, the largest and most prominent being the vertebral body (figure 2.1), a cylindrical bone in which blood, fat, bone marrow, and certain fluids reside. At the top and bottom of each vertebral body are the *vertebral end plates* (figure 2.2), which are prone to fracture (often unrecognized) and are therefore one source of back pain. Connecting the posterior bony part of the vertebral body at either side of the spinal canal are tubelike bone structures called *pedicles* (figure 2.2). The spine takes its name from the *spinous processes* (figure 2.1), those familiar knobs you feel beneath your skin at the midline of your back. The base of the spinous processes and the *lamina* (figure 2.2), a thin plate of bone, complete the spinal canal's ring.

The bones of the spine also possess facet joints, which are susceptible to the same diseases as the joints of your fingers, hips, and knees. They have a *joint capsule* that contains joint fluid, or *synovial fluid* (figure 2.5). Therefore, they are synovial joints. If all this seems a bit dry and academic, do not worry. It will soon add up to a new understanding between you and your back.

THE LUMBAR DISC

Between the vertebrae sits the famous—or infamous—*lumbar disc.* The lumbar disc has an outer structure called the *annulus fibrosus,* which consists of a tough intertwining bundle of collagen fibers. The center of the disc contains less-organized jellylike collagen, the *nucleus pulposus.* The structure is similar to a jelly-filled doughnut (figure 2.3). The disc attaches to the vertebrae via the annulus peripherally and a thin cartilaginous end plate centrally. When all the intervertebral discs are measured relative to the bony vertebrae, together they constitute approximately one-third the length of your spine. The discs are also the largest organs in your body without their own blood supply. In fact, you "grow" taller while sleeping

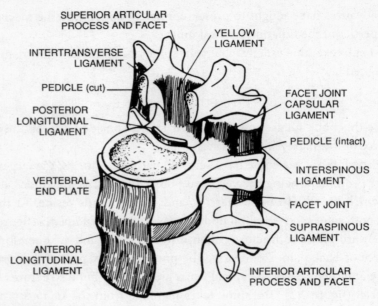

FIGURE 2.2. Ligaments of the Spine

In addition to the disc, about seven ligaments connect one vertebra to the next. The ligaments help to control the motion of the spine and prevent excessive motion. Because of their elasticity, a certain amount of motion is allowed. (*REPRODUCED WITH PERMISSION FROM WHITE, A. A., AND PANJABI, M. M.: CLINICAL BIOMECHANICS OF THE SPINE, 2ND ED., J. B. LIPPINCOTT, 1990.*)

at night, as the discs swell and accumulate water when your back is *not* subjected to the gravitational and mechanical forces in addition to the vibratory stress of your erect posture while performing daily activities. In the daytime, you "shrink" back to your normal height as this accumulated water is gradually forced out of the discs by the above-mentioned forces.

This process of daily fluid exchange serves to aide in both disc nutrition and removal of metabolic by-products. The health of the disc is dependent upon this process. The relative fluid accumulation in the disc is more pronounced in the weightless state, as our astronauts found out to their discomfiture. During their missions into space, they actually "grew" as much as two inches taller. Their height returned to normal when their spines were subjected to the normal physiologic loads and gravitational forces upon their return.

Since you probably do not need to worry about zero gravity conditions, let us get back to what concerns you. Of note, there are certain mo-

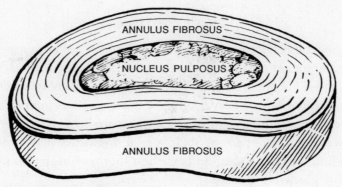

FIGURE 2.3. The Intervertebral Disc

Here we see an isolated drawing of the intervertebral disc. The central portion is the gel-like nucleus pulposus, which contains a large amount of water. The concentric layered rings are known as the annulus fibrosus. These structures change with age. The nucleus tends to dry out, and the annulus tends to become disorganized and less elastic. Any combination of the nucleus and the annulus can herniate into the spinal canal, causing pain in the back and/or leg.

dalities being advertised on television and in newspapers suggesting that the gravity-free state can be reproduced in their office using a device. One must view these claims with caution. There is evidence that biochemical changes in the disc can increase its moisture content, causing pain. Since emotional stress is reported to change body chemistry, some researchers have theorized that such may be the mechanism whereby stress produces backache. Could the effects of mental strain on disc swelling provide a partial solution to the old philosophical problem of how the mind affects the body? Possibly! More research is required.

In any case, much of the spine's strength and resilience come from the disc, especially its main structure, the annulus fibrosus ("ring of fibers" in Latin). The annulus fibrosus, composed of a tough lattice network of crossed collagen fibers, is directly attached to the bone around the periphery of vertebral end plates of the adjacent vertebrae, providing mechanical strength. The nucleus pulposus—a more elastic, soft, less-organized collagen in the center of the disc—is contained by the elliptical annulus fibers and the adjacent vertebral end plates. The beauty of this elegant structure is that the disc is designed for efficient energy absorption. It is the spine's "shock absorber," which we will discuss further in the biomechanics section of this chapter.

FACET JOINTS

The gliding joints between the vertebrae, along the posterior aspect of the spinal column, are called the facet joints, or facet articulations. (See figure 1.1.) They are important for spine mobility and stability. The mechanics of your spine depend heavily on these relatively small joints. The angles and orientation of these sliding joint surfaces are important determinants in the way your spine moves. Their special mechanics play a role in the normal function of the spine and may be a source of back pain if they are injured or affected by disease.

The body protuberances of these joints are covered on each side with smooth, slick *cartilage*, like the gristle on a chicken bone. These joints are covered by a joint capsule that contains sensitive synovial cells that produce joint fluid, which nourishes and lubricates the joints. The joints can become irritated or inflamed and cause back pain. Synovial joints can be every bit as troublesome as the joints in the rest of your body, lending themselves to be affected by the full spectrum of arthritic diseases. (More about this in chapter 3).

LIGAMENTS

Ligaments, as you may know, are strong bands of fibrous tissue that bind bones, or other body parts, together (figure 2.2). We will not discuss all of the ligaments of the spine in detail; however, there are several that are very important to review for those of us that are backache sufferers. One is the *posterior longitudinal ligament,* which, as its name suggests, runs down the length of the spinal column behind the vertebral bodies. Because this ligament is narrow at the level of the disc, some doctors have proposed that it increases the danger that the disc may protrude back into the spinal canal and cause nerve irritation. More about this later.

Another potentially troubling ligament is the *ligamentum flavum* (Latin for "yellow ligament"), a generous bundle of highly specialized fibers that run along the back of the spine from the base of the spinous process and corresponding lamina, then attach to the adjacent laminae (figure 2.2). They are like elastic roof shingles between the vertebral arches. The yellow ligament is the most elastic structure in the human body. It aids in covering neural structures in the spaces between the posterior bony vertebral arches, contributing to the formation of the spinal canal. Unfortunately, this ligament loses its elasticity as you grow older. The yellow ligament can become inflamed, thickened, and calcified, and can bulge into the spinal canal. These changes are usually associated with facet joint arthritis and bulging of the disc. The end result of these combined structural alterations in the spinal anatomy is a frequently painful condition of narrowing, stricture, or crowding of the neural structures in the spinal canal. Doctors call this condition *spinal stenosis*.

MUSCLES

The back muscles are quite complex. The basic biochemical principle is that your overall level of fitness and muscle tone, including the supporting abdominal wall musculature, are crucial to your lumbar spine's stability. The major players are the abdominal muscles, the *iliopsoas,* and the erector spinae musculature (figure 2.4). The abdominal muscles include the *rectus abdominis, transversus abdominis, external oblique*, and *internal oblique*. These layers of flat muscles cover the front and sides of the abdomen wall, or lower trunk. The rectus abdominis is the group of muscles that give the athlete the often-described "six-pack." The iliopsoas muscle is actually the confluence of two muscle groups, the *iliacus* and the *psoas*. It runs along the front and side of the spine from the lumbar area, around the inside of the pelvis (*ilium*), to just below the hip joint. There it attaches to the thighbone. (In the steer, this muscle is underworked; it provides the delicate filet mignon steak, tenderloin, and beef Wellington.) The erector spinae, also referred to as the *sacrospinalis,* is a complex bundle of muscles that course along both sides of the vertebral column down to the sacrum. These muscle groups play a major role in spinal support and biomechanics.

Covering all these muscle tissues is a specialized fibrous tissue called the *fascia,* which has been thought by some to be a source of back pain syndromes. In Japan, surgeons have actually removed part of this sheath of fascia in the hopes of relieving pain. The procedure has never been popular in the United States; however, there is considerable interest in *fibrositis* and *fibromyalgia,* which some physicians think may be causes of back pain. These conditions are reviewed in the next chapter.

NERVES

Ah yes, let us not forget those ever important *nerves,* the bane of back pain sufferers' existence. Most of the anatomic structures we have just discussed possess a nerve supply and thus have the potential to transmit pain (figure 2.5). Although these spinal structures serve to protect the neural

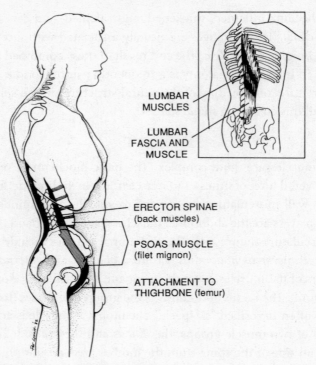

FIGURE 2.4. Muscles of the Spine

It is very important to understand this picture. First of all, it shows the important erector spinae muscles (see muscles and fascia in insert), which are the firm, prominent muscles that you can feel in the lower part of your back on either side of the midline. These muscles can be so painful when they are tensed and cramped up in spasms. (Spasms are intensely contracted, painful muscles.) On the front of the spine, there is the psoas muscle, which attaches to the front and sides of the lower back and goes down and across the hip joint to attach to the near part of the thighbone (femur). When strains are imposed on this muscle, tremendous forces are exerted on the lumbar spine. These forces can be very irritating to the low back. In a number of places in the book, you will find these muscles to be a key factor in back pain. I hope that we have made the anatomy clear to you, as it will help you to understand and relieve your backache.

elements, it follows that injury to any of these important structures via physical or chemical irritation can produce what this book is all about: backache.

As discussed, these structures protect the spinal cord. The cord itself

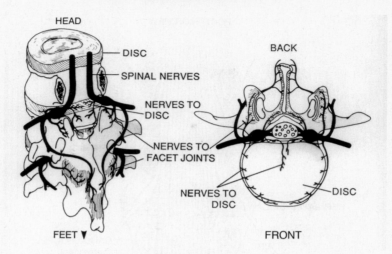

FIGURE 2.5. Neural Structures of the Lumbar Spine

This picture demonstrates that there is a generous nerve supply to most of the anatomic structures in the lumbar spine. To the left, we have a look at the back of the spine, with one of the structures removed to show the nerves. On the right, there is a cross section (horizontal, or axial, section) of the spine, which gives us a look right down the spinal canal. This is the kind of view physicians see on a CT scan or MRI scan. The major important structures shown here are the nerves to the capsule of the facet joints and the nerves to the intervertebral disc. However, we must remember that almost any of the structures can be a source of spine pain because of their ample nerve supply. *(REPRODUCED WITH PERMISSION FROM WHITE, A. A., AND PANJABI, M. M.: CLINICAL BIOMECHANICS OF THE SPINE, 2ND ED., J. B. LIPPINCOTT, 1990.)*

ends at the top of the lumbar spine. From there down, the spinal canal is filled with a bundle of nerves called the *cauda equina* (Latin for "horse's tail") (figures 2.6a and b). These nerves not only control the muscles of the legs, bladder, bowel, and sexual function but also carry sensation from the hips and legs to the spinal cord and brain. Therefore, when the cauda equina is encroached upon by abnormal structures protruding into the spinal canal, the result is a problem known as spinal stenosis. Back and leg pain may ensue. (By the way, if you ever wanted to insult someone in Latin, you could refer to him as a cauda equina. It means horse's tail, but that is pretty close to being a horse's . . . !)

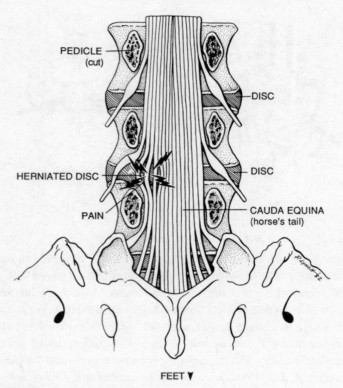

FIGURE 2.6A. Spinal Anatomy

This is a view of the lumbar spine from behind with all of the *posterior bone* removed and the *dura* (which contains the nerve structures and spinal fluid) opened up, to show the relationship of the neural elements to the adjacent spinal structures. The purpose is to demonstrate that many nerves come through here. The picture shows that a bulging or herniated disc in this area can irritate the nerve going down into the leg and/or the combined group of nerves known as the cauda equina.

THE SACROILIAC JOINT

Some readers may recall the song "The Hucklebuck," recorded by everyone from Louis Armstrong to Frank Sinatra to the orthopedist's best friend, Chubby Checker. One of the lines goes, "Start a little movement in your sacroiliac." In fact, there is some motion possible across the *sacroiliac joint*, although it is limited. Back when I started practicing medicine, this joint

CROSS-SECTION VIEW

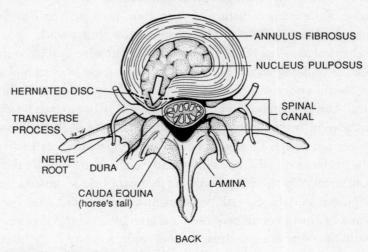

BACK

FIGURE 2.6B. Spinal Anatomy

This is another view, this time looking down the spinal canal to show how a herniated or bulging disc can irritate the nerve. Figures 2.6a and b are showing essentially the same thing from two different perspectives.

was the number one scapegoat for back pain. The sacroiliac joint is located between the sacrum (just below the lumbar spine) and the larger, "winged" ilium region of the pelvic bone. Nowadays, it receives too scant attention. Certainly many of our patients point to just that region when they localize their backache.

Because it is a synovial joint, with a membrane prone to irritation and inflammation, the sacroiliac joint can be affected by any kind of arthritis. One type, known as *ankylosing spondylitis*, can provoke deformity, a rigid spine, severe pain, and inflammation. This condition is sometimes associated with actual bony growth across the sacroiliac joint. We will further discuss ankylosing spondylitis and other kinds of arthritis in chapter 3.

Spinal Mechanics

Now that you understand the rudimentary anatomy of your lumbar spine, it is time for a primer in back mechanics. How do all of these parts work together? Not unlike the preceding anatomy lesson, you can simply refer to this section as your glossary of biomechanical terms, particularly if you feel like reviewing the terminology. If you want to further expand your knowledge of the intrinsic nature of your spine, read on! You may find it quite intriguing, especially if you like to know how things work.

Mechanical laws are reliable and consistent if we're dealing with automobiles or building roads. But when we apply these laws to biological systems, they do not work quite so precisely, although they can help us a great deal. Unfortunately, the physical behavior of bones and ligaments is quite different from that of inorganic materials like steel. For example, an engineer can design a bridge if he knows the span, the weather conditions, the bridge materials, the number and weight of the vehicles that will cross, and so on. Now, if you can imagine that same bridge constructed out of biological materials, the task becomes much less predictable. The biological materials will not all have the same strength, nor will they respond to stress in the same manner. Imagine that as the loads of the vehicles increase or decrease, the bridge responds by becoming stronger or weaker. In addition, if one structure becomes damaged (diseased), it may suddenly fail without warning.

The point to take home with you is this: Inanimate objects such as metals follow clear engineering laws, but you probably would not want to have an inert, fixed, steel-like spine. Biological systems are living cells with mechanical properties that are in a state of constant change. That means they can *adapt* or *respond* to changes in the environment, including biomechanical stress, disease processes, and traumatic injury. For example, your bones and muscles respond to the stress of exercise by becoming denser and stronger. It is ultimately helpful that your living bones and ligaments are more mercurial and adaptive than the parts of a bridge. Anatomic structures have the ability to heal.

You may be surprised to learn that much of the pioneering work in biomechanics was in fact performed by analyzing the spine. Much of this early research was concerned with the collection of data on vertebral strength. Why? During the 1940s there was a major focus of attention on two of the "four horsemen," war and disease. When fighter pilots had to escape from a doomed aircraft, they ejected from the cockpit. The ejection seats basically functioned by igniting an explosive under the cockpit seats. Needless to say, this applied considerable impact forces to both the derriere and spine. Effective and safe ejection seats required knowledge of the biomechanical tolerance limits of the vertebrae when subjected to the applied forces.

The other early biomechanical studies were performed by Swedish researchers led by the late Professor Carl Hirsch and, subsequently, his protégé, Professor Alf Nachemson. They were motivated by more humanitarian and clinical aspects of survival. The pervasiveness of low back pain, its impact on job absenteeism, and its high cost to society lent impetus to the expanding science of orthopedic biomechanics of the spine. Here are some of the things that we have learned . . .

POSTURE

It would make a fascinating master's thesis to analyze cocktail parties and other social events by observing the posture of the participants. Such an analysis would perhaps allow for an assessment of the relative influence of biology and culture. Who might you notice? Perhaps someone with a spinal deformity like scoliosis, the sideways curvature of the spine. Other individuals in the crowd might include an erect-standing military person, an athlete, a dancer, a short man who is stretching, or a tall woman slouching. An assertive person may be leaning over his interlocutor, or a timid person may be cowering. A seductive woman in a tight sweater is standing in such a manner as to reveal her charms, while a come-hither male is lounging in tight pants. All of the partygoers have their characteristic posturing, and I recommend posture analysis as a pastime to take your mind off your backache at a party.

Of course, posture has its physiologic considerations as well. As we have discussed, the spine has its natural anatomic curves. An individual will have a normal posture as long as these curves are neither exaggerated by excessive or inappropriate muscle activity, or congenital or neurological conditions, nor deformed by laziness, slack muscles, or social dynamics. (Those of you with teenagers will understand the last point.) Good posture is a matter of holding the shoulders level and slightly back and carrying the chin slightly tucked in, while moderately flattening the lumbar *lordosis* (swayback) by rotating the pelvis forward (figure 2.7).

In the relaxed standing posture, the muscles should not have to work too vigorously, for it's the job of the spine's ligaments to hold it in the proper position, allowing the muscles relative rest and relaxation. However, the erector spinae muscles that span along the posterior aspect of the spine, as well as the abdominal muscles do contract when we stand. The psoas major muscle also contributes. When it comes to sitting, our muscles do the same job, though the erector spinae muscles must work a little harder.

GOOD   BAD

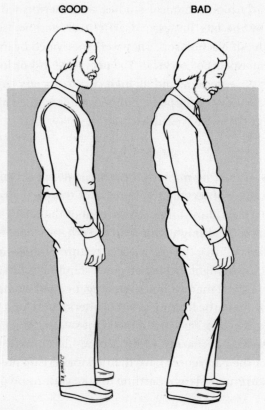

FIGURE 2.7. Posture

"Good" and "bad" posture are demonstrated. The spine on the left is in the less swayback, or extended, position; it is straighter. The spine in this position tends to be better balanced and distributes the forces in a more even manner. Theoretically, this is a less painful, more therapeutic position for the ailing back. There is room for legitimate disagreement on this issue. The posture issue may be no more than aesthetics. When the spine is extended in the swayback position shown on the right, there may be excessive forces and irritation of the posterior joints. There may also be disc bulging, which can be irritating to the nearby nerves.

MOVEMENT

When a prospective spinal fusion patient asks, "How much will I be able to bend after surgery?" he or she is usually concerned with something we doctors call *flexion*, or bending forward (figure 2.8). Whenever you bend forward, the bending or rearrangement of your lumbar vertebrae accomplishes the first sixty degrees of the movement, then your hip joint takes care of an additional twenty-five degrees. If you undergo a surgical spinal fusion of two adjacent lumbar vertebrae, the motion between these bones is eliminated. Fusion of two lumbar vertebrae will result in a loss of approximately ten to fifteen degrees of flexion motion, compared to the normal spine. However, because of hip mobility and the motion of the remaining unfused vertebral segments, this restriction of motion is rarely perceptible in most patients.

A second important motion of the spine is *extension*: This is the medical term for arching your back, bending it backward as a diver does (figure 2.8). Such spinal motion is crucial not only to lovers everywhere but also to dancers and athletes—especially gymnasts, divers, football players, wrestlers, boxers, and tennis players. Here our erector spinae muscles really count.

We do have some choice in how our spine is positioned. Our posture can be affected by bracing, but also by the manner in which we sit, stand, and play sports. We have just mentioned flexion; as we extend or bend backward, the intervertebral disc bulges slightly backward about 1.5 millimeters. A degenerated disc bulges even more with extension. This may possibly cause trouble because either the disc itself gets pinched or it impinges on nearby nerves. When we get to the section on backache dos and don'ts (chapters 5 and 9), I'll tell you how to protect your spine when you play sports.

Lateral bending, or bending to either side, is another movement your spine often performs (figure 2.8). As you might guess, the muscles on the side toward which you are bending contract and, therefore, are more active than the corresponding muscles on the opposite side. The disc can bulge in a similar manner on the bending side. Lateral bending can also cause pain by stretching the facet joints on the side opposite the bend or by compressing/impinging on those on the bending side.

Axial rotation is another phrase that your back doctor may mention. Imagine an invisible line passing vertically through the center of your body. That line represents the longitudinal axis. Now, if you rotate your body around that axis, you get a picture of axial rotation (figure 2.8). The erector spinae muscles on the side toward which you turn are active, as are the small rotator muscles on the opposite side. The *gluteal muscles* in your buttocks are also mobilized to stabilize your hips and pelvis. Back sufferers

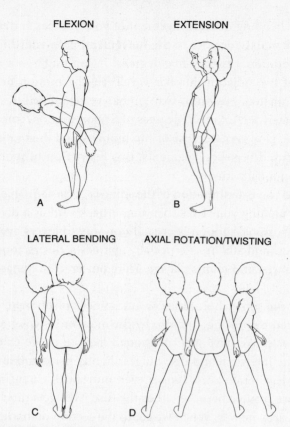

FIGURE 2.8. Motion of the Spine

(A) Flexion: The loads on the spine in this position are great, and diseased spines are certainly likely to be irritated by this position. (B) Extension: The extension, or swayback, position can also be painful to the diseased spine because of irritation of the posterior (facet) joints and disc bulging. (C) Lateral bending: This can sometimes be painful on one or both sides due to irritation of the facet joints. (D) Axial rotation, or twisting: Twisting motions, axial rotations, or torsional loading on the spine are key movements in a number of sports.

should learn about axial rotation (even if it does sound like something occurring in interstellar space!), because it can result in the application of a particularly dangerous stress to the disc. (See page 241.)

Sources of Mechanical Problems

MUSCLE SPASM

When the spinal structures are irritated or diseased, the related back muscles, especially the erector spinae muscles, oftentimes go into spasm. Perhaps this spasm reaction is a reflexive splinting mechanism intended to prevent further injury as well as reduce motion and diminish further irritation. Anyone who has ever had a muscle cramp, or any skier, runner, or swimmer who has suffered a charley horse, knows the agony of muscle spasm. Our introduction to the way the muscles constantly monitor the spine's movements should prepare us for the fact that pitching a ball, or even climbing out of the bathtub, could irritate a sick spine and cause a sensitive muscle to spasm. Any contraction or stretching can produce spasm in a vulnerable muscle. That is why rest, heat, braces, massage, and medications that diminish inflammation and relax your muscles have been a reliable conservative course of treatment for low back pain sufferers for years.

DISC MECHANICS

Here's where we get to what, for many of you, is the crux of backache. If you read the first part of this chapter, you already know that the disc is a tough, fibrous, layered organ with a gelatinous center that absorbs a great deal of water in its young, healthy state. Moreover, just as it is inexorable that we will develop laugh lines and gray hair, our discs become less resilient. The disc becomes less mobile and narrower, and the cells lose fluid content. Of course, this natural disc aging process need be no more pathological than gray hair. Nevertheless, since your discs can sometimes give you a hard time, a basic course in disc mechanics to better your understanding of shock absorbing and weight bearing is essential. So here we go!

Most of the initial disc pressure studies performed on living human beings were carried out on rather heroic Swedish medical student volunteers. They agreed to have needles inserted through their backs and spinal canals into the centers of their intervertebral discs. From their humane and entrepreneurial volunteerism, we gained a tremendous amount of information regarding the different mechanical pressures on the disc. (These subjects and others did in fact receive a tax-free payment for their time

and efforts. To my mind, however, this does not detract from the courage
they demonstrated.)

From these interesting human studies, the following all-important
facts stand out: When you sit, the forces on the lumbar spine are almost
50 percent greater than when you're standing. When you lie on your side,
the lumbar spine is subjected to forces 25 percent *less* than standing pressures. When the subjects in this study were lying supine (on their backs)
with hips and knees flexed, the forces were the least of all. The supine pressures were measured to be a mere one-third of that with erect standing
posture.

Now, we have already mentioned that as fluid pressure builds up inside the disc, it becomes stiffer, less energy absorbent, and possibly painful
and subject to injury. When we lie in bed at night, less force is exerted on
the intervertebral disc. As a result, it absorbs more fluid. This may be the
answer to the perplexing problem of morning back pain. The good news
is that nocturnal disc fluid accumulation equilibrates itself in two hours or
less. All of this has a bearing on back care, as we will see in chapter 5.

As your automobile gets older, its shock absorbers tend to wear out;
the same is true, more or less, of your discs. As their shock-absorbing powers wane, various mechanical problems may occur. Scientists have not yet
figured out why some aging discs become painful and others do not. Several new theories suggest that chemical irritants associated with the degenerative changes may be the culprits. Here we will mention how some of
your daily activities, which have names you probably never expected, can
adversely affect the disc.

- **Vertical compression loading:** Picture stacking weights on top of your
  disc. This is essentially what happens when you pick up your child, your
  groceries, your briefcase, or your paycheck. Compression loading alone
  will not actually make the disc herniate, but it can make it bulge into
  the spinal canal, and degenerated discs bulge more than normal ones.
  The most frequent compression loading injury is a fracture of the vertebra's end plate, which, by the way, often does not show up on an X-ray.
- **Torsional loading:** Think of this one as a twist to the disc. If you were
  to twist a rope by holding one end firm and turning the other along
  the up-and-down axis, you would have torsion. When it comes to your
  back, perhaps the most serious mechanical threat comes from lifting
  something heavy while twisting to the side. Doctors' offices are full of

patients who relate the onset of back pain to this ominous lift-with-a-twist movement, often describing a loud snap or pop that most likely means a rupturing disc. It comes as no surprise that sports that involve twisting motions (for instance, bowling, golf, and baseball) produce a fair share of back pain and sciatica patients.

THE PSOAS MUSCLE

One of the basic mechanical principles of back function is that a tense, highly stressed psoas muscle tends to irritate the back. The psoas is a long muscle that originates from the front of the lumbar spine, traverses the inside of the pelvis, and attaches to the thighbone (the femur) just past the hip joint. This muscle is shown in figure 2.4. You should understand that a relaxed psoas muscle is good for the bad back, and I will be demonstrating this repeatedly in chapters 8 and 9.

THE YELLOW LIGAMENT

This ligament (also known as the ligamentum flavum), lying in the most posterior aspect of the spinal canal, deserves some comment here (figure 2.2). In the very early phases of a spinal segment's motion, only a slight force permits extensive stretching of this ligament. However, as the motion continues, more force is required. In the later phase of motion, the ligament becomes very taut. With continued loading, such as gardening for an extended period in the forward flexed posture, the prolonged force can permanently stretch or rupture this ligament. These biomechanical properties are true for all of the other ligaments in the back. When the very elastic yellow ligament loses its elasticity, as can occur with aging, it sometimes bulges into the spinal canal, contributing to back and leg pain. This compromising of the spinal canal, usually in conjunction with the bulging of other structures, can compress important neural elements, resulting in what we call spinal stenosis.

ABDOMINAL MUSCLE MECHANICS

You probably do not realize how important your abdomen is to your back. When we hold our spines erect or bend slightly forward, the back muscles must contract and exert tremendous forces to maintain balance and equilibrium. In addition, these muscles must work at a considerable mechanical disadvantages because they apply their forces close to the center of motion. (Remember your high school physics lessons on levers and pulleys?) The net result is that strong forces are applied to the discs, vertebrae, and other spinal components. The spine is very sensitive to anything that shifts the center of gravity forward and adds to its mechanical disadvantage. Obesity, pregnancy, and carrying a heavy object in front of you are three noteworthy examples (figure 2.9, 3.11, and 5.3, respectively).

However, your spine has an excellent ally in the abdomen. Strong abdominal muscles that create good turgor in the trunk (stomach and chest) can share some of the spine muscles' work. The result is less pressure on the spine and less danger of damage or irritation. It is important to note that in both health and disease, but particularly disease, the spine is highly sensitive to even the most subtle mechanical factors. This fact will help you to look after your bad back, as we will see in chapter 5.

Now that you know everything (well, just about everything) about your spine's anatomy and mechanics, you are almost ready to tackle your bad back. Here you have learned how it is all put together and how it functions. In the next chapter, you will find out about some of the ways in which this exquisitely complex part of you can go awry.

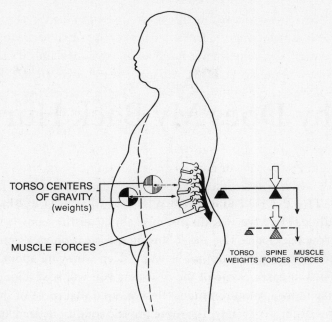

FIGURE 2.9. Weight Gain Affects Spinal Mechanics

This figure shows how obesity shifts the center of gravity forward. Compare the different forces operating on the spine in a fat man and a thin man: The erector spinae muscles (represented by the dark area) in back of the spine must contract and exert forces to hold the person erect. In a fat person, the center of gravity is moved forward; in the diagram, this is indicated by the circle with dark sections, which is shifted more anteriorly. In this case, the erector spinae muscles must work harder and exert a greater force to keep the spine erect. When this occurs, there is a great deal more force and pressure within the structures of the spine at both the facet joints and the disc. This is irritating even to a normal spine, and certainly it can cause difficulty for an abnormal spine. If we look at the center of gravity that is closer to the spine, as shown by the circle with the gray quadrants, we see that the erector spinae muscles do not have to work quite as hard to counterbalance the center of gravity; the forces within the spine are not as great and therefore not as irritating or painful. This is one of the important reasons that staying as lean as possible is thought to be helpful for those with back problems. *(REPRODUCED WITH PERMISSION FROM WHITE, A. A., AND PANJABI, M. M.: CLINICAL BIOMECHANICS OF THE SPINE, 2ND ED., J. B. LIPPINCOTT, 1990.)*

CHAPTER 3

Why Does My Back Hurt?

HERE IS THAT CHAPTER FOR WHICH YOU HAVE BEEN PA-
tiently waiting. Here we will discuss just about all the known medical
causes of low back pain. Use the following information as a convenient
reference. However, please do not lose any sleep worrying about serious
or mysterious diseases. Some of the disorders you will read about in this
chapter may indeed sound ominous. Rest assured that most of the really
bad diseases occur very rarely. The more prosaic conditions are likely to be
causing your malaise. When physicians consider possible diagnoses, the
phrase *common things occur commonly* is at the forefront of their thought
processes. While I cannot urge you strongly enough to get a proper evaluation, diagnosis, and treatment of any pain that stays with you for more
than three or four weeks, take comfort in the knowledge that even persistent backaches seldom spell dire disease.

This long inventory notwithstanding, we must face the disquieting
fact that the exact cause of backache all too frequently remains incognito.
As a matter of fact, in the strict scientific sense, modern medical science
can definitely diagnose the cause in only about 15 percent of the acute
cases. (Beware the "practitioner" who quickly examines you and says, "I
know exactly what is wrong and I will cure you!") On the positive side,
modern clinical skills are quite effective in diagnosing herniated discs,
fractures, certain types of arthritis, infections, tumors, and spinal stenosis when they cause low back pain. Back pain secondary to a lumbar
muscle-ligament strain is quite common. We doctors are actually better at
managing your back problem than we are at finding its exact cause. Now,
onward.

Disc Diseases

DISC DEGENERATION

Degeneration is an unfortunate term, but do not let it dismay you. You have already learned that your intervertebral discs will inexorably age, gracefully or ungracefully, along with the rest of your anatomic structures. In the case of your disc, the aging process means that it gradually loses water, becoming less springy, smaller, and less effective as a shock absorber from about age thirty on (figure 3.1a). With advancing age, the disc can become calcified. Furthermore, on rare occasions, bony spurs bridge across the disc and fuse together.

We do not understand why some degenerating discs cause a lot of trouble for their owners, while others that look virtually identical on an X-ray, MRI scan, or physical exam are completely painless. As we will see,

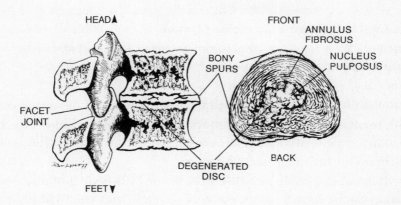

FIGURE 3.1A. Degenerative Spinal Changes

Cross section of the vertebra that shows the severe degeneration of a disc and the adjacent vertebrae. (*Left*) You're looking at a side view of two vertebrae that have been cut in half vertically, with a disc sandwiched between them. We see these changes as a virtually normal process of aging. However, in some people, it seems to be associated with a great deal of back pain. Patients may have symptoms of simple back pain, or back and leg pain. If you compare the disc shown here with the more normal disc in figure 2.3, you can appreciate the changes of degeneration. (*REPRODUCED WITH PERMISSION FROM WHITE, A. A., AND PANJABI, M. M.: CLINICAL BIOMECHANICS OF THE SPINE, 2ND ED., J. B. LIPPINCOTT, 1990.*)

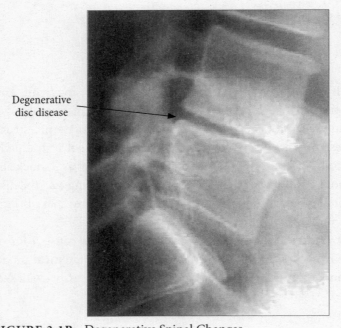

Degenerative
disc disease

FIGURE 3.1B. Degenerative Spinal Changes
The above X-ray is a side view of the lower lumbar spine that reveals degenerative changes with narrowing of the disc space.

episodes of low back pain *without* sciatica (irritation of the sciatic nerve, with resultant pain from your buttocks to your foot) can sometimes foreshadow actual sciatic symptoms caused by disc herniation. This will be discussed further in the next subsection.

It is not easy to be sure that an X-ray or MRI finding of disc degeneration can be considered the cause of your low back pain. Usually, these findings are blamed when there are no other apparent causes and there is a localized area of wear that seems to have progressed beyond the disc itself. The diagnosis can perhaps be clarified with the use of an X-ray or CT scan in conjunction with *discography*, a moderately painful test in which a special dye is injected into the disc before the "picture" is snapped. The injection also serves to stimulate the disc in an effort to re-create the pain, therefore aiding in localizing the pain generator. There is an ongoing debate surrounding both the clinical accuracy and cost-effectiveness of discography.

Unfortunately, there is no magic formula for preventing disc degeneration. Good health practices plus proper bending and lifting, exercises,

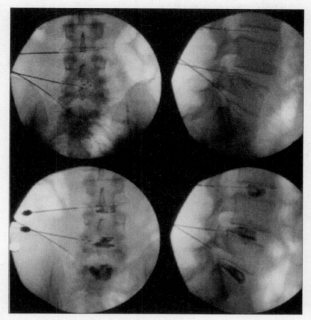

FIGURE 3.2A. Lumbar Discography

This figure reveals images obtained during a discogram. Needles are placed into the discs of interest, followed by injection of a contrast material. The injection allows for assessment of both the structural integrity of the disc and the pain response.

and general back care (described in chapter 5) can help by cutting down on mechanical wear and tear. Treatment consisting of rest, medication, and the use of good body mechanics should have you upright and pain-free again in about two months or less. Ninety percent of patients recover within three months.

SCIATICA/HERNIATED DISC

If you have ever suffered from sciatica, you are probably familiar with its annoying symptoms in your lower back and legs: numbness or abnormal sensitivity (when even a light touch is painful), tingling, or "pins and needles" in the leg.

The sciatic nerve runs from your buttocks down your leg to your foot. When something compresses it, sciatica can be the result. The sciatic nerve lies close to the intervertebral disc. When part of the disc bulges, protrudes, or ruptures and becomes dislodged from between the vertebrae,

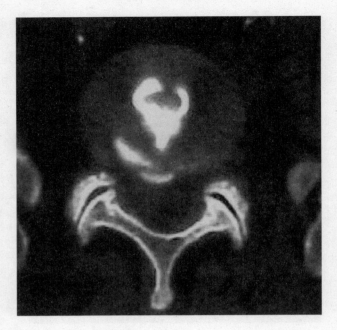

FIGURE 3.2B.　Lumbar Discography

A CT scan following discography can be utilized to ascertain the structural integrity of the disc. This figure reveals a leaking of dye from the disc, consistent with an annular tear.

it can impinge on the adjacent nerve. This condition is called *disc herniation* (see figures 2.6a and b and the glossary). The first documented case was reported in England in 1911. In 1934 two Harvard professors, William J. Mixter, a neurosurgeon, and Joseph Barr, an orthopedic surgeon, published their classic report on disc herniation, documenting the disease clinically and by microscopic description. Thanks to them, we can now tell you a great deal about how your disc is behaving when it acts up.

Before moving on, here is the answer to the question patients often ask: What causes the disc to herniate? Here is a scientific answer: Engineers studied human disc specimens and produced herniation by flexing, lateral bending, and applying a sudden compression load (figure 3.3). Obviously, the situation shown in the diagram is not the way it happens in real life. However, bending forward then twisting to one side associated with sudden lifting (compression) can do the job. We also know that a disc can herniate gradually, and as a result of other types of repetitive forces and movements.

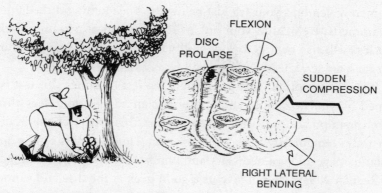

FIGURE 3.3. Mechanics of Injury

A mechanism of disc herniation is shown here, somewhat facetiously, but the point can be made. Using fresh human spine specimens with the posterior bone removed, the specimen was manipulated as shown in the figure. It was flexed, bent forward, and twisted to the right side, and then a sudden compression was applied to it. The man in the picture who has bumped his head against the tree theoretically is at risk for rupturing his disc on the left side and developing sciatica, or left leg pain. (*REPRODUCED WITH PERMISSION FROM WHITE, A. A., AND PANJABI, M. M.:* CLINICAL BIOMECHANICS OF THE SPINE, *2ND ED., J. B. LIPPINCOTT, 1990.*)

How can you tell if you have disc disease? This and the following several paragraphs will tell you how we diagnose a disc herniation. You will usually feel significant low back pain *before* the onset of leg symptoms. The symptoms may begin as severe pain or a superficial ache. Often coughing, sneezing, or straining during bowel movements will make the pain shoot down your leg all the way into your toes. Sometimes the leg pain, especially if you are an athlete, may start by mimicking a charley horse or pulled muscle. The misery of sciatica may run the gamut from sharp, precise pain to hazy aches. Patients may describe it in myriad ways. You may find that bending or twisting around aggravates your symptoms.

An important part of your clinical evaluation is the physical examination conducted by your doctor. The entire physical exam will not be reviewed here, but a few salient points will provide you with useful background information as you encounter this aspect of your evaluation. The physician will look for changes in your reflexes about the knee and ankle (knee jerk and ankle jerk). They will be tested using a neurologic reflex hammer, which taps your leg just below the knee joint and the large tendon immediately behind your ankle. The strength of certain muscles in your legs will also be tested. Your ability to resist certain manipulations of your toes, ankles, knees, and hips will be assessed.

It is also important that the straight leg test be done. This test is performed as you lie supine and the physician carries your legs through several manipulations. Please be aware that this aspect of the exam can sometimes temporarily aggravate your pain. However, this causes no particular damage and is a necessary and important part of the examination.

Regular X-rays do not give us a good peek at the disc and cannot really diagnose the disease. Beware of needless X-rays. A routine set of spine X-rays in a young woman, for example, has a radiation effect on her ovaries equivalent to chest X-rays administered daily for sixty days.

Magnetic resonance imaging (MRI) can generate pictures of spinal anatomy when the body is scanned while passed through a large magnet. Because of the safety and image quality, MRI has almost completely replaced myelography (which involves a spinal injection of dye) and computer tomography (CT scans) as a technology of choice to diagnose a herniated disc. This technology has developed numerous additional capabilities. The MRI scanner can also be useful in evaluating fractures, infections, tumors, and vascular abnormalities. Intravenous administration of a contrast medium, gadolinium diethylenetriaminepentacetic acid (DPTA, Gadolinium), combined with MRI, brings out anatomic detail and may help in recognizing the distinction between scar tissue and recurrent disc herniation. Gadolinium is not required for all cases and should be used selectively. Patients with a history of kidney disease who are exposed to gadolinium are at increased risk of developing a condition called nephrogenic systemic fibrosis. For them, other imaging modalities should be considered.

An example of an MRI of a herniated lumbar intervertebral disc is shown in figure 3.4a. One thing to keep in mind as you and your doctor evaluate your imaging studies is the fact that 30 percent of disc herniations, although present, are not the cause of pain. Therefore, you want to be certain that in addition to the imaging evidence of a disc herniation, you have the other clinical characteristics of a herniated disc. Certainly before considering surgery or other invasive procedures, you want to have the appropriate indications. These are presented in detail in chapter 7, "To Operate or Not to Operate."

Prior to the more general availability of MRI, we used CT scans and

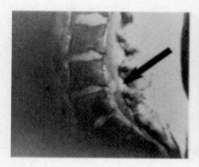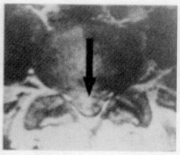

FIGURE 3.4A. MRI of Disc Herniation

(A) This is a lateral view of an MRI scan. Note large disc herniation posterior to the disc space between L5 and S1 or the fifth lumbar and first sacral vertebrae (arrow, HNP = herniated nucleus pulposus). (B) This is a horizontal view. The disc is seen protruding into the canal slightly to the left of the midline (arrow).

myelography to confirm the diagnosis of herniated discs. Myelography is sometimes used alone or in conjunction with a CT scan to evaluate a complicated disc problem. In this test, a needle is inserted into the sheath around the nerve, in the spinal canal. A dye that will show on an X-ray is then injected, which allows the doctor to visualize the neural structures in the spinal canal. Do not cringe yet. While you may have heard a lot of scary stories, some patients do not find myelography particularly painful. However, in addition to being most likely painful, this procedure is associated with risks such as infection and headaches. Therefore, do not jump into myelography unless you and your doctor have decided to go ahead with surgery if the test is positive.

The CT scan-myelogram still has a place in our diagnostic tool set when complicated or unusual clinical problems are being evaluated. For example, patients who have had a spinal fusion with instrumentation and have sustained a new injury may require this approach.

Individuals that have had procedures that will be adversely affected by the magnet in the MRI will also be candidates for a CT-myelogram. This would include patients with metallic implants such as pacemakers and/or defibrillators, cardiac or vascular stents, inner ear implants, and brain aneurysm clips. If the MRI can affect the function and/or position of a medical device, then it should be avoided. In addition, patients who have a history of kidney disease or allergic reactions to intravenous contrast

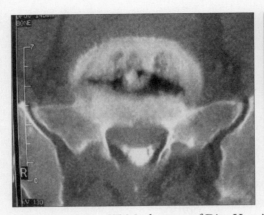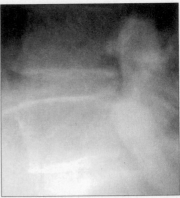

FIGURE 3.4B. CT-Myelogram of Disc Herniation

This figure reveals the appearance of a disc herniation with the use of a CT scan and myelogram. On the left is a horizontal view. The view on the right is lateral.

should avoid the myelogram. A CT scan alone is helpful, but the study provides limited information. The CT scan can sometimes present a false impression that a disc herniation is present. These and all clinical evaluation studies should be combined with the patient's history, physical exam, and personality evaluation for the most accurate diagnosis and treatment plan.

Electrodiagnostic studies including electromyography (EMG) and nerve conduction studies (NCS) can be very helpful. During an EMG, very fine needles are placed in the muscles to record electrical activity. Certain abnormal readings suggest nerve irritation or damage that may be caused by a herniated disc. Nerve conduction studies measure the speed with which the nerves carry out various functions. An abnormally slow conduction rate may indicate nerve damage from an impinged nerve by an abnormal disc. These tests are helpful when there is no clear clinical evidence of which nerves are compromised or when there may be multiple nerves involved.

How do you avoid a herniated disc in the first place? There are many exotic and elaborate answers to this question, but the scientific evidence supports this answer: Simply nurture your general health, do not smoke, do not drive or ride around in motor vehicles for more than two hours per day, and avoid back stresses such as lifting in awkward positions that can provoke disc herniation. Certain sports (see chapter 9) are probably hard on the spine, lowering your threshold for disc herniation. If you already have a herniated disc, see chapters 5 and 6 for a discussion of conservative treatment options. If these conservative treatments fail, surgery may be necessary (chapter 7).

Arthritic Disease of the Spine

Any type of arthritis that attacks the joints elsewhere in your body can also affect your spine. Whenever we have inflammation of the joints, we have arthritis. The inflammation almost always brings pain, and is associated with engorgement of tissues and high concentrations of inflammatory cells such as white blood cells. Arthritis can settle anywhere on the spectrum from very subtle (for example, frequent *bursitis* or occasional aches and pains in the joints) to the crippling, deforming disease we hear about on telethons.

The intervertebral joints in your spine are synovial joints, as you learned in chapter 2, and this synovial lining is sensitive to a number of chemical, immunologic, and other disease processes. Would that the Creator had never wrought a synovial tissue, since it plays such a large role in causing pain in our joints. Of course, having no synovial tissue would aggravate the energy crisis. Without the lubricating fluid it produces, we would have to oil our joints, and change the oil, too, no doubt!

Several arthritic diseases are thought to be based on some kind of allergic or autoimmune response, in which the body's immune system attacks its own tissue. The fibrous tissue called *collagen*—which makes up a large part of your bone, cartilage, and ligaments—is affected in the so-called collagen diseases. This category includes rheumatoid arthritis, degenerative arthritis, and ankylosing spondylitis. Other systemic collagen diseases, for the record, include systemic lupus erythematosus, periarteritis nodosa, and scleroderma, but we won't discuss them in this book. So back to the back.

Laboratory tests are usually necessary to reveal the immunologic factors involved in collagen disease. Then, too, the general manifestation of the disease, including associated skin problems and other disorders, can help a careful internist, orthopedist, rheumatologist, or dermatologist tell you what you've got. Sometimes it is no easy matter to determine which of these diseases is hurting your spine.

SPONDYLITIS (DEGENERATIVE ARTHRITIS)

Normal wear and tear in the spine can cause pain and inflammation. Technically this is called *degenerative arthritis*. But that sounds so unsavory that we can instead use the term *spondylitis*, Greek for "inflammation of the vertebra." Don't let these terms depress you. The normal use of the spine results in certain alterations in the cartilage around the bony tissues, sometimes producing pain. We're speaking primarily of the intervertebral facet joints, though the joints between the vertebral bodies can also act up. Consult chapter 2 on back anatomy if you need to. While this wear and tear afflicts nearly all spines as they age, only some people appear to have pain associated with the changes.

How can you tell if you are suffering from spondylitis? When wear changes show up on the X-ray and nothing else is found to account for your pain, spondylitis is usually implicated. What does the X-ray reveal specifically? Osteophytes, or bony spurs, can be observed, as well as minor deformities of the vertebral bodies (figure 3.1a).

You can ask yourself: Is your pain worse after inactivity—for example, when you get up in the morning? Does it gradually subside as you move around? Does your back ache more when the weather is cold or damp or the barometric pressure changes? By the way, now you know why Grandpa could predict the weather by the state of his joints. Is there a limit to full motion, and pain at the outer edges of motion? Do bending, lifting, prolonged sitting, twisting, or riding in cars or planes hurt your spine? If the answer to many of these questions is yes, you may be a spondylitis sufferer.

Do not despair. The good news is that regular, gentle exercise, good muscle tone, and normal weight maintenance can keep wear changes from causing back pain. And when your back does hurt, aspirin and other nonsteroidal anti-inflammatory drugs (NSAIDs) are helpful.

Nonsteroidal Anti-inflammatory Drugs (NSAIDs)

GENERIC NAME	BRAND NAME
aspirin	Bayer, others
celecoxib	Celebrex (COX-2 inhibitor)
diclofenac	Voltaren
diflunisal	Dolobid
etodolac	Lodine

ibuprofen	Motrin, Advil
indomethacin	Indocin
ketoprofen	Orudis
meloxicam	Mobic
nabumetone	Relafen
naproxen	Aleve, others
oxaprozin	Daypro
piroxicam	Feldene
sulindac	Clinoril
trisalicylate	Trilisate
fenoprofen	Nalfon
flurbiprofen	Ansaid
ketorolac	Toradol
meclofenamate	Meclomen
salsalate	Disalcid
tolmetin	Tolectin

Another class of NSAIDs includes cyclooxygenase-2 (COX-2) selective inhibitor. Like the traditional NSAIDs, COX-2 inhibitors are effective in reducing inflammation, with the added benefit of a lowered gastrointestinal risk profile (gastritis, ulcers, or bleeding). Celecoxib (Celebrex) is the only COX-2 drug available in the United States. Cardiovascular risk factors led to the withdrawal of rofecoxib (Vioxx) and valdecoxib (Bextra) from the market. Patients with liver or kidney disease may have to avoid NSAIDs. Occasionally a brace may be recommended to support a degenerative lumbar spine. On the rare occasion when the degenerative changes are confined to one area, foster abnormal motion, and are clearly the source of a patient's backache, a spinal fusion can be considered.

ANKYLOSING SPONDYLITIS

Spondylitis, as we've said, means inflammation of the spine, and *ankylosing* means stiffening. Put them together, and you have stiffening of an inflamed, painful spine, the hallmark of this disorder. This is the disease, by the way, that *Saturday Review* magazine editor Norman Cousins reportedly cured in an unorthodox fashion: with "laughter therapy." In a book called *Anatomy of an Illness as Perceived by the Patient,* he recalls how he checked into a hotel room and watched many solid hours of videotapes of *Candid Camera* and other comedy shows, then emerged with a reanimated will to live and a more comfortable spine. Mr. Cousins may have felt better because he stimulated his body's production of natural painkill-ers, endorphins (see chapter 4). A positive attitude is crucial to healing, of course, but in this chapter we'll discuss more conventional treatment.

This very painful form of arthritis commonly afflicts males in their twenties and thirties. As the spine stiffens, the connection between the ribs and the thoracic (middle) spine sometimes becomes so rigid that the pa-tient can barely expand his chest. With a stiff neck and upper spine, he may walk around in a slight crouched position, and in severe cases, major deformity may result.

In the earliest stages, though, these changes may not be so clear-cut. When ankylosing spondylitis starts as low back pain, it will actually turn up in the neighborhood of the sacroiliac joint. The sacroiliac joint is be-tween the lower back and the pelvic bone, remember? The pain may even be referred to the hip and thigh, confusing the diagnosis with interver-tebral disc disease. The case history usually comprises pain in the major joints of the spine and perhaps transient pain in other joints, such as the shoulder, hip, knee, ankle, elbow, or wrist. Characteristically, however, an-kylosing spondylitis will eventually settle in the spine.

If your doctor suspects that you have ankylosing spondylitis, he or she will perform a few lab tests. The rate at which your red blood cells settle to the bottom of a test tube generally increases with this disorder. This mea-surement is called the erythrocyte sedimentation rate (ESR), commonly referred to as the "sed" rate. It is one clue of active inflammatory disease. The diagnosis is supported by a positive result from another special test, called HLA-B27 (human leukocyte antigen B27), which measures the pres-ence of certain immunologic protein markers on the surface of your cells.

Unfortunately, we doctors know of no way to prevent this ailment. But once the diagnosis is made, it is very important for you to exercise regularly, although severe pain may make it difficult indeed. You should also wear a brace, if necessary, to forestall major deformity. When the de-formity is severe and incapacitating, the patient may choose to have his bony spine (not the spinal cord) cut through and straightened surgically. Since it is a rather awesome operation, it should be done by an experi-enced surgeon in a hospital with a reliable spine service. Even so, since one out of every ten or twenty patients dies or suffers major complications, you should contemplate surgery only when you simply cannot tolerate a life limited to seeing only the ground a few feet ahead and never the horizon. Refer to chapter 7 for further discussion.

RHEUMATOID ARTHRITIS

This is the bogeyman, the form of arthritis that is most often synonymous with *crippling arthritis* and gives the disease its bleak reputation. While it usually afflicts the knee, hip, hand, and wrist joints more than the back, rheumatoid arthritis (RA) can also hit the lumbar spine. Actually, rheumatoid arthritis is not just a disease of the joints; it can perform its dirty work on almost any system of the body. For some reason, it's more common in women than in men. The disease inflicts joint deformity, usually making it easy to diagnose. In the United States, the annual incidence is approximately 70 per 100,000 people. Confirmation comes from laboratory tests that detect the *rheumatoid factor* in the blood. Additional blood tests include a complete blood count (CBC), metabolic panel, ESR, and antinuclear antibody (ANA). These tests, if positive, are indicators of inflammatory arthritis.

Nobody knows what causes rheumatoid arthritis, but doctors suspect an autoimmune response is to blame. That is, your immune system forms antibodies against its own tissue as if it were a foreign invader. You might think of it as the body turning around and attacking itself. Any joint in the body can be affected, including the spine.

Medical treatment of rheumatoid arthritis focuses primarily on three type of pharmacologic choices, or medicines. The first are nonsteroidal anti-inflammatory drugs (NSAIDs), which reduce acute inflammation and pain. (See the list on page 46.) They help but do not alter disease progression. The second class of pharmacologic agents is corticosteroids, such as prednisone (Deltasone) and methylprednisolone (Depo-Medral). These agents have both anti-inflammatory and immunoregulatory effects. Side effects of chronic corticosteroid use include weight gain, elevated blood pressure and blood glucose, increased incidence of cataracts, accelerated osteoporosis progression, and avascular necrosis of bone.

The third class of agents is the disease-modifying antirheumatic drugs (DMARDs). They include:

Disease-Modifying Anti-rheumatic Drugs (DMARDs)

GENERIC NAME	BRAND NAME
methotrexate	Rheumatrex
sulfasalazine	Azulfidine

GENERIC NAME	BRAND NAME
leflunomide	Arava
etanercept	Enbrel
infliximab	Remicade
adalimumab	Humira
abatacept	Orencia
rituximab	Rituxan
anakinra	Kineret
antimalarials	
gold salts	
d-penicillamine	Cuprimine
cyclosporin A	Sandimmune
cyclophosphamide	Cytoxan
azathioprine	Imuran

These agents improve symptoms associated with active RA and have been shown to alter the course of the disease, improving outcomes. They are often started soon after the diagnosis has been confirmed. Gentle, active exercise and appropriate braces can help prevent progressive deformity, however.

Spondylolisthesis

This tongue twister (dare even your orthopedist to say it fast!) comes from the Greek term for "slipping vertebrae." In this condition, a defect in the bony structure of the back part of one vertebra allows the front parts of the vertebra to move forward and out of alignment with the rest of your spine. Picture a child stacking blocks. If the second block from the bottom were to slide forward, three or more blocks on top of it will tilt, too, right? And that is essentially what happens in spondylolisthesis. When one vertebra slips forward, several vertebrae above it tend to pitch forward as well (figure 3.5a).

This defect, in addition to being common in Eskimos, is seen frequently in several groups of athletes: gymnasts, interior linemen (in American football), sumo wrestlers, weight lifters, soccer players, and javelin throwers. These sports all require lots of flexion-extension activity or heavy lifting, moving from a flexed to extended position. The defect is created by a type of fatigue break in the bone. This break occurs as a result of many repeated forces on a bone (accumulated impact loading), none of which individually would be strong enough to break it. This is analogous to the march fracture seen in the metatarsal (forefoot bone) of the military recruit who has not done much walking before basic training. No one blow breaks his bone, but the long marches eventually do. A bone scan (see page 77) is useful in diagnosing this "overuse" condition.

Here's an interesting bit of low back trivia. Now that you're in "the club," these little anecdotes have a place in your conversations with fellow "low backers." If you study contortionists, you will discover that they can be divided into two groups: those who contour by bending forward (flexing), called Klischnigg contortionists, and those who contort by bending backward (extending), known as Caoutche contortionists. The defect of spondylolisthesis is seen only in the the extenders. They subject their backs to extreme lordosis when bending backward. So, in order to cause the fa-

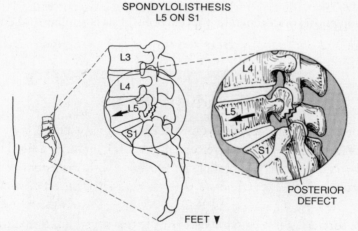

SPONDYLOLISTHESIS
L5 ON S1

POSTERIOR
DEFECT

FEET ▼

FIGURE 3.5A. Spondylolisthesis

This is an example of a defect in the posterior bony part of the L5 vertebra, causing it to slip forward (see arrow) in relation to S1. This slip is called spondylolisthesis. This problem is found in a variety of different patients for different reasons. The levels shown are the lumbar 3, 4, and 5 vertebrae and the first sacral vertebra. The spondylolisthesis is at L5/S1. That is where it most commonly occurs, although it can sometimes occur at the junction between L4 and L5. The defect in the posterior bony structures can occur due to a congenital defect (spondylolysis, or pars defect) or a fracture. Facet joint degeneration can also lead to this problem, as seen in figure 3.5b.

tigue failure of the portion of your spine shown in figure 3.5, you have got to bend backward with force, the way the gymnasts and the Caoutche contortionists do. The end result is, generally, severe low back pain and pain in the hips and thighs, and when there's nerve root irritation, sciatica develops, usually in both limbs. Younger people may suffer from spasms or tightness of the hamstring muscles in the backs of the thighs, producing stooped posture, an odd gait, and considerable pain. The defect in the back of the vertebra does not itself cause pain unless it is the result of a fracture. But it does expose you to some risk of developing the slippage we just discussed. The slippage can be seen on an X-ray.

Spine pain due to spondylolisthesis that does not respond to conservative therapies like painkillers and braces can usually be alleviated by surgery. You and your doctor may elect to proceed with a spinal fusion (*arthrodesis*) of the lower part of the involved segment of the spine. If there is a neurological deficit from an irritated sciatic nerve, it may be necessary to remove a portion of the vertebra to relieve the irritation from the root of the nerve.

A diagnosis of degenerative spondylolisthesis is similar to the nonde-

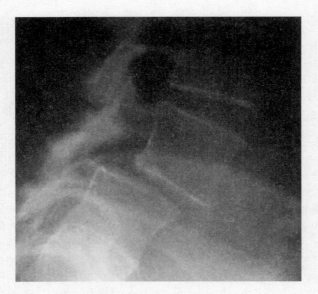

FIGURE 3.5B. Degenerative Spondylolisthesis

This figure demonstrates anterior displacement (spondylolisthesis) of L4 on L5 due to degenerative changes between the two adjacent vertebrae.

generative kind, except that the forward slipping shown in figure 3.5b occurs for a different reason. It happens not because of a defect in the bone
but rather because of a deformation: molding, or yielding of the bone
around the joints as a result of wear-and-tear changes. This condition occurs four times more frequently in people who have diabetes than in those
who do not. The reason may be related to relatively weaker ligaments in
the diabetic patient, which could be due to deficiency in the production of
collagen, the major component of ligaments.

Spinal Stenosis

Stenosis is the narrowing, constriction, or compression of a structure. Spinal stenosis is problematic because it closes off sufficient room for the
spinal cord, cauda equina, and/or nerves (figure 3.6). The causes vary. Actually, a herniated disc results in a type of spinal stenosis. It is not usually called that, because the clinical picture tends to be different. You see,
anything that encroaches on your all-important spinal canal can lead to
stenosis. Examples are bony spur formation around the vertebral bodies; wear-and-tear changes and distortion around the intervertebral facet
joints; swelling of the joint capsule; displacement and/or enlargement of
the yellow ligament; and thickening of the vertebrae's thin bony plate, or
lamina (figure 3.7). Spondylolisthesis can also result in spinal stenosis. The
spinal canal may also simply be constricted by congenital malformation.
You might wish to refer back to our lesson in chapter 2 to recall each of
these mysterious parts of your anatomy.

People over fifty are the most common stenosis victims. Symptoms include substantial back pain with variable leg pain and weakness when you
walk. But the nerve deficit symptoms—weakness, pain, pins and needles,
coldness, or loss of sensation in the limbs—have a more generalized and
irregular pattern than in disc herniation. Do you have pain after walking,
and does it diminish when you walk uphill or worsen when you go downhill? When you stop and rest, does the pain stay with you? Does squatting or sitting, leaning forward, and bending your back help with the pain?
Have you noticed that you are relatively more comfortable pushing a gro-
cery shopping cart? This position tends to open up the canal space. A study
of figure 3.7 will help you to understand this point better. Does coughing,
sneezing, or straining during bowel movements aggravate your discomfort? These afflictions hint that you may have stenosis. Unlike disc disease

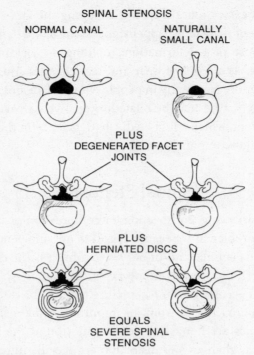

FIGURE 3.6. Spinal Stenosis

This figure shows an axial cross-sectional view of a number of spines, emphasizing the shape and size of the spinal canal. Spinal stenosis is a disease in which the spinal canal is encroached upon in various ways. The space available for the cauda equina or the nerves as they pass along the canal becomes inadequate. The top two pictures show a normal canal (*left*) and (*right*) a canal that is compromised as a result of individual development (congenitally small). The next set of pictures shows how degenerative changes of the facet joints and the vertebral bodies can compromise the space available, particularly in the congenitally small canal on the right. The next two illustrations show that a bulging or herniated disk further compromises the space available in both circumstances. These pictures explain the essence of the disease known as spinal stenosis. (*REPRODUCED WITH PERMISSION FROM WHITE, A. A., AND PANJABI, M. M.: CLINICAL BIOMECHANICS OF THE SPINE, 2ND ED., J. B. LIPPINCOTT, 1990.*)

and other kinds of backache with an intermittent course, spinal stenosis generally gets progressively more painful.

How does your doctor know if you have stenosis? Your history, phys-

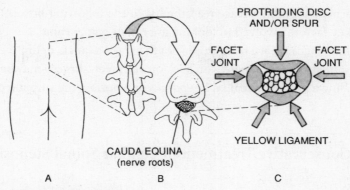

FIGURE 3.7. Spinal Stenosis

(A) is a posterior view of the back of patient with lumbar spinal stenosis. (B) is a view of L3, L4, and L5 lumbar vertebrae, those most commonly involved in lumbar spinal stenosis. Vertebrae are rotated ninety degrees to allow us to look down the spinal canal, where we see the cauda equina, which is a collection of all the nerve roots that run down the canal within the dura. Some of the nerve roots exit at each level to go into the legs. (A) shows the cauda equina from the back with the back of the spinal column (spinous processes, laminae, and facet joints) removed along with the dural sheath, which covers the nerve roots. (C) is a schematic representation of the spinal canal and the compressed dural sheath and nerve roots. From the front of the canal, the disc and/or a bone ridge (osteophyte) encroaches on the canal. From the back, the yellow ligament, which has lost some or all of its elasticity and become scarred and thickened, protrudes into the canal. From either or both sides, a deformed, scarred, and possibly swollen facet joint may encroach on the space available within the canal. These are the culprits that collectively bring about pain, weakness, and other signs and symptoms of lumbar spinal stenosis.

ical findings, and X-rays can usually uncover the disease. Sometimes myelography or a CT scan or MRI can help evaluate the exact state of your spinal canal.

I must acknowledge that physicians have yet to discover how to prevent spinal stenosis.

Treatment of this disease consists of rest (lying on one's side with hip and knees bent as in figure 5.12), painkillers, and anti-inflammatory drugs, together with support from a flexion corset or brace and gradual, appropriate exercise. You may notice that most of the back problems we are discussing do not get cured miraculously but require patience and tincture of time for recuperation. Please read the list in the following box, a synopsis of the key factors involved in looking after your spinal canal.

What you can learn from this is not to expect a quick, definitive cure. If all these treatments fail to get you back on your feet, surgery may be the answer. Using a procedure called *lumbar decompression,* the surgeon operates

Conservative Treatment of Lumbar Spinal Stenosis

Medication
- Aspirin and other NSAIDs; corticosteroids given orally (Medrol dose pack prescribed by MD) or via injection (epidural steroids).

Rest
- A brief period of bed rest, no greater than two days.

Orthosis
- Effective thoracolumbar spinal brace, which keeps the spine in some flexion.

Exercise
- Stationary bicycling—lean forward slightly.
- Physical therapy and back mechanics education.

Behavior Modification
- *Do* use a pushcart when shopping, leaning forward on the cart. This allows you to walk farther with a greater degree of comfort.
- *Do* stop, sit, lean forward gently. This relieves pain by opening the spinal canal somewhat.
- *Do* take side-lying position (see figure 5.12, page 116). This, too, relieves pain by opening up the spinal canal.
- *Don't* involve yourself in prolonged standing, heavy lifting, or any extension of the spine, including tennis serves, swimming the breaststroke or butterfly, and kneeling in a church pew.
- *Don't* sleep flat on your back without having pillows under your knees.

on the spine from the back and frees the nerve roots as they exit through their tunnel from the spinal (main) canal through a smaller canal (*neural foramen*) and into the legs. The structures forming the back of the spinal canal—including the spinous process, lamina, and yellow ligament—must be removed to make room for the nerves. In some cases, spine fusion is also necessary. The decompression may include one or more of the following: *laminotomy, laminectomy, partial facetectomy, foraminotomy,* and possibly *discectomy.* We will discuss surgical treatment later in chapter 7, along with a new technique whereby a spacer is placed between adjacent spinous processes to increase the volume of the spinal canal.

A few other diseases can cause spinal stenosis. Among them are: *Paget's disease,* a disease of unknown origin that causes abnormal growth and distortion of a number of different bones; and *fluorosis,* due to excessive fluoride exposure. This results in thickened bones and can contribute to stenosis when there is a preexisting narrowing of the spinal canal. In some cases postsurgical problems, like the formation of scar tissue or bony overgrowth of a fusion, can lead to stenosis as well.

Scoliosis

You may recognize this condition and perhaps have referred to it in lay terms as "curvature of the spine" (figure 3.8). Not all scoliotic spines are painful, but some are. Pain on the inner side of the curve is believed to be due to degenerative or arthritic changes. The outside of the curve may hurt as well. Standing, bending, or doing heavy work usually makes the back hurt more. But pain is not the only problem. Sometimes scoliosis can progress to a severe deformity, such that the patient's abnormal posture may even interfere with the working of the heart and lungs.

It is vital to be on the lookout for scoliosis in young people, especially teenage girls. Many communities have formal scoliosis screening programs—an important innovation, since early treatment with a brace can help avoid surgery later. However, you can do your own at-home screening too. Does your child's hemline hang differently on one side of her body? Is there a discrepancy in the height of her shoulders, or the protuberance of her breasts or rib cage? Does she have a slight rib hump? Have your child bend over as shown in figure 3.9. If the answer to any of these questions is yes, take her (or in some cases, him, for boys are not im-

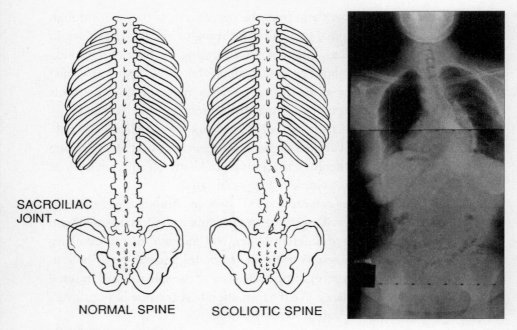

SACROILIAC
JOINT

NORMAL SPINE   SCOLIOTIC SPINE

FIGURE 3.8. Scoliosis

This figure depicts the major curvature, or deformity, in a scoliotic spine. This curvature is mainly in the lumbar region. Scoliosis occurs most often in the thoracic spine as seen in the X-ray on the right. The curvatures most commonly associated with low back pain are in the lumbar region.

mune) to a qualified orthopedist. There is evolving technology that may improve our understanding of the genetics of scoliosis and risk factors for curve progression.

Treatment? A brace and/or a good exercise program may help slow progression or may even partially reverse scoliosis; nevertheless, a spinal fusion may be necessary in more serious cases.

Osteoporosis

Here we move from adolescence to a later stage of life. Osteoporosis is probably the world's most common bone disease, for it is almost universal in older women, due to postmenopausal hormonal changes, age, and a decrease in activity. Half of all women over forty-five have some X-ray evidence of osteoporosis, and by age seventy-five that proportion soars to

THORACIC SCOLIOSIS AND RIB HUMP

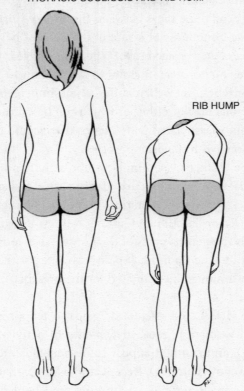

RIB HUMP

FIGURE 3.9. Scoliosis

This drawing provides a brief but reliable screening test for recognizing thoracic scoliosis, which is more common in girls. If you suspect a curvature, have your child bend forward. If a slight rib hump is seen or a slight difference in the prominence of the rib cage or the muscles in the lumbar spine is evident, you should suspect scoliosis and have your youngster examined by a physician. Other hints of scoliosis are difficulty in balancing or adjusting a skirt at the waistline or hemline. It is important to recognize scoliosis early, when it can be treated most effectively.

90 percent. As the median age of the U.S. population shifts upward, osteoporosis will probably become epidemic.

Bone is made up of large protein molecules known as collagen and a mineral structure built of a calcium-phosphorus complex. The latter is what gives bones their hardness. Aging, hormonal changes (which can be accentuated by nutritional problems), and inactivity cause bone to lose a great deal of its calcium, weakening the mineral structure. The average person reaches peak bone mass between the ages of thirty and thirty-five. We begin to lose bone mass at a rate of 0.5 percent per year. In women, bone loss occurs at an average rate of 3 percent per year for the first seven to ten years after menopause. It slows to 0.5 percent to 1 percent in later decades. The vertebrae may then suffer small, imperceptible fractures or large, more obvious breaks, either of which can be excruciating. Note that if this severe pain is associated with a fever, there could be an infection in the vertebrae along with the osteoporosis.

As the bone weakens, seemingly minor activities such as carrying a grandchild, (mis)stepping off a curb, or trying to lift a stuck window can fracture the back. Home preventatives include applying nonslip stick-on tiles in the shower or bathtub and adding railings to bathtubs, stairs, and other potentially dangerous parts of the house. Also, loose rugs can be removed or tacked to the floor. Back pain associated with exertion or a fall in an elderly person must be evaluated for the presence of a *vertebral compression fracture*.

There is no guaranteed safeguard against osteoporosis. Whether you are a man or a woman, a good diet, plenty of activity (including free-weight training), and sunlight appear to be beneficial. Sunlight exposure increases the level of vitamin D. Recent studies show that athletic training programs (low-impact aerobics, swimming, and light weight lifting) increase bone density in the young and the elderly. Premenopausal women are encouraged to remain active athletically so as to "store up" extra bone mass. Consequently, when they reach menopause and begin to gradually lose bone mass, they will have some protective reserve. This is the "warehousing" concept, or preventive medicine with regard to postmenopausal osteoporosis.

Some physicians recommend estrogen replacement therapy for postmenopausal women. The attendant risks of uterine cancer with its use can be reduced if progesterone is also utilized. The associated risks of breast cancer and venous thromboembolic events (blood clots in your legs that may travel to your lungs) are also of increasing concern. The decision to use postmenopausal hormonal treatment should be made with a physician who will then prescribe and supervise the therapy. Family medical history is a significant factor when making these decisions.

Other factors and agents that may help in the treatment of osteoporosis are fluoride, calcium, vitamin D, calcitonin, androgens, and the bisphosphonates: alendronate (Fosamax), risedronate (Actonel), ibandronate (Boniva), zoledronic acid (Reclast), and recombinant parathyroid hormone teriparatide (Forteo). Some patients develop gastritis (an upset stomach) with bisphosphonates. Certain forms may be given at widely spaced intervals to minimize side effects. New evidence suggests that treatment with certain bisphosphonates should be time limited because additional benefit may not be achieved after two to five years. There is also evidence suggesting that Forteo may improve rates of bone healing after a fracture. You need a physician's advice in determining your treatment. Such treatment is undertaken in conjunction with yearly bone densitometry (DEXA scan: dual-energy X-ray absorptiometry) studies to assess patient response. There is increasing interest in using certain blood or urine tests (markers) to assess bone metabolism in response to treatment. Such tests may help to determine how long an affected patient should take these types of medication.

The DEXA scan measures bone mineral density (BMD). As discussed above, the average person reaches his or her peak bone mass between the ages of thirty and thirty-five. The DEXA scan results are reported in two ways: a T score and a Z score. The T score represents your measured BMD compared to that of a person in the years of peak bone mass; in other words, how you compare to the normal thirty- to thirty-five-year-old person at his or her best. The Z score represents your measured BMD compared to a group of individuals of similar age. Osteoporosis is determined to be present if the T score has a standard deviation (SD) of greater than 2.5 below the mean. In other words, if your T score is −2.5 SD or worse, you have osteoporosis. A T score measurement of −1.0 to −2.49 SD is deemed *osteopenia,* the precursor to osteoporosis. A Z score that is one standard deviation below the mean (−1.0 SD) doubles the risk of fracture. Whenever possible, the osteoporosis patient should not be confined to bed. Why? Staying active, perhaps with the aid of a painkiller, not only seems to head off further osteoporotic weakening but also protects against blood clots and lung complications, which often go hand in hand with too much time in bed.

Infections

VERTEBRAL INFECTIONS (OSTEOMYELITIS)

Did you know that bacterial infections can lodge virtually anywhere in your body? Obviously, a penetrating wound or an open fracture that exposes the bone can lead to an infected spine. We know that after surgery, one or two out of every hundred patients develop an infection in the area operated on. Other possible sources of vertebral infections may surprise you: A simple boil on the skin may spread bacteria throughout the bloodstream, and so can, believe it or not, chronically infected teeth or gums. Drug addicts or anyone else who uses unsterile needles may also come down with a vertebral infection. Do not lose sleep over these very rare complications; we are simply presenting the whole truth in this book.

Infections of the bladder and kidneys can spread to the spine, because the large network of veins draining these areas is in intimate contact with your vertebral circulation. Finally, diabetics tend to have a lowered resistance to infection in many parts of the body, including the back.

Diagnosis of the particular type of bacteria that is invading your spine requires either a *needle biopsy* or an *open surgical biopsy* of the vertebral body, done under general anesthesia. With the patient asleep or under local anesthesia, a needle is skillfully inserted in the region of the suspected infection and a sample is taken. An X-ray fluoroscopy or CT scan may guide the doctor. Once the specific bacteria are identified the infection is treated with the appropriate antibiotics. Sometimes, surgical decompression, or *debridement* (thorough wound cleansing, removing all pus, dead bone, and foreign particles), is necessary. The more the infection has spread, the more extensive the surgery. That is why infection is important to mention here, even though it is not a very common source of back pain. It is easily overlooked, and that, as we have seen, becomes dangerous.

DISCITIS

Sometimes one disc (occasionally two) of the lumbar spine becomes inflamed and extremely painful, a condition known as *discitis*. People of all ages get it, though it's much more common in young people under twenty, and its cause remains puzzling. A viral or bacterial infection could be the villain, or discitis may simply be a baffling hypersensitivity or inflammatory response.

In any case, discitis will usually show up on an X-ray in the form of a narrowed disc space or *sclerosis,* a local increase in bone density that shows up on a conventional X-ray as a white spot. MRI can be of assistance in making the diagnosis. Treatment is a matter of rest—maybe even immobilization with a body cast—and careful observation as the disease runs its course. Discitis can last several weeks to several months, depending on its cause. Steroids, like cortisone, have been used with varying success. Antibiotics are effective if a bacterial infection is the cause. Staphylococcus aureus is the most common bacterial agent in spine infections. There is increasing concern regarding resistant bacterial organisms that are sometimes more challenging to treat.

Fibrositis, Fibromyalgia, Myofascial Pain

For practical clinical purposes, and for the purposes of this discussion, we can lump this trio of diagnoses together. These three diagnoses are controversial and largely unproven; nevertheless, there is a considerable quantity of published papers describing various clinical aspects of these conditions.

Fibrositis means inflammation of the fibrous tissue (fascia), the usually thin, strong, low-friction material that separates muscles from each other and from other tissues. *Myalgia* is muscle pain. *Fibromyalgia* is pain in the fibrous tissue and the muscle. *Myofascial pain* is pain in the same tissues, but listed in reverse order; that is, *myo* (muscle) and *fascial* (fascia).

Here are several serious comments about this clinical issue: The problem is more likely to be found in women between twenty and fifty years of age. There is back pain associated with unresolved emotional concerns, sleep disturbances, viral illness, and immune disorders (sensitivity reactions). At present, the cause of this condition is unknown. There are thought to be changes in the normal physiology of nerve function and changes in the muscles. The beginning of the problem may be an injury, followed initially by back pain in the upper and outer part of the buttocks and pain in the legs. The big feature of this condition is the existence of *trigger points.* These are points in the body that are very tender; when touched, they may elicit vague regional pain. The American College of Rheumatology's formal criteria for a diagnosis of fibromyalgia require that tenderness be demonstrated in at least eleven of eighteen specific locations.

Patients are thought to be helped through trigger point injections, applying anesthetic spray, massages, or manipulation. Studies show that this group of patients is probably different from those with the common non-specific low back pain condition. There is much to be learned about this entity, for while some competent physicians think that this is a definite, distinct, diagnosable, and treatable disease, others are highly skeptical. If you are curious about what my patients are told, here it is: "Do not spend much time or money on the fibrositis, fibromyalgia, and myofascial pain syndromes unless you're absolutely certain that it's worth it!" Time and research will tell us if this is another fad or a substantive recognition of a fully characterizable disease entity. It usually improves once a patient is re-assured that it is *not* a serious, permanent, crippling condition.

Tumors: Benign and Malignant

The first, most noteworthy message here is that tumors of the spine are *extremely* rare. Probably fewer than one in ten thousand backache patients has cancer in the spine, so why should you be a part of this tiny minority? Do not let your mind wander to malignancy whenever your back hurts. Simply make sure that you have a thorough medical evaluation if you have been laid up for more than several weeks.

Since this is a complete guide to backache, we should not exclude tumors. A tumor, or *neoplasm*, is a growth, of abnormal tissue. There are two basic varieties: *benign* (noncancerous) and *malignant* (cancerous). If left untreated, a malignant tumor can grow larger and potentially spread to other locations. Spreading to other locations is called *metastasis,* which in some situations may cause very serious illness or death. Benign tumors tend to grow more slowly and usually are not crippling or fatal. Some benign tumors can behave aggressively, however.

A tumor can involve or arise from any of the spine's structures: bone, ligaments, nerves, muscles, or synovial tissue. Symptoms are variable, but unlike the pain of a disc problem, for instance, which may come and go, tumor pain is generally continuous. Particularly in the case of malignancy, the condition steadily worsens, unrelieved by bed rest or respite from activity.

Primary spinal tumors are those that originate in the spine, while *metastatic spinal tumors* migrate from a primary malignancy elsewhere in the body and seed the spine, most often in the bone. Cancers of the breast, thyroid gland, intestine, and kidney not infrequently metastasize to the spine. Tumors of the lymphatic system (lymphoma) and a disease called *multiple myeloma* (cancer of the bone marrow) can also spread to or originate in the spine, causing pain. But a note of reassurance: It's quite uncommon for metastatic tumors to show up first in the spine; more often the initial symptoms point to the site of origin. So while metastatic tumors of the spine are slightly more common than primary ones, it is still improbable that your backache is an undiagnosed cancer.

The diagnosis is ultimately made with X-rays, MRI, CT scan, and/ or bone scan. *Angiography,* injection of a special radiopaque dye into the blood vessels for viewing purposes, may also be performed. If a tumor does show up, of course, your doctor must find out whether it is benign or malignant. This is usually accomplished with a biopsy. Some tumors have a characteristic appearance on the imaging studies. However, the definitive diagnosis may require a tissue sample obtained only through biopsy. Biopsies can be performed by needle aspiration, surgical incision, and removal of a portion of the mass, or complete excision of the tumor. The specimen is sent to a pathologist for examination under the microscope. Sometimes it takes several days to obtain an answer, particularly if the specimen contains bone. Specimens that contain bone require special preparation in order to make the slides to examine. Certain lesions can be assessed by analyzing blood or urine samples.

Whenever possible, a primary tumor is removed along with a margin of normal tissue to ensure that all of the malignancy is caught. This can be a challenging surgical procedure, so make sure that you are in experienced hands. Clear communication between the surgeon, pathologist, and oncologist is of great importance. A metastatic tumor may also be treated surgically, especially if it turns out to be a solitary secondary tumor. However, if the tumor has already spread to several other sites, total tumor removal becomes less pressing. Radiation therapy and chemotherapy (anticancer drugs) can help vanquish both primary and secondary tumors. Lymphoma, as well as metastatic tumors from the breast, prostate, and thyroid, typically respond well to radiation and chemotherapy.

Then comes the important necessity of carefully planned surgical reconstruction of the spine. During and after surgery, the spinal cord and nerve roots must be protected. Such is an important consideration when the method of reconstructing the excised structures is devised. Some of the support structure for the spine may be removed during excision of the tumor. The reconstruction may involve the use of a bone graft harvested from another location on the patient's body (*autograft;* for instance, from the hip bone or the calf bone) or from the bone bank (*allograft*). Metal implants, polymers, or bone cement may be utilized as well to re-construct the spine. Obviously, if you have a spine tumor, you'll want to seek an experienced, knowledgeable surgeon and cancer specialist at a large regional hospital or medical center. A medical team of experts is nec-essary for these complex medical problems.

Meanwhile, please be assured that most of the other conditions we list in this chapter are much more likely back pain culprits than cancer.

Back Injuries

Of course, your spine is far from invulnerable. As you move about, jog, or lift bureaus, office typewriters, or toddlers, you run the risk of pulled mus-cles, sprains, torn ligaments, or fractures of the spine.

MUSCLE AND LIGAMENT INJURIES

The back muscles and many of the ligaments you learned about in chap-ter 2 can be injured or irritated (figure 3.10). What may do you in is that sudden movement in the heat of a tennis match, a game of touch football, or a fall, twist, or sudden muscle contraction to avoid a fall. To us orthope-dists, life sometimes looks like an obstacle course full of potential pitfalls for the back. These can result in a strain or sprain to the ligaments, a pulled muscle, muscle strain, or charley horse. All of which can make you mighty uncomfortable.

Sudden pain usually follows a clear-cut injury, although there may be a delay of hours or even a day or two. Specific movements tend to ag-gravate the pain, and muscle injury may bring with it a palpable muscle spasm. Muscle spasms can also happen *without* muscle injury, as a reflex phenomenon from irritated deeper structures, including torn ligaments, infections, tumors, chronic disc irritation, or herniation. The way you move, your posture, and other tests permit your doctor to separate a pri-mary muscle spasm from that caused by some underlying disorder.

How do you prevent muscle and ligament injury? Warm-up and stretching exercises before sports or heavy labor are critical, as is proper training in lifting. (Chapters 5 and 9 give more detailed advice.) Treatment most often consists of rest, ice (for the first forty-eight hours), heat, mas-sage, warm showers or baths, and aspirin to combat both pain and inflam-

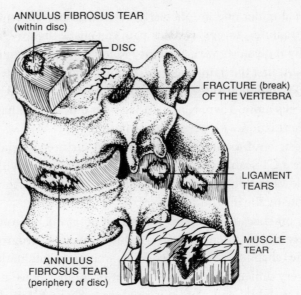

ANNULUS FIBROSUS TEAR (within disc)

DISC

FRACTURE (break) OF THE VERTEBRA

LIGAMENT TEARS

MUSCLE TEAR

ANNULUS FIBROSUS TEAR (periphery of disc)

FIGURE 3.10. Common Back Injuries

This picture is to remind us of the various structures in the spine that can be impaired by injury. These structures, when injured, may cause acute low back pain problems. We recall from figure 2.5 that there are plenty of nerves around to supply most of these structures; when they are damaged, we can expect to have some real pain problems. *(REPRODUCED WITH PERMISSION FROM WHITE, A. A., AND PANJABI, M. M.: CLINICAL BIOMECHANICS OF THE SPINE, 2ND ED., J. B. LIPPINCOTT, 1990.)*

mation. After a time, as your backache subsides, you can gradually resume activity.

Take solace in the thought that the muscle and ligament injuries are *not* often the prelude to a life flat on your back. The odds are excellent that you will recover fully and spontaneously in about two weeks or less.

VERTEBRAL END PLATE FRACTURES

When you study back anatomy, you can see that the vertebral body sports a bony plate at both top and bottom. If you wish, you can visualize the vertebral bodies as a stack of tin cans separated by jelly doughnuts, the discs. In this scheme of things, the cylinder of the can is the vertebral body and the covers at either end are the vertebral end plates. When the end plate cracks or fractures, severe low back pain can ensue (figure 3.10).

Usually it all starts with an injury followed by an abrupt spell of low back pain. At first the pain is severe, then it gradually subsides after two or three weeks, although some residual discomfort may haunt you for three or four weeks more. There is not any leg pain unless there happens also to be a disc herniation with nerve root irritation.

Lab tests tend to show a totally normal picture. Special X-ray techniques like a CT scan, bone scan, or MRI may be required. These imaging studies allows the doctor to see the bone in slices or accentuate a recent break, allowing the diagnosis to be made.

Safety practices are the only prevention program. Treatment? Bed rest in the early phases, then, as your symptoms permit, progressive activity and muscle rehabilitation exercises. When muscle rehabilitation seems unlikely or very difficult, a reinforced corset or lumbar brace may help. Undiagnosed vertebral end plate fractures are fairly rare, but since they can cause perplexing pain, exposure to special X-ray may be warranted. Of course, if you suffer from osteoporosis, infections, or tumors, a very slight injury can crack the end plates. Sometimes, the end plates become gradually deformed and parts of the disc protrude up into the vertebral body. This condition, called Schmorl's node, shows up on an X-ray and is not generally thought of as a cause of back pain.

OTHER SPINE FRACTURES

Unlike end plate fractures, other spine fractures readily reveal themselves on an X-ray. Only when the fracture is not obvious, your doctor may order a bone scan or MRI to determine if it is a new fracture or an old one. Fractures that are more than three to four months old may have healed and are therefore pretty quiescent on a bone scan.

The same important precautions we keep harping on will help you prevent spine fractures. Treatment may dictate a brief period of bed rest and the use of a brace. Bracing of a spine fracture is utilized until the fracture has healed. Persistent pain associated with a vertebral compression fracture may be treated with *vertebroplasty* or *kyphoplasty:* the injection of an acrylic bone cement into the fracture site. These procedures have been shown to potentially benefit the patient by diminishing pain associated with the fracture. Kyphoplasty and vertebroplasty are not without significant risks. In severe fracture cases, surgery may be necessary to relieve the pressure on the nerves or to realign and stabilize the spine with special stainless-steel rods, plates, and screws, or wires with rods. These spine implant devices help align the vertebrae and protect them from further injury. Bone grafting to aide in healing the fracture may also be required. Physical therapy is the usual sequel. Surgical treatment will be discussed further in chapter 7. Once healed, the formerly fractured back generally goes on to function magnificently and painlessly, even when its owner plays rowdy sports or does heavy chores.

Is it not perplexing when you ponder the case of a patient with no X-ray evidence of fracture who nonetheless complains of incapacitating backaches? All I can say is that the perception and expression of pain can be subjective. We doctors still have something to learn about the biomechanical, genetic, psychological, and even economic factors that affect back pain.

Pregnancy

Of course, pregnancy is *not* a disease. When patients have a back condition and ask about getting pregnant, I almost never advise against the desire to bring a child into the world. But I do prescribe certain medications, and I virtually never recommend elective surgery for back pain in pregnant patients. However, there are reports in the medical literature of disc herniations during pregnancy, with severe progressive neurologic deficits, that were safely treated surgically. We must try to exhaust conservative measures in the typical cases. There are ways that you, your child-to-be, and your back can cope rather well through this uniquely glorious process.

Pregnancy is indeed a blessed event; nonetheless, it does cause some mechanical derangements of the spine, as the pregnant woman's increased bulk shifts her center of gravity forward. To maintain equilibrium, as we have said previously, the lumbar spine must carry heavier-than-normal stresses. Therefore, pain or actual damage can result (see figure 2.9 and chapter 5). If that were not annoying enough, during pregnancy, hormones are released that loosen the pelvic ligaments. Levels of the hormones relaxin, estrogen, progesterone, and cortisol all increase during pregnancy. Unfortunately, these hormones alter the mechanics of the sacroiliac and other joints. Relaxin has been implicated in pregnancy-related low back pain due to its effect of increasing ligament and joint laxity in the pelvis and lumbar spine. Such an effect results in greater joint mobility and diminished ligament tensile strength. This effect is believed to be enhanced by estrogen through mechanisms not clearly understood.

The effect of these changes culminates in an undermining of the back's mechanical strength. Mother Nature has her excellent intentions. The purpose of these hormone-mediated changes is to relax the pelvic ligaments as well as promote expansion of the cervix and uterus in preparation for delivery of the baby. Of course, a flexible pelvis allows the fetus's head to travel through the birth canal. It has been theorized that this effect may also serve to minimize the expectant mother's fracture risk due to a fall or other trauma during pregnancy. During the third trimester, there is greater fluid retention and pressure placed on the aorta and vena cava by the gravid uterus. The resultant fluid and metabolic shifts may exacerbate the low back pain. Sleeping on one's side using a wedge-shaped pillow to support the abdomen, wearing support stockings to improve venous return, massage, and sacroiliac belts may be of assistance. Women who are more physically fit prior to pregnancy have a lower incidence of low back pain. Additional risk factors include maintaining a rigorous work schedule, smoking, a history of multiple abortions, and low back pain during previous pregnancies.

Even a normal spine, not to mention one already prone to problems, can suffer during pregnancy. Some of the symptoms can even become chronic, outlasting the pregnancy. Add to this the fact that a pregnant

Checklist for Pregnant Women

- Understand why you're experiencing pain (more weight, more leverage, loose joints).
- Learn and practice the ergonomic principles for back care during and after pregnancy.
- Do your regular exercises and abdominal strengthening and other exercises prescribed by your obstetrician or midwife.
- Get a corset support if you cannot find relief.
- Virtually all basics in this book apply to you except that the medications that you can take are limited, and surgery for your backache is typically avoided.
- Be patient. You will get through it and enjoy the pleasures of motherhood.

woman no longer has good control of her abdominal muscles, the back's hardworking colleagues, and you get the picture.

We're frequently asked several key questions about back pain and pregnancy. Here are the answers. The questions will be obvious.

- The position of comfort while pregnant is lying on your side, whether relaxing or making love. See figure 8.3 on page 234.
- Sit in the reclining position for relaxation.
- Generally, your muscle strengthening, relaxing, and breathing exercises are best done on your back.
- If you find positions that are comfortable yet different from my recommendations, by all means go with what feels best for your back.
- The pregnant woman's prevention program consists of an exercise program tailored for expectant mothers, plus good posture and body mechanics and proper lifting (see chapter 5), and enough rest to cut down on spine stress. Conscientious, regular exercise (walking, biking, or swimming) to maintain erector spinae and general muscle tone is probably the best thing a pregnant woman can do to prevent back pain.
- Wearing shoes with good arch supports and low heels is another important preventive measure.
- A corset like the one shown in figure 3.11 can help with severe pain.
- Heat, massage, and tender, loving care from family and an understanding mate cannot be overprescribed.

Severe back pain during pregnancy must be evaluated to ensure that the fetus is viable as well as to rule out premature labor, urinary tract infections, kidney stones, or any other related medical conditions. Naturally, the use of X-rays is usually avoided, particularly during the first trimester. However, a major injury or trauma may require an X-ray to facilitate proper treatment. The risk to the fetus is minimized by altering the technique; however, we want to reduce all risks. You should not ignore persistent or worsening pain. Contact your physician.

Other Diseases That Hurt Your Back

Sometimes when your back cries for help, it may be a symptom of a medical problem in another organ system as remote as the kidneys, gastrointestinal tract, heart, lungs, or major blood vessels. Here is a list some of the

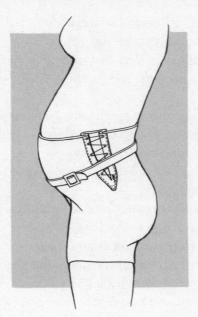

FIGURE 3.11. Corset

This is a special corset for back pain in pregnancy. If we refer back to figure 2.9, we can observe how, as with obesity, pregnancy shifts a woman's center of gravity forward. The idea of this brace is to provide some additional
support to help the hardworking muscles, and also to shift the center of gravity backward so that the erector spinae do not have to work so hard and the
forces on the spine are not as great. When the corset can achieve this, the
mother-to-be is more comfortable and has less back pain.

systemic diseases that can be associated with back pain, although the spine
is not the main culprit.

VISCERAL DISEASES

Some diseases of the abdomen and pelvic region can manifest as spine
pain. Here we will outline several such conditions. There is one caveat,
however: You must beware of a psychological phenomenon known as
"medical student's disease" or "sophomore-itis." As medical students pe-
ruse their textbooks, they may become stricken with a record number of
strange symptoms, which tend to cluster around whatever ailments they
are currently studying. Of course, male students cannot suffer from ovar-

ian cancer symptoms, nor do female students come down with all the signs of prostatitis, since they do not respectively possess the corresponding organs. Nonetheless, virtually any symptom that the student reads about in the medical textbook may find its way into his or her subconscious, leading to potential somatic manifestations of a "disease" that is not present. One "cure" is to consider whether the aches and pains you are feeling are related to those you just have read about here. If they were not around before, then the sudden appearance may suggest "sophomore-itis." As an alternative, when you get weary of your current "disease," select a set of symptoms that seems more interesting and less inconvenient and read about it for a while.

By the way, the healthy, robust secretary with whom I work mentioned that whenever she typed parts of this book, she got a slight backache. Presumably, you, the reader, already have a real backache and need not worry about a hypochondriacal one. However, if you happen to be a backache-free reader, forewarned is forearmed!

Now let us proceed.

Usually, pain caused by abdominal disease is independent of the kinds of activities that stimulate true spine pain. And neither rest nor the maneuvers that relieve pain in the spine do much to alleviate visceral backache. But because it can be hard to tell whether back pain is coming from your back or from deeper inside the body, it's important to have any persistent backache carefully and thoroughly checked.

Roughly one in ten adults suffers from gastrointestinal or stomach *ulcers,* which do not *usually* cause low back pain. They typically bring about abdominal pain and sometimes involve the chest. Yet, an ulcer may occasionally reveal its presence as a deep pain in the upper lumbar spine area, either at the midline or on either side. If your ache is due to an ulcer, you can expect it to be irritated by chili, curried chicken, southern barbecue, peppers, spaghetti, pizza, and other spicy foods. The symptoms can be soothed by milk, cream, ice cream, and antacids. Medications such as ranitidine (Zantac) or omeprazole (Prilosec) may be used. Ulcer pain can occur during or after eating a meal. Gallbladder-related pain from inflammation (cholecystitis) or gallstones can have a similar presentation. If the pain were caused by an abdominal tumor, it probably would not have these clear-cut eating-related and other temporal patterns. Coughing, running, bending, lifting, and other actions that exacerbate other sorts of backache have little bearing on ulcer pain. These abdominal disorders should be evaluated by your primary care physician for proper diagnosis, treatment, and possible referral to a gastroenterologist.

Diseases of the large intestine, such as inflammation, ulceration, or tumors, can sometimes lead to complaints of lower back pain. Again, this kind of pain tends to be deep, severe, and unrelated to rest or activity. Sometimes it is affected one way or another by bowel movements. Diseases of the upper abdominal structures, like the pancreas and regional lymph nodes, can also cause back pain that may radiate into the hip or thigh as well. Next, we must mention the *kidneys* and *urinary bladder* as possible, though improbable, sources of low back pain. Urinary tract infections that reach the kidneys can be associated with back or flank pain, as can kidney stones. Here again, be suspicious of deep pain. Other signs and symptoms that must be properly evaluated include: difficulty in urinating; changes in frequency, color, smell, or strength of the stream; and the presence of blood and/or discharge from the penis or urethra.

In men, chronic *prostate disease* can cause back discomfort. The prostate gland is a walnut-size, male-only gland at the base of the body. It surrounds the small urethra tube that exits the bladder and goes into the base of the penis. Urinary problems such as difficulty in starting or maintaining the stream, relative sexual impotence, or penile discharge are important signs of a prostate problem (i.e., prostatitis, prostate hypertrophy, or cancer). Cancer of the prostate or rectum can also produce some of these symptoms. Evaluation by a urologist may be in order.

In women, menstruation can provoke pelvic and back pain. Many back patients suffer most at midcycle or at the onset of their periods. A retroflexed uterus has been associated with back pain during menses. Back pain may indicate the presence of disease in the female sex organs. An infected fallopian tube, ovary, or uterus may be reflected in the lower back. In *endometriosis,* the endometrial tissue lining the uterus attaches to other structures, usually in the pelvis, causing painful inflammation. A *prolapsed uterus* and tumors of the sex organs can also cause backache. All of these tend to be felt as deep pain unaffected by physical activity.

Please, dear reader, do not suffer sleepless nights contemplating these remote dangers. If you are in good health and your pains have been with you for only two or three weeks, you probably have no reason to worry.

BACK PAIN ARISING FROM THE HIP

We must also include the possibility that disease of the hip is affecting your back. Arthritis, fracture, infections, or a tumor of the hip could be to blame. A fracture usually occurs after some form of trauma, most often a fall. We discussed arthritic diseases of the spine earlier in this chapter, and the same diseases can affect any joint, including the hips.

A rare disease called avascular necrosis, in which the ball at the top of the femur (thighbone) loses its blood supply, can also mimic back problems. Hip diseases usually cause pain in the groin and can be recognized during a thorough physical exam and X-rays.

VASCULAR DISEASE

I imagine that you never suspected that so many parts of your body can affect your back! Bear with me, please; we are almost to the end of our list.

To the tally of all the other obscure and not-so-obscure diseases you have already waded through, we must add diseases of the blood vessels. Blockage of either the iliac vessels, which travel into the hips and legs, or the aorta can produce back pain. Most of the time, these vessels are occluded by calcified cholesterol-laden deposits called atherosclerotic plaques.

Vascular patients generally have back and leg pain that gets worse with walking. The faster or farther they walk, the more pronounced the pain. The pain generally subsides if the patient stands and rests. These aches are not exacerbated by coughing, sneezing, bending, prolonged sitting, and so on. A deep muscular pain in the leg and, more likely, a pins-and-needles sensation similar to that of a limb that falls asleep may be the predominant symptoms.

The diagnosis is made on the basis of a medical history, which may include smoking or sexual impotence in men. Pulses may be sluggish at the foot or ankle, behind the knee, or sometimes at the femoral artery in the groin. *Arteriography,* a test in which a radiopaque dye is injected into the arteries, followed by X-rays, may ultimately be required to reveal the extent of the vascular disease. Treatment depends on the severity of the disease. The regimen may include a strict diet, regular exercise, and vasodilator drugs to improve circulation. Balloon angioplasty and/or placement of a stent to keep the vessels open may be required, along with blood-thinning medications. In more serious cases, bypass surgery may be performed.

Leg-Length Inequality

This one is tough to pin down because of the great difficulty of making accurate measurements. Nevertheless, I for one have resisted the idea that leg-length differences may be a source of persistent aggravation of low back pain. Those who believe differing leg lengths cause pain have varying opinions on how big a discrepancy in length causes pain. Some say very little—less than 1 centimeter. Others say there would have to be at least a 2-centimeter difference. If a patient with back pain and leg pain on the same side as the long leg consistently measures a 2-centimeter to 2.5 centimeter difference, we think that there is no risk in trying a shoe lift of ½ to ¾ inches on the short leg. Studies have shown that there is not only a poor correlation between leg-length inequality and low back pain, but a similar poor relation exists when scoliosis is examined.

"It's All in Your Mind"

You may not realize just how intimately your body and mind affect each other. We will scrutinize the emotional underside of back pain in greater detail in chapter 4. For the moment, let us just say that separating bodily aches from the more ethereal aches of the soul is a less straightforward matter than you might think. Every physical pain impinges on your mind, and psychological pain in turn sends messages to every corner of your body. Therefore, to complete our round-trip journey through the causes of backache, we cannot neglect the following:

DEPRESSION

It is not that rare for severely depressed patients to focus on the lower back as the source of their pain. These patients are neither faking nor carping, for their hurt *feels* absolutely real, although no organic cause may be found.

If you have a thorough physical and your doctor suggests that your backache may have its roots in your mind, do not feel angry or ashamed. Of course, doctors aren't infallible, and it is possible your doctor has overlooked a hard-to-diagnose physical problem. Of course, even depressed or severely disturbed patients can have real organic disease. On the other hand, an experienced physician is *usually* capable of recognizing when a back problem is due largely to depression. Certainly, before you rush into surgery for a back disease that does not really exist, get a second opinion.

HYSTERIA

The word *hysteria*, translated from its original Greek form (*hystera*), means "wandering womb." In ancient Greece, this uncontrollable psychoneurotic condition was thought to be due to an odd displacement of the female organs. Nowadays, in medical parlance, the term is applied to men as well, for a "disease" based more on emotional imbalance than organic disturbance. When it comes to back pain, some patients may be confined to bed in order to retreat from emotional stress, avoid lovemaking, win sympathy from others, or for any number of *subconscious* reasons.

Even though it is fortunate that hysterical backache is usually short-lived, treatment is not always easy. Tranquilizers and painkillers are often ineffective, and in many situations they should not be used. In any case, psychiatrists, psychologists, social workers, members of the clergy, and others adept at dealing with the mind are more appropriate managers for this "backache" than orthopedists or neurosurgeons.

Remember that hysterical symptoms often look and feel very real. The afflicted individual is *not* a mere malingerer or complainer.

CAMPTOCORMIA

While you are not likely to be suffering from this dramatic hysterical disorder, it belongs on our list of emotional ills. Classic cases of *camptocormia* have reached epidemic proportions in the military. A typically young soldier comes to the doctor complaining of severe back pain. His posture may be so tilted as to make the hunchback of Notre Dame look like a West Point plebe by comparison. The treatment? The doctor may say, "You have a back condition that, though deforming at the moment, will improve. But your condition makes it inappropriate for you to remain in the military, so we will let you go home as soon as your spine straightens up a little." The patient usually straightens up completely within a week or two.

Compare this situation with that of a worker who drudges at an ill-paid, boring, unsatisfying job and comes down with a back injury that can earn him workmen's compensation for life. In such cases, even the backache sufferer himself may be confused about how much the pain is in his back and how much it is in his head. More about all this in chapter 4.

MALINGERING

In a sense, all malingering is a form of "compensation-itis," though the disability payments may be in the form of exemption from military service, escape from burdensome responsibilities, or extraordinary attention from doctors or family members. It is generally distinguishable from an unconscious behavior pattern such as hysterical paralysis. The differences, however, can be murky and the degree of sophistication with which patients present their symptoms varies across the board. More about malingering later.

The Backache with No Name

Medical books call it *idiopathic back pain,* but do not let the lofty term impress you. It is really medical jargon for "Who knows?" It might seem a bit ironic to end our comprehensive chapter on the causes of back pain on a note of bewilderment, but the fact is that some backaches never do yield a clear-cut cause.

Eloquent testimony on the pervasiveness of idiopathic back pain is the fact that in December 1980, a workshop on this subject was organized by the National Institutes of Health, the American Academy of Orthopaedic Surgeons, and the Orthopaedic Research Society. Epidemiologists, psychologists, psychiatrists, anatomists, bioengineers, neuroscientists, orthopedic surgeons, rheumatologists, sports medicine and occupational medicine experts, and anesthesiologists all convened to plan a multidisciplinary attack on this mystery. The focused research program that resulted helped us to develop a disciplined scientific approach using new technology for future studies.

A follow-up workshop was convened in 1989 by the same organizations. This second meeting was published by the American Academy of Orthopaedic Surgeons in the book *New Perspectives on Low Back Pain.* The full citation is listed in the bibliography at the back of this book. That publication is intended for the biomedical scientist, but it can be useful to anyone interested in the best, state-of-the-art scientific information. (See bibliography under "Chapter 3.")

CHAPTER 4

Pain and the Mind

*Man is chastened with pain upon his bed and with
continual strife in his bones, so that his life loathes bread,
and his appetite dainty food.*

—JOB 33:19–20

IT SEEMS LIKE A DOWNER TO START THIS CHAPTER WITH ONE of the bleakest biblical tales. But the seeming senselessness of Job's woes brings us to a central problem of pain. Job was a pious man who feared, respected, and followed God. Yet, he suffered plague, blight, and boils as well as the loss of loved ones, and he could not understand why. After many well-meaning but not-too-helpful suggestions from friends and neighbors, Job finally got a message from God that said, in effect, "Keep the faith, my son." This answer may be as good as any with respect to why pain occurs: Sometimes, it is simply our lot. However, like Job, if you can keep the faith, be patient, and remember that back pain alone, no matter how dreadful, never killed anyone, then you are well equipped to move forward. Armed with this knowledge, faith, and a positive attitude, you are definitely ahead of the game.

Why do some people suffer and others do not? Is there something that they can do about it, or are they doomed to be passive victims? There is plenty that you can do to help yourself, and you are by no means a doomed victim. Read on with renewed faith and hope.

In the Brain

Pain is not as simple as it may seem. First of all, your pain is not actually *in* your lower back; in a very real sense, it is in your brain. That is where the nerve-transmitted signals from all painful stimuli are processed.

Here are a few true stories that will serve us well in this discussion.

The first story takes place in 1967. The setting is a one-story framed building housing the large, open orthopedic wards of the Fort Ord Army Hospital in Monterey County, California, where Vietnam War veterans were being treated and where I served as a medical officer.

A twenty-three-year-old recruit lies in one of the beds. He sustained a gunshot wound to his right hand while engaged in combat six months earlier. Soon after the injury, his wound was thoroughly surgically cleaned and debrided (washed with sterile water and all the dead, damaged, and dirty tissue removed). Unfortunately, despite these measures, this soldier went on to develop an infection. He was treated at a medical facility in the Philippines, where the infection was successfully treated, prior to transfer to Fort Ord.

Like many of his fellow injured Vietnam veterans, the young man became depressed, frustrated, and hostile. An aspiring electrician, he worried that his maimed hand might interfere with his career. As his frustration heightened and his depression deepened, he became progressively more uncooperative and combative. His hand was strangely changing right before his eyes. The hand and arm began to swell. The skin became very slick and discolored, fluctuating between extreme wetness and extreme dryness. Of greater concern was that his arm became so sensitive to pain that the mere movement of air across the skin triggered sheer agony. Traffic in his room had to be kept in "slow motion" to minimize air turbulence.

All of these changes developed despite the fact that his infection had obviously cleared up! What was occurring and why? The young man suffered from something that doctors have termed *causalgia, reflex sympathetic dystrophy (RSD),* and *complex regional pain syndrome (CRPS),* leading to nerve-generated, or *neuropathic,* pain. Such a hypersensitive pain syndrome can occur following major or minor injuries. It is a clear-cut example of how emotional distress greatly exaggerates an initially organic problem, heightening pain sensitivity out of proportion to what is anticipated. Its treatment consists of psychiatric help, a supportive environment, physical therapy, and frequent Novocain blocks of one of the sympathetic nerve centers in the neck region. As I was completing my assignment and preparing to leave the hospital, the young man was moving his arm and hand with little pain and was well on the road to recovery.

Now let us journey to the other end of the spectrum. This time our story takes us to Vietnam.

An army colonel, who had been evacuated forty-five minutes earlier from the battlefield (the medical evacuation system in Vietnam was the best in history), was alert and talkative and did not complain of pain. At first, a doctor would have thought him normal but for the fact that he was a little excited. A quick glance at his feet, however, revealed that the left one was hanging from the leg by a couple of tendons and muscle fibers. The exposed bone was packed with more mud than I had ever seen in the prior six months of treating multiple very severe war injuries. A few days later, when the colonel was medically stabilized, he was able to relate what happened. His tale was confirmed by several of his men.

While on a search-and-destroy mission, the soldiers had been cleverly ambushed. The colonel witnessed several of his men get wounded. As the ambusher started to retreat, the colonel caught sight of him. His anger and frustration gave way to elation, and he set off in pursuit of the enemy, only to step on a medium-size land mine, which exploded and blew off his foot. Amazingly, undaunted, or unaware, he continued the chase for three or four minutes. Although his men noticed he was running with a limp, it was not until he had collapsed from shock and blood loss that they caught up with him. Only then did they discover the cause: an almost completely severed and dangling foot. This seasoned colonel did not deny his pain but said that in the heat of the moment it had felt more like a sprained ankle.

These are two dramatic examples of how pain is filtered through the mind. In one case, the patient's negative emotions intensified his pain; in the other, the peculiar élan of the battlefield dimmed what should have been agony. It turns out that these perplexing "psychological" phenomena may be partly physiological, rooted in some tricks of human biochemistry, as we will see later.

Another, more typical example of the subjectivity of pain is demonstrated here. Let's say that you and your coworker are production managers for two different product lines for a small company. The company president informs both of you that your respective production teams will have to work additional hours to ready product for an upcoming international sales push. Both production teams go to work at once. The effort requires a long stretch of fourteen-hour days.

Consider two different subsequent scenarios. In the first, the president of the company returns to congratulate you both for your hard work. The sales presentation was a success, resulting in multimillion-dollar international contracts. He tells you both, "We are closing early today, and I have reserved an entire restaurant for all of the employees so that we can celebrate." You go to your desk to tidy up a few things before you leave. As you back away from your desk, you trip and fall over your coworker, spraining your lower back as you land hard on the floor. You have already been subjected to the stress of the long hours that you have been working. But with the good news of success, you are on an emotional high. You get up from the floor, with you and your coworker both eager to be the first to say "I'm sorry" and help each other. Although your back is sore, you go to the celebration. You later take aspirin, and within two weeks, the back pain is a forgotten memory.

Now consider scenario number two. The president informs you that despite the long hours, the sales push was not successful. He informs you that three-quarters of your team will have to be laid off, including you. He expresses sorrow over bearing bad news and hands you the pink slips to distribute. You later go to your desk to gather your belongings. As you back away from your desk, you trip and fall over your coworker and land on the floor, resulting in a lower back sprain. And, yes, you have already been subjected to the stress of the long hours that you have been working.

Rather than an emotional high, you have the added stress of having just lost your job. Instead of offering a sincere "I'm sorry" and helping your coworker up, you exchange several unpleasant words. Your back is sore, and you storm out of the workplace. You later take aspirin, which provides only minimal relief. You are out of work for months, and the back pain lingers. The injury that occurred is identical in both scenarios, but the emotional landscape differs.

You do not have to be a recuperating soldier or stressed at the workplace to witness the subjectivity of pain. There may even be social and cultural differences in the pain reaction. Scandinavians, New Englanders, and the Irish are purported to behave stoically in the face of pain, while people from Jewish, Italian, and other Mediterranean cultures are traditionally much more vociferous in their complaints of pain, often curbing their activities in response. Then there is the stereotype of Asian reticence regarding the expression of pain. Granted, these are generalizations that may or may not apply to each unique individual.

There may also be gender differences that affect how much pain a person feels. In our culture, for instance, it is less acceptable for men to cry than it is for women, perhaps making it harder for men to deal with pain.

Also, when men become dependent because of back disability and pain, it may cause them a great deal more tension, anxiety, frustration, hostility, and guilt than it does for women in our society. Again, these are generalizations that may not apply to the single mother who works two jobs to support her family.

The point is this: Your psychic structure at any given time—including your personal philosophy, religion, or cultural conditioning—can elevate or lower your pain threshold. Obviously, organized medicine lacks a "pain-o-meter" to objectively measure pain intensity. We have to take the patient's word for how much he or she suffers.

Now, *why* do we have pain in the first place? First of all, pain is a mechanism to alert us that an injury has occurred, so that we can react appropriately and usually in a protective manner. We move our hand instantly away from a hot stove. When we severely sprain an ankle or break a leg, we usually know instinctively not to continue bearing weight on the affected extremity. In contrast, diabetics can develop a condition called *peripheral neuropathy,* which robs their feet of sensation. Patients affected by this abnormality may injure a foot without realizing what has occurred, leading to further damage or infection in the absence of the normal protective response to a painful stimulus. Pain can also be a signal that something more subtle is wrong. We may find that a long drive sitting in a car without stopping to rest makes our back ache. Certain foods can cause heartburn that could later lead to stomach ulcers. Pain can serve as a subtle or overt warning sign that prompts you to avoid further injury.

Another, more philosophical theory of pain is that it places our experience of pleasure in perspective. Without pain, the philosopher asks, to what can we compare pleasure? Plato, in his allegory of the cave, felt that one could not appreciate light until one had experienced darkness. I have always objected to this idea. Not unlike most, I would be perfectly willing to accept the challenge of appreciating intense pleasure without any reference to pain whatsoever!

The Gate Control Theory of Pain

What happens to us physiologically when we feel pain? If you touch a hot stove, for example, the nerves in your skin are vigorously stimulated, and they send high-magnitude impulses along the nerve fibers into the spinal cord. These impulses enter the spinal cord along nerve pathways, then cross over from one side of the spinal cord to the other, and ascend into the midbrain: the center of your brain. The transmitted pain signals seem to stop in a part of the brain called the *thalamus*. The interaction between the thalamus and the convoluted outer *cortex*—the "thinking" part of your brain—is still quite mysterious. What is the connection between the transmission of nerve fibers in the thalamus and our ultimate "Ouch!" exclamation—or, perhaps, a less reserved exclamation—initiated in the outer cortex of the brain?

Now we come to the gate control theory of pain (figures 4.1a and 4.1b). It suggests that a "gate" somewhere in the spinal cord closes to slow or stop pain transmission and increases pain intensity by opening. According to this theory, the closed-gate and open-gate signals emanate from one of four places: the brain's outer cortex, the midbrain, the spinal cord, or nerve fibers peripheral to the spinal cord. The peripheral pain transmitting nerve fibers include but are not limited to those in the skin, muscle, the sheathlike covering of the bones (*periosteum*), and joints of the back and limbs. As it happens, smaller-diameter nerve fibers, or *S fibers,* which carry impulses from the peripheral nerves into the spinal cord, *do* open the gate, freely transmitting pain messages. Conversely, larger-diameter *L fibers* close the gate. Other fibers, thought to send messages from the midbrain down into the lower parts of the central nervous system, can also close the gate.

Let us examine the "Ouch!" of low back pain. Nerves run throughout your lumbar spine, so virtually any of them can transmit pain. If arthritis of the facet joints is the pain source, the nerves that carry the "Ouch!" impulse from the affected joint into the spinal cord can be destroyed in a procedure called a *neurectomy.* The result? No nerves, no pain. Another way to close the pain gate is with a *spinal fusion*, which gets rid of the "Ouch!" by basically eliminating the joint and removing the possibility of abnormal painful motion.

If the intervertebral disc is at fault, and you remove all or part of the disc (discectomy), the mechanism irritating the nerve is gone. A wide variety of surgical procedures similarly block pain transmission somewhere between the original "Ouch!" source and the brain. The closer these procedures come to the brain, the more radical they are. We just mentioned neurectomy, in which a nerve is effectively cut just before it enters the spinal cord. Moving higher up the nervous system, a *tractotomy* cuts the nerve within the cord itself. There also have been operations in which certain nerve tracts *within the brain* have been severed.

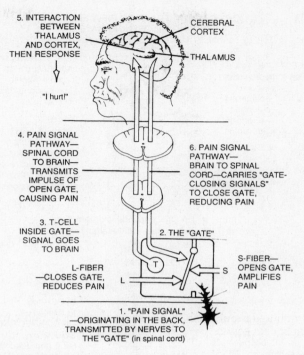

5. INTERACTION BETWEEN THALAMUS AND CORTEX, THEN RESPONSE

CEREBRAL CORTEX

THALAMUS

"I hurt!"

4. PAIN SIGNAL PATHWAY— SPINAL CORD TO BRAIN— TRANSMITS IMPULSE OF OPEN GATE, CAUSING PAIN

6. PAIN SIGNAL PATHWAY— BRAIN TO SPINAL CORD—CARRIES "GATE-CLOSING SIGNALS" TO CLOSE GATE, REDUCING PAIN

3. T-CELL INSIDE GATE— SIGNAL GOES TO BRAIN

2. THE "GATE"

L-FIBER —CLOSES GATE, REDUCES PAIN

T

L

S

S-FIBER— OPENS GATE, AMPLIFIES PAIN

1. "PAIN SIGNAL" —ORIGINATING IN THE BACK, TRANSMITTED BY NERVES TO THE "GATE" (in spinal cord)

FIGURE 4.1A. Gate Control Theory

This somewhat complex diagram explains a great deal about pain. You can benefit from this book without tackling this illustration. However, I urge you to study this diagram because it will considerably improve your understanding of pain. Figure 4.1a illustrates the theory and 4.1b the theoretical mechanisms through which a broad variety of clinical phenomena may occur. Let's begin with Figure 4.1a. First, at the bottom of the figure is a pain signal, or stimulus, that (1) originates somewhere in your back and is (2) transmitted by the nerves to the "gate," which opens, triggering the T cells (3) that send the pain signal up the spinal cord (4) to the thalamus in the brain. There is an interaction between the thalamus and the cortex of the brain, and the pain signal is interpreted. (5) You respond, "I hurt!" The brain can produce signals that travel down the spinal cord to close the gate (6). The structure of the nervous system is such that even without such signals from the back or the brain, other nerve fibers (S fibers and L fibers) can affect the intensity of the pain. The S fibers tend to open the gate wider, amplifying the pain signal, while the L fibers tend to close the gate, reducing the pain signal. Therefore, pain signals sometimes are not transmitted to the brain, or are only weakly transmitted (remember our colonel in Vietnam). Another thing to bear in mind is that the spinal cord and midbrain can produce endorphins, chemicals that reduce pain either by acting on the gate, on the brain, or sometimes on both.

CORTICAL AND THALAMIC INFLUENCES
BLOCKING OR OPENING GATE

BLOCKING GATE
pain medications
tranquilizers
placebos
meditation
euphoria
endorphins

OPENING GATE
anxiety, depression
sadomasochism
memory of pain
life-situation crisis
chronic pain

OPENING
OR BLOCKING
cultural factors
personal philosophy
feeling about work
feeling about sports
monetary factors

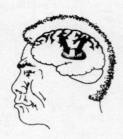

"I hurt!" or "I'm OK!" depends on interactions
between cortex and thalamus.

CORD LEVEL
BLOCKING
dorsal column
stimulator
tractotomy
endorphins

PERIPHERAL
BLOCKING STIMULI
acupuncture
electrical stimulation (TENS)
heat, cold, massage
traction, manipulation
salves and ointments

THE "GATE"

BLOCKING,
ELIMINATING
OR CORRECTING
SOURCE
facet neurectomy
discectomy
spine fusion
chymopapain
anti-inflammatory drugs

FIGURE 4.1B. Gate Control Theory

In this figure, we find suggestions regarding how pain may be stimulated or suppressed by events taking place in the brain. Also presented is an example of how peripheral events can cause or suppress pain. The endorphins may work at both sites. Might I suggest that you examine this figure once again after you've finished this chapter. You may glean more from it the second time.

But there are nonsurgical ways to close your pain gates. The L fibers, the gate-closing nerves, can be stimulated instead. How? Acupuncture, transcutaneous electrical nerve stimulation (TENS), heat and ice massage, and regular massage all probably send stimuli to the cord and midbrain via the peripheral nerves, telling the midbrain to fire the L fibers that close the pain gates. So may traction, manipulation, and mildly irritating or soothing salves and ointments. You may remember the dorsal column stimulator (also known as a spinal cord stimulator) that was popular in the 1960s.

It is now being revisited as a tool for pain control for certain conditions. In this technique, an electrode implanted in the epidural space overlying the spinal cord sends electrical signals to close the gate. The common denominator of all these methods is that they interrupt pain messages between the back and the brain.

And let us not forget about the use of medications. Where do they work in the central nervous system to block pain messages? The answer, of course, is in the brain itself. Analgesics, tranquilizers, and muscle relaxants, for example, probably interfere with communication between the cortex—your "thinking cap"—and the deeper thalamus. NSAIDs can block the production of inflammatory mediators and substances that can affect nerve-ending sensitivity. Actually, you do not have to take a drug to change the way the cortex and thalamus commune. Transcendental meditation, hypnosis, and other relaxation techniques appear to work at this site, as does the famous *placebo effect*. The placebo effect dictates that one in every three people will have real pain relief from a fake painkiller. All that is necessary is that they *think* it is a real pain pill, though it may be a simple sugar capsule.

Again, you see how the psyche operates in pain perception, perhaps even changing the way parts of our brain and peripheral nervous system "listen" to one another and transmit signals. On the darker side, anxiety, depression, and other negative emotions intensify pain, either lowering the threshold for pain sensitivity or altering the brain's interpretation of the signal. The reason chronic pain is such a tough nut to crack is that the memory of pain tends to lower your pain threshold, resulting in a more intense response. And, for good or ill, life crises—like divorce, the death of a loved one, a job change, or even a promotion or high honor—change pain perception. Even finances obtrude. A person with modest savings who is about to retire may find it difficult to return to work with a disabled back. But another person, who must attend a rigorous business meeting to close a multimillion-dollar deal, is likely to be more successful at closing the "Ouch!" gate. Take a few minutes to study figure 4.1b. Then think of ways that you can control your own pain gate. Drugs are best considered temporary, short-term gatekeepers.

Natural Painkillers

During the 1990s, we were able to add one more piece to the pain puzzle. Several years ago, scientists were startled to discover that our bodies produce their own painkillers, called endorphins, the natural version of morphine. Different mechanisms can stimulate the brain to produce endorphins. Stress, acute injury, and aerobic exercise are just a few mechanisms. In fact, the once-puzzling pain relief afforded by acupuncture, meditation, and the placebo effect seems to be due to these chemicals. Endorphins attach to receptors, or target sites, within the brain, spinal cord, and peripheral pain-transmitting nerve endings, dulling the pain. There are several theories regarding how these substances work, but one study indicated that they block the release of irritating chemicals from nerve endings. Other studies have shown that opiates bind to the same receptors.

There is good reason to believe that emotional and cultural factors also influence the amount of endorphins you produce. Even natural childbirth—wherein training, relaxation, and concentration can make the brain block or reinterpret pain—may depend on endorphins. The "jogger's high" and the strange analgesia of the colonel with the severed foot owe something to these morphinelike chemicals.

Much of what we've just discussed can be explained as follows: Whatever closed the gate stimulated the body's natural painkillers. Bear this phenomenon in mind when we talk about how to treat your own back pain. There is evidence that the body's ability to make endorphins is diminished when opiates (morphine, for example) are administered.

The Relaxation Response

I assume that you are sitting or reclining as you read this book. Take a moment now and really get comfortable. Now breathe in a relaxed, ordinary way and mentally repeat the word *one . . . one . . . one . . .* If other thoughts intrude, gently ignore them, continuing to think *one . . . one . . . one . . .* Go on repeating *one . . . one . . . one . . .* while softly placing all other thoughts out of your mind. Concentrate and continue this for four or five minutes. You may close your eyes if you wish, and continue for another five minutes. But do not go to sleep. You have just experienced what my friend and colleague Dr. Herbert Benson, of Harvard Medical School in Boston, has coined the "relaxation response."

According to Dr. Benson, the relaxation response is at the core of the prayer practices of many of the world's religions. Its elements include a relaxed position, concentration on breathing, and the repetition of a particular statement, prayer, or syllable while keeping extraneous thoughts out of the mind and staying awake. If you have tried Transcendental Meditation or another meditative practice, you will recognize this exercise as virtually identical, except that repetition of the word *one* replaces the mantra or prayer.

While some of the profound effects of the relaxation response remain rather mysterious, it is obvious to doctors and laymen alike that it reduces stress. Thus, it can make pain patients a great deal more comfortable. Here again, the brain and spinal cord may be secreting their own internal opiates, the endorphins, when you put yourself in a relaxed state.

Biofeedback is a close cousin of the relaxation response. Usually, an electronic sensor is set up to pick up the electrical responses from a muscle that contracts in association with tension. The patient learns to relax him- or herself and the muscle as a voluntary controlled response. This process, if effective, reduces the pain experience.

Mind as Ally—or Enemy?

Are you wondering why we are spending so much time on parts of you other than your aching back? Does our discussion of pain gates and internal opiates strike you as obscure? Well, the next chapter will give you very precise instructions for dealing with the physical side of back pain: how to prevent it, how to heal it. This chapter is devoted to *emotional* care.

Now you have learned how your body and mind work together when it comes to pain. Pain will be around to challenge mankind for a long time. You can get considerable help from outside sources, including doctors, family, friends, and relatives. However, you will ultimately need a strong dose of self-discipline and optimism to overcome your disease. This is no abstraction. If you learn to draw on your mind's latent healing powers, it will make a huge difference to your back.

How can you make your emotions work for you instead of against you? Get involved in something "outside yourself." Pursue a hobby, volunteer, exercise, explore music and the arts, to give just a few examples. We know that people who have "something better to do" do not suffer as much.

Coloring Your World (Get a Mission in Life!)

Here we will talk about the virtues of a positive attitude. Do not let the Norman Vincent Peale (*The Power of Positive Thinking*) overtones turn you off. This section may even be the most important part of this book.

As a doctor, I am often struck by the fantastic rehabilitative abilities of certain groups of patients. Again and again I have noticed that amateur and professional athletes, people who own their own businesses, and individuals in leadership positions (executives, teachers, coaches, school principals, community leaders, and so on) make amazingly fast and thorough recoveries from their back ailments Why? It is simple. These individuals possess high motivation and a positive mental attitude. That is not to say that *all* executives embody such praiseworthy traits, or that nonprofessional, nonexecutive people are not capable of great optimism under stress. The point is not the occupation or the socioeconomic status, it is the mind-set.

Here is the take-home message: Make up your mind, here and now, that you want to get well. Take action and commit yourself to cooperating conscientiously with your treatment. If you do, there is little doubt that you will do much better.

Dear reader: The next three sections may contain the most important and helpful message in this book. Read them again and again. Read the whole chapter again if you do not understand or agree with these statements.

Now that I have begun to preach a bit, let me warn you about the other side of the coin. Two frequent tragic figures, in my experience, succumb to the deadly duo of backache and a negative mental state. I have dubbed them the "poor soul" and the "compensation tragedy," but in real life, there is considerable overlap between the two.

I do not expect to dazzle anyone with any psychiatric elegance here; I simply draw from my own clinical experience with these unfortunate individuals. Some of you may suspect that you fall into one of these categories. If so, I hope you will feel that you are being treated fairly in this section.

Moreover, you may possibly find the impetus to recognize yourself and turn your situation around before you reach the point of no return.

The Poor Soul

We have noted that pain is a spectrum ranging from something primarily organic with a faint psychological overlay to the primarily psychological with a hint of real disease. The poor soul can start anywhere on the spectrum. No matter where he begins, however, he soon becomes rewarded, consciously or not, by persisting in his pain-behavior pattern. How can pain be rewarding? Well, it may mean *escape* from sexual intimacy, otherwise deemed the "Sorry, not tonight, dear" syndrome. Relief from responsibilities at home or on the job may be achieved. It may be a weapon to threaten, punish, blackmail, manipulate, or prevent a bad relationship from dissolving. It may gain the attention or sympathy of someone who otherwise would not give you the time of day. It may serve as a "reason" for not achieving a personal goal in life. "I would have been a great ballplayer, but I injured my back": How many times have we empathetically listened to that type of story?

The pain pattern persists at both conscious and unconscious levels, perhaps becoming ever more unconscious. The patient arrives at his doctor's office so depressed, hostile, guilty, or determined to maintain his pain behavior that diagnosis and treatment may be very difficult if not impossible. And yet, he keeps going back to the doctor to document the disease, elicit sympathy, and alleviate guilt. Sometimes he will refuse to communicate his symptoms clearly or follow his doctor's advice. He may even become outright hostile toward physicians and other practitioners.

Sometimes there is a clear-cut diagnosis, followed by transient improvement or actual deterioration. At other times, there is an imprecise diagnosis, and surgery or other invasive tests may be performed. These procedures almost always aggravate the poor soul's overall condition. However, no matter what happens, the poor soul returns for more and more therapy and, appropriately or not, opts for one or more operations. It is a fact of life that if a patient complains of a backache long enough and vigorously enough to enough people, including a number of surgeons, sooner or later he will end up on the operating table. So the cycle goes on. The poor soul's reward system may be reinforced, or it may break down at any point, due to his own frustration or the frustration of those around him, leaving depression in its wake. This pain pattern can run for two, fifteen, or twenty-five years.

How do you recognize a poor soul? Usually he lacks animation and facial expression, rarely makes eye contact, and may hobble, limp, or walk with crutches, a cane, or a walker in a dramatic fashion. He may be obese or dramatically emaciated. For him, life has no joy. Over the months or years, as his all-consuming pain behavior isolates him from friends and family, his only contact with the world may be the games he plays with health professionals. Games that no one wins.

Why do we take the time to paint the poor soul's portrait? Such a portrait merely serves as a warning. I want to remind you that, just as a positive attitude can work miracles, a negative attitude can permit a back problem to dominate and devastate your life. If you think that you resemble the poor soul in any respect, turn around right now and run as fast as you can in the opposite direction. Start by discussing your problem openly and frankly with your doctor, or anyone else who will listen.

The Compensation Tragedy

If this section prevents just one compensation tragedy, then it is worth much more than the time and space allotted.

Let us start with the unlikely subject of pirates. Some of the following information comes from a lecture by compensation expert Rodney Beals, MD, presented at the 1979 meeting of the American Academy of Orthopaedic Surgeons in Philadelphia.

Pirates had a fairly standard system of operation. Expenses included costs of the ship, provisions, a surgeon, a shipwright, and a compensation for disability. After subtracting operating expenses, they divided the profits. The disability costs included scheduled and unscheduled benefits. Examples of scheduled compensations are as follows, expressed as pieces of eight:

Right arm	600	Left leg	400
Left arm	500	Eye	100
Right leg	500	Finger	100

Examples of unscheduled compensations are described:

Our surgeon (evaluated) the wounded (finding) four crippled and six hurt, to whom we gave six hundred pieces of eight a man and a thousand to those who were crippled, as was our custom.

Some people question whether contemporary compensation laws have evolved much from those developed by the pirates. While workmen's compensation, whereby the employer bears the cost of a job-related disability, serves an obvious purpose, our present system also prolongs disease instead of promoting health. One study of patients hospitalized for back injuries revealed that compensation patients received 200 percent more physical therapy than noncompensation patients, even though they had 33 percent less impairment.

New Zealand provides us with an example of how compensation laws can affect patterns of disease. The laws New Zealand passed in 1979 were considered the most comprehensive in the world. They allowed a worker injured on the job to stay home with pay for one week. When they went into effect, absenteeism rose decidedly. Many workers with minor injuries who would have previously continued to work immediately after first-aid treatment instead began going on compensation for an entire week.

And, as you might guess, the number of tests and X-rays is directly related to your insurance coverage. The consequences? First, unnecessary X-rays mean needless radiation exposure, and tests like myelography pose even more serious risks. An MRI scan is a noninvasive and useful tool, but quite expensive when not utilized appropriately. These diagnostic tests can represent "documentation" of a real disease in the patient's mind, when there may be only a minor or nonexistent problem.

The cost to society is only part of the compensation picture. The other, more ominous cost is not financial. There are data to show that backache patients receiving compensation do not respond as well to treatment as patients cared for under another system. The appeals process, which allows patients to appeal a case after it is closed in hopes of getting a better award, lifts recuperation to another level of complexity.

Sometimes we see patients who have had ten or twenty back operations and are still suffering. They are on full disability, but do you think they are happy? Enough myelograms, and surgical procedures can themselves result in an organic basis for pain.

And remember that pain behavior is complex and tricky. Do not naively assume that once your case is settled and you are compensated, you can turn off your ailment at will. It might not work out that way. Somewhere along the line, the chronic pain patient loses touch with reality, and his whole life revolves around his disability. To compound his misery, even the most compassionate doctor, nurse, or therapist, put off by the patient's hopelessness or hostility, may covertly avoid him.

The lawyer is literally a limited partner in this venture. Remember, what may be good for the "case" may not be good for your health. Once the settlements are made or not made, the lawyers, insurance adjusters, and others withdraw. You may be left with a less-than-healthy mind and body, weary family and friends, and a growing acquaintance with the druggist.

You should view an injury on the job just as you would if it occurred at home. The treatment and recovery should be similar. Never forget that your number one priority is to get back to normal as soon as possible. Endeavors to beat the system subvert that goal, and you risk becoming the pawn of your employer, insurance company, lawyer, doctor, or other practitioner.

The Unbroken Circle

YOUR REAL BACKACHE AND YOUR
SPOUSE OR SIGNIFICANT OTHER

Having just traced a saga of family manipulation and medical-legal tangles, let me now seek to exonerate the patient with a real backache. It is one of the most excruciating and disabling illnesses around. The pain is comparable to that of a severe toothache, with several important differences. A toothache sufferer's activity limitations usually include adherence to a soft diet, with perhaps the use of medication to deaden the pain. A backache victim may not be able to walk, run, ride, swim, make love, dance, or move around at all. In addition, you may not receive much sympathy for a disease that cannot be diagnosed or treated with certainty. Backache can be chronic and unpredictable, with a typical course of transient improvements and setbacks that can severely tax family members. So let us address the patient's family for a moment. The key words are *patience, sympathy, understanding,* and *practical adjustments*. Here are some undesirable scenarios that can occur without the above.

Let us examine, for example, the back patient who is the wife of a busy professional man who depends on her behind-the-scenes productivity in order to devote his full energies to work. Now she is laid up, and he resents the desertion of his able assistant. Many men who gallantly adjust to a wife's acute illness become intolerant of a chronic disability. Even when finances allow some domestic help, the husband may complain of the stranger's way of doing things. Basically, he may assume that his wife's problem is not real. He may even indulge in the paranoid fantasy that she is punishing him with her affliction.

How does he react? He may either discourage her from seeing doctors or push her around from practitioner to practitioner. He may pressure her into inappropriate surgery or oppose a needed operation.

Now let us change the identity of the patient. This time the patient is the breadwinner.

At first, his wife may welcome his unaccustomed presence at home, the time for casual discussion, newspaper reading and television watching à deux, and so forth. Yet, as his condition becomes chronic, the backache sufferer quickly gets depressed, angry, guilty, or afraid, and is no longer such a pleasant companion.

What can you do if you are the spouse of a backache victim? First of all, do not propel your partner around to multiple practitioners, although sometimes a second opinion is desirable. Above all, do not badger him/her into unnecessary surgery: Think how you would feel if the operation backfired and made your spouse worse in some way. Do not deny your partner's pain. Be patient. Although you cannot feel a tumor in his/her back, thank heavens, acknowledge that there *is* a disease there. Be sympathetic. Remember your spouse's fine track record. He/she certainly does not want to fail you now but is profoundly disabled. Be understanding.

If you work, consider telling your colleagues or superiors about your home situation, explaining that you may have to be less productive than usual. Perhaps specific adjustments can remove some of the pressure: more assistance on the job, changed deadlines, or new strategies, such as performing some work at home. Be practical.

You and your spouse might take several one- to two-hour "vacations" from each other during the day. As the pain becomes tolerable, invite some close friends in once or twice a week. Feel free to discuss the disease's course and prognosis, but do not let the conversation revolve completely around your mate's disability. When possible, go out for a walk or a ride. Walking and getting some fresh air can be quite therapeutic. The backache sufferer can sit or lie in a reclining seat, perhaps in the backseat of the car.

If lying down is more comfortable, then sit up to see the scenery at intervals. And now is the time for some loving sexual ingenuity (see chapter 8).

As your back ailment becomes chronic, the challenge intensifies. Careful communication, understanding, and mutual support are crucial. If your family life becomes severely restricted, it may be a good idea to step back and talk to the physician, a social worker, or some other advisor about such possibilities as retraining for an alternative career. Whatever you do, *please* do not fall into the saga of the eternally treated, multiply operated-upon poor soul or miserable compensation patient. Be positive. Take charge and plan the next stage of your life, given the limitations that your back condition has presented. If you were a heavy manual laborer, then you may need to seek a new career. One of my patients shared with me that he used his back injury as a catalyst to leave heavy construction work and "go back to college and pursue the business degree I had always dreamed of but never thought I had the time for."

Remember to nurture your spirit as well as your back. As we said at the beginning of this chapter, your body has its own internal control mechanisms for pain. You merely need to help it work. If marshaling your own dormant recuperative powers means meditation, positive thinking, acupuncture, biofeedback, psychiatric or psychological help, family counseling, or any combination of the above, then do it! Just remember that relatives, friends, doctors, other medical personnel, and the whole health care system can help, but ultimately *you* are the most important ingredient in the successful outcome.

CHAPTER 5

Basic Back Self-Care

A Program of Prevention and Home Treatment

AHHHH, YOU HAVE FINALLY ARRIVED. THIS IS THE CORE chapter of the book, especially for those of you who are impatient with the arcana of spine ailments and just want to know how to take care of your back. These are the pages that should be read, reread, and assimilated into your lifestyle. They contain what I consider the most reliable information, culled from sound scientific research and my own full career of experience with patients. You will be told precisely how to put it into practice. The underlying formula is maximum comfort and minimum harm. The "first physician," Hippocrates, whose two-thousand-year-old oath new doctors still repeat, advised, *"Primum non nocere,"* or, "First of all, do not harm." Not a bad place to start. We are all aware that medical and pseudomedical procedures can do harm. When you get to chapter 7, you will hear much about possible surgical harm. But, as your own physician, you can also harm yourself if you are not properly informed. By mastering the ABC's of back care, you will begin, I hope, to solve some of the problems of your back.

Now, not all of you are alike and, of course, everyone does not have the same disease. Certain suggestions will work for some readers while selected recommendations are better for others. Hang on to those that work well for you and forget about the ones that do not.

The first section of this chapter deals with specific preventive measures that should become your constant companions over the years. But if you are already lying flat on your back and want to get to the straight talk about healing, read on.

How to Prevent Backache

Now you are a student at our "low back school," the goal of which is to nurture your back in your daily life. Presumably, most of you have had backache, so prevention may seem academic right now. But "it ain't necessarily so." After you recover from this bout, you will be highly motivated to head off a recurrence. It would not be unusual, either, for you to become a back care evangelist, lecturing friends, lovers, and family about how to prevent a first attack.

Some prevention principles are covered elsewhere, but let us review the basics: rest, proper nutrition, ample exercise, and weight control.

STAYING SLIM AND WORKING OUT

Shedding excess pounds reduces the load that your beleaguered spine must carry around. Unhappily, there is no magic diet. Sorry to break the news so ungently. Albert Einstein said, "Energy is neither created nor destroyed." In your body's terms, the weight you walk around with represents the calories left over when you subtract the calories used up from those consumed. These facts of the physical universe may seem self-evident, but fad diets tend to obscure them. We must admit that although there is a wealth of data to support the assertion that avoiding obesity is good for you in many ways, the statistics reviewed in chapter 1 do not *prove* that if you are overweight, your back is more likely to hurt.

Regular exercise not only burns up your adipose (fatty) tissue, it also maintains muscle tone, good circulation, and mobility. We have noted in chapter 2 that good muscle tone is essential to a robust spine. When additional weight is in the form of fat rather than muscle, it tends to be distributed so as to shift your center of gravity forward. This is hardly a fine state of affairs for your back.

The bottom line is that any physical exercise more strenuous than merely sitting on your derriere has some value, especially if performed at least two to three times a week. Chapter 9, devoted to sports and the back, lists the risk factors of various sports. If you have a serious back problem, of course, you should not take up a high-risk game. Again, sticking with the facts, although some studies show that being in shape protects you from backache, there are some that fail to show any benefit.

GOOD ERGONOMICS

We learn algebra and history in school, and we may have even dabbled in Greek or ancient Aramaic. But how many of us, unless destined for a career in a white coat, learn even the rudiments of our own anatomy? Few of us get enough health education. How many mothers teach their small children that the way to sit, ride in the car, sleep, and lift things affects the spine directly? Since you are now converts to back care, you already realize that factors such as a sedentary life, driving long distances, and lifting objects way out in front of you or with a twisting motion threaten your back. Right?

Under the upcoming do's-and-don'ts section, we will give ergonomics lessons for a number of occupations, including homemaking.

BACK CARE ON THE JOB

Industries can help tremendously by redesigning work environments. Better-designed secretarial chairs, desk and worktable arrangements, and motor vehicle seats, for example, would spare many employees' backs. It would also be nice if basic back education for high-risk workers and supervised exercise programs became part of the wave of the future. A simple but critical innovation is to minimize the number of times a worker must lift something off the floor. By starting from at least two feet *above* floor level, the employee can avoid dangerous bending.

Our hospital has a safety committee, which consulted me about office chairs. One zealous member wanted to change all the institution's chairs "to wipe out backache." Of course, back pain is so multifaceted that better seats alone would not eradicate it as the Salk vaccine all but wiped out polio. But why not start by describing the perfect desk chair, since a new chair is a relatively easy modification.

The ideal seat is adjustable to the optimal height, permitting you to sit with your feet flat on the floor, your thighs resting comfortably on the seat, and your knees bent about ninety degrees. It should support your lumbar spine with a good adjustable backrest, with its most prominent part at the middle with the lower back, right at its point of greatest inward curvature. The backrest should have a rigid spring soft enough to let you lean back ten to twenty degrees but stiff enough to support you in the upright position. It is also nice if the stiffness or resistance of the backrest (its ability to "go back" or change its angle) is adjustable. Swivels and wheels? Both would benefit an individual who must sit and alternately face several different directions, like a Hindu goddess, and move small distances. The ideal chair should be upholstered with a material that permits heat transfer and does not allow too much body slippage (figure 5.1).

Of course, in the best of all possible worlds, we would be all be sitting in individually molded chairs that precisely fit the contours of our backs. But in a world of limited resources, taking a tip from this chapter's recommendations will be sufficient. We can at least expect a comfortable chair that supports, and does not irritate, our lumbar spine. We will talk more about supportive seats toward the end of the chapter.

What if your job requires heaving lifting? Well, you can take a hint from weight lifters and use a large belt or small abdominal corset for additional support. This precaution, based on the concept of intra-abdominal pressures described in chapter 2, also has the added psychological benefit

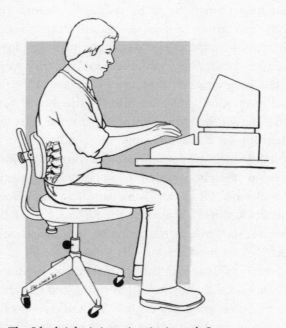

FIGURE 5.1. The Ideal Administrative Assistant's Seat

Note the back support just at the level of the lumbar spine. It is flexible, so that the assistant can lean back, yet supportive. There is good support for the thighs. The feet are flat on the floor, the knees are bent at ninety degrees. Although the chair can be supportive, the rigidity of the backrest should be adjustable to the individual's needs. Small armrests are a nice addition.

of reminding you to think before you lift. Evaluate your work environment and proceed with your tasks in a manner that reduces the mechanical stress on your back.

Dos and Don'ts for a Happy Back

Now let's take a stark look at exactly what you do at home and on the job. If you are scrupulous about heeding the following dos and don'ts as they apply to you, perhaps your backache will take a long vacation or even divorce you.

FOR HOME WORKERS

DO step on a box while ironing, and station one foot on the base of the cabinet when washing dishes. Remember the bar rail (figure 5.2).

DO use a high (above waist level, at least) table for changing the baby's diapers, to avoid undue bending while lifting.

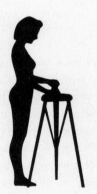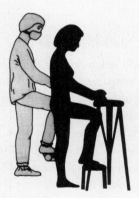

FIGURE 5.2. Benefits of the Bar Rail

This picture demonstrates the mechanical benefits of a bar rail or similar modality in other settings. On the left, we have a swayback (extended) spine with full stretch of the psoas muscle. On the right, we see a woman ironing and also one working at the operating table. In both cases, one foot is on a foot stool (bar rail) to flex the hip, relax the psoas muscle, and relieve back pain. This important principle of ergonomics has been recognized by successful drinking establishments for a long time. *(REPRODUCED WITH PERMISSION FROM WHITE, A. A., AND PANJABI, M. M.: CLINICAL BIOMECHANICS OF THE SPINE, 2ND ED., J. B. LIPPINCOTT, 1990.)*

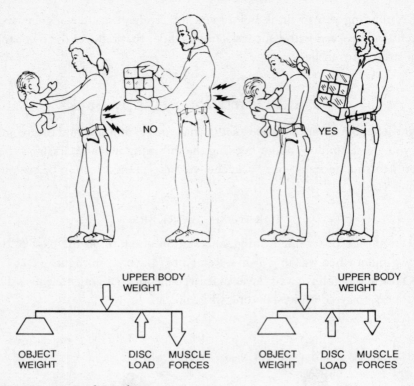

FIGURE 5.3. Back Mechanics

This picture will enhance your understanding of back mechanics. First, you must simply compare the *no* picture on the left with the *yes* picture on the right. Even if you are not interested in *why*, simply remember to lift and carry objects and babies as close as possible to the body. A study of the lever system shows that the forces on the back (the disc) depend upon (1) the weight of the object lifted, (2) the weight of the upper body, (3) muscle forces, and (4) lever arms. The *no* picture creates larger lever arms, requiring large muscle forces. The result is considerable force on the disc. In the *yes* picture, the lever is shorter and the muscle and disc forces are reduced. *(REPRODUCED WITH PERMISSION FROM WHITE, A. A., AND PANJABI, M. M.: CLINICAL BIO-MECHANICS OF THE SPINE, 2ND ED., J. B. LIPPINCOTT, 1990.)*

DO carry the baby as close to your body as possible, against your shoulder (figure 5.3).

DO bend your knees and keep objects (or babies) close to you when lifting; let your legs help you lift (figure 5.4). Don't lift the way a man does in figure 5.5.

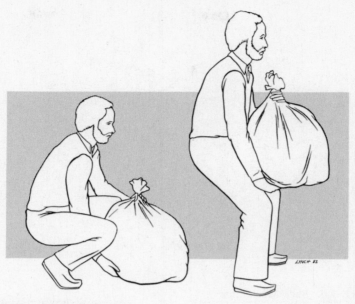

FIGURE 5.4. Back Mechanics

This is the classic proper lifting picture. The main points are (1) bend down with your hips and knees, *not* with your back, (2) lift with your legs, *not* with your back, and (3) keep the object *as close as possible* to your body.

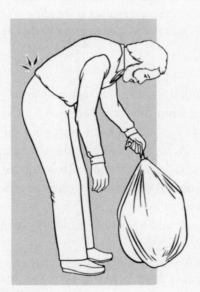

FIGURE 5.5. Back Mechanics

This is the classic wrong way to lift!

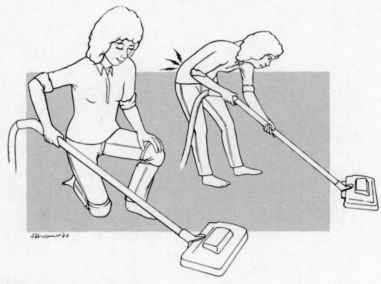

FIGURE 5.6. Back Mechanics

This technique helps to protect home workers with backache from what is probably their most threatening task. With a fresh new backache, this job simply ought to be avoided. Otherwise, it should be performed *not* in the usual manner of bending at the waist but *down on one knee*. If your knees are sensitive, get some sponge-rubber knee pads from any sports shop—a worthwhile investment. (The alternative is standing erect, moving your feet to advance in the direction that you want to move the vacuum to avoid bending and twisting.)

DO use a long-handled vacuum cleaner and kneel on one knee instead of bending over from the waist (figure 5.6). Use sponge-rubber knee pads. Always use your hands to support yourself when you must bend from the waist. According to my patients, vacuuming is one of the most notorious backache irritants. To maintain good posture, move your feet in the direction you wish to advance the vacuum, rather than bending and twisting.

DO use shopping carts and helpers as much as possible when loading and unloading groceries.

DO use care in lifting packages out of the car trunk. Position the package close to your body before lifting.

DO kneel down for gardening and break it up into five- to ten-minute intervals. Don't bend at the waist.

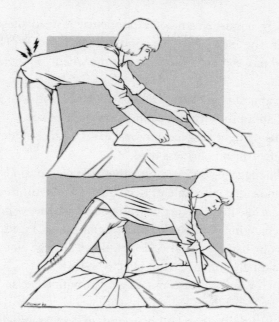

FIGURE 5.7. Back Mechanics

The home worker can avoid a lot of back pain irritation by simply support-ing the upper part of the body on the hands and knees when making the bed. It's better to have both sides of the bed away from the wall, so that you do not have to reach as far across the bed.

DON'T vacuum for long periods at a stretch. Break up the job into five- to ten-minute periods, with several hours or days in between. If you have back pain, have someone else do the vacuuming.

DON'T bend over to make a bed. When you can, kneel on the bed with one knee. Brace yourself with your arm to take pressure off your back. Another useful technique is to kneel on the floor at each side of the bed to straighten or tuck in sheets (figure 5.7).

DON'T try to open a stuck window if it is too tight; get help.

DON'T jerk-lift anything, stuck windows included.

FOR EXECUTIVES

DO get an appropriate chair.

DO get enough exercise to counter your sedentary work.

DO consider a chest-high or waist-high working surface as a part-time al-ternative to sitting.

DO occasionally hand-deliver correspondence instead of sending it by messenger. The exercise will be good for you.

DO get up and move about from time to time when you dictate or talk on the phone.

DO break up car and plane trips. Get out of the car and walk a bit at intervals; walk about the airplane cabin every hour or so.

DO consider using light luggage and briefcases with shoulder straps. This can be a lifesaver on business trips.

DO balance the luggage you carry on either side of your body. If your load must be one-sided, alternate it. Keep luggage to a minimum.

DO use a collapsible luggage carrier with wheels whenever possible.

DO consider changing your workstation organization, location, and so on to meet your back's special considerations. It need not compromise, and may actually enhance, your effectiveness.

DON'T overload your briefcase and *do* get one with wheels.

DON'T drive long distances without rest stops.

DON'T go all-out on the baseball diamond, or on any athletic field of endeavor, when you've been sedentary and out of condition. Work up to it gradually.

DON'T play golf unless you are aware of the risks and are willing to accept them (unless you are one of the lucky low back golfers who can get away with playing golf; see chapter 9).

DON'T have surgery just to get back to work two or three weeks sooner. Give bed rest and nonoperative treatments a good chance to help you.

DON'T hesitate to get up and move around the boardroom after prolonged sitting.

FOR ADMINISTRATIVE ASSISTANTS

DON'T arrange your desk so you're frequently twisting from one position to another.

DON'T bend over files for extended periods.

DON'T, if you happen to wear heels higher than 4.5 centimeters (1¾ inch), walk around in them all day. Keep a spare low-heeled pair in your drawer.

FOR HOSPITAL WORKERS

DO wait for help in lifting patients. Yes, everyone's busy, but they will be even busier if you are home from work with a bad back.

DO use transfer boards when possible to transfer patients from bed to stretcher, and so on. If it is not an emergency, it's worth the time.

DO put your foot on the bottom of the operating table or hospital bed (like a bar rail) to relax your psoas muscle while attending to an operation or caring for a patient at bedside (figure 5.2).

DO sit down to make a difficult vein puncture or a blood pressure reading rather than bending over the patient and struggling for several minutes.

DO sit in an appropriate chair when reading or studying.

DO remember that pushing a hospital bed or stretcher is better for your back than pulling it.

DO transfer your weight from one foot to the other when standing for long periods of time (more than several minutes).

DO raise the patient's bed to a comfortable level—waist level—when working with him/her.

DON'T assume you have cancer. We medical people always assume the worst when we get sick.

DON'T assume that, unless you keep working when you should be resting your bad back, all your patients will die. Someone else will take good care of them for you.

DON'T fail to be as careful and conservative with yourself as you would be with a patient.

DON'T lift improperly because you think nothing can happen to *you*.

DON'T climb up on a patient's bed with your knees when trying to lift him/her.

FLIGHT ATTENDANTS

DO pay special care to your lifting techniques.

DO maintain good overall muscle tone, especially in your abdomen and legs.

DO use wheels and carts to help transport your luggage. Maybe other travelers will learn from you.

DO get help from colleagues for difficult lifting.

DO look around you and suggest changes in work requirements and cabin design that could destress your back.

DO push rather than pull serving carts up and down the aisles.

DO keep your back straight and bend from the knees, and keep objects close to your body when lifting beverage kits and other heavy objects.

DO take time and care in stowing and retrieving things from under seats. Always get as close as possible to the object and avoid jerking motions.

DO bend from the knees and keep your back straight when removing and passing trays. If your back is bothering you, just pass the first tray to the aisle-seat passenger. Then, while leaning one arm on the back of the seat in front, pass the tray with the other. This will avoid the stressful position of bending at the waist and holding something way out in front of you.

DO, when carrying trays, pile them one on top of another when possible. Carry no more than three at a time, close to the body, with your elbows straight.

DON'T try to lift heavy objects into the overhead compartments.

DON'T make long reaches with a food tray—delivering a tray over two passengers to the one in the window seat, for instance. Chapter 2 explains why this maneuver is dangerous. Some friendly passengers may be willing to pass the tray to their neighbor.

DON'T reach above your head or out from your body to lift even moderately heavy objects.

FOR PILOTS AND COCKPIT CREW

DO get up and walk through the cabin a few times if security regulations permit. The kids will love it, and it will be great for your back.

DON'T sit the whole time on long flights. Get up and stretch if you can.

FOR HEAVY LABORERS

DO look for ways to reduce the injury potential in your workplace. Everything that needs to be lifted should be two feet off the floor.

DO put a priority on good abdominal, leg, and general muscle tone. A recent study of Los Angeles firefighters showed that good conditioning *prevented* back injuries.

DO ask for assistance from coworkers in heavy-lifting situations.

DO consider wearing a small back support or a large belt if you're doing lots of lifting. Although it remains unproven, this idea is theoretically sound.

DO use all available lifting aids whenever possible.

DON'T push yourself to do too much too soon during your convalescence from a back problem, but **DO** get back into the work environment and routine as soon as you can.

FOR EVERYBODY

DO be patient. You *will* get better.

DO what you can to control stress, depression, and anxiety in your life.

DO be considerate of your back when making love.

DO get adequate exercise, especially for strengthening your abdomen.

DO change position often if you're sitting a lot. Sit on one hip for a while, then the other, then both. Then slouch a bit before sitting erect for a while.

DO rest your arms on armrests when available, or on your lap when they're not.

DO try to use a chair that supports your lower back and has the potential to recline to about a 120-degree angle. Its seat should be wide enough for you to move around in it, and it should have armrests.

DO put a blanket, towel, or lumbar support behind your lower spine while driving. Place two pillows under your passenger-side arm as an armrest if the car does not have one. Rest your other forearm on the armrest built into the driver-side door. If none is present, improvise one there too.

DO obtain and use a cruise control in appropriate conditions when driving. This gives you more freedom to move about, shift your weight, and change your back position.

DO use a footstool or foot rail when standing for long periods (such as when ironing, working at the kitchen sink, or sitting at a bar.) Now you know why bars have bar rails.

DO get a long shoehorn if bending forward to put on your shoes aggravates your pain.

DO try to balance the load you're carrying on each side.

DO perform exercises that strengthen your stomach muscles. Stomach-tensing (isometric abdominal) exercises are better than sit-ups if you already have a bad back. Also, it is a very good idea to strengthen the back muscles. (See the exercise section of this chapter.) Just two precautionary notes: (1) Don't become a fanatic about exercise, and (2) don't take your conscience on any long guilt trips about not doing them.

DO exercise when you sit for prolonged periods in planes, trains, buses, and cars. See figures 5.8 and 5.9 for your "Olympic-class" seat exercises.

DON'T sit for extended periods.

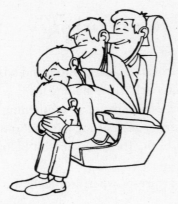

FIGURE 5.8. Seated Exercises

Draw the stomach in fully. Bend forward at the waist until the chest touches the thighs, then *gently* take your upper torso back to the upright position. Use your hands to help push yourself up. Do this twenty or thirty times about every two sitting hours. This is not for those of you with a sharp new back pain. It's good for all the rest of us. Remember this rule, however: If it hurts, don't do it. The advantage of this exercise is that it stimulates circulation and prevents stiffening. *(FIGURE REPRODUCED WITH PERMISSION FROM THE* SAS IN-THE-CHAIR EXERCISE BOOK, *BANTAM BOOKS INC., 1979.)*

DON'T bend over at the waist to pick up anything—or for more than a few seconds for any reason.

DON'T hold packages away from the body with your arms extended. Keeping the load close to the body reduces the burden on the lower spine.

DON'T do any vigorous back activity first thing in the morning, when your discs are more injury-prone because they have absorbed extra fluid while you were lying down asleep.

DON'T jog on very hard surfaces, especially if you're overweight and lack good jogging shoes. The combination of hard surface, poor footwear, and a bulky, awkward body can upset an already sensitive spine.

DON'T do exercises that involve excessive twisting and turning. Remember what we said of twist-induced back pain during Chubby Checker's heyday?

DON'T work standing on a hard surface if you can avoid it. If you can't, invest in some thick crepe or soft rubber soles and heels to absorb some of the impact.

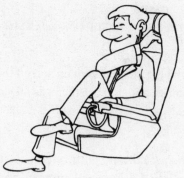

FIGURE 5.9. Seated Exercises

Lift the left and right knees alternately toward the opposite elbow. Reach a bit toward the opposite knee with the elbow. This is good for circulation, and it imparts a very slight and well-controlled axial rotation to the lumbar spine. This prevents the stiffness in the knee joints and the spine that can occur with prolonged sitting. Repeat the exercises fifteen times in each direction for every two hours of sitting time. *(FIGURE REPRODUCED WITH PERMISSION FROM THE SAS IN-THE-CHAIR EXERCISE BOOK, BANTAM BOOKS INC., 1979.)* The more inquisitive reader may ask, "Why is he advising me to bend forward as in figure 5.8 and to use my psoas muscle to twist a bit in figure 5.9?" The reason is that when you sit in one position a long time, your spine needs a bit of motion and stimulation. So you should do these two exercises, but slowly and gently.

DON'T become an unhappy compensation cripple.

DON'T carry your wallet in your back pocket if you have back pain and sciatica, as the wallet presses on the sciatic nerve when you sit or drive, aggravating your condition. This is an example of what we in medicine call a "pearl of wisdom," and I learned it from a truck driver patient of mine with sciatica! It certainly makes medical sense, since we doctors press on the sciatic nerve, just as a back wallet does, when we test for sciatica.

DON'T give up! It takes time. Follow this book, and *you will* get better.

An additional note for airline travelers: Prolonged travel with extended immobility has been associated with an increased risk of developing a deep venous thrombosis (DVT). If such a blood clot forms in your legs, it can break off and travel through the bloodstream into a lung, resulting in a potentially life-threatening pulmonary embolism (PE). There are conflict-

Summary of Preventive Measures

- Stay in shape by working out regularly.
- Learn and practice good ergonomics both on and off the job.
- Learn these do's and don'ts, and practice them, as they relate to you.

ing reports regarding the actual risk, with references made to predisposing factors such as a previous DVT, recent surgery, pregnancy, taking oral contraceptives, malignancy, restricted mobility, and genetically acquired clotting abnormalities. If you have any of these risk factors, please consult your physician prior to travel. If you have a long trip, stay hydrated, get up and walk around, stretch your legs at regular intervals, and wear loose-fitting clothing. Some physicians advise using support hose or compression stockings to reduce swelling and encourage blood flow in the deep veins. Those with risk factors may be prescribed the blood thinner heparin by their physicians. Although there is no objective data to demonstrate its efficacy, taking aspirin is sometimes advised as a preventive measure.

How to Treat Your Own Backache

Okay, you just did something to your back. You hit a beautiful topspin serve. Or you lifted a tire out of your car's trunk and twisted around to set it on the ground. Or perhaps you simply bent over from your chair to pick up a paper clip.

In any case, the pain hit. Maybe it was a mild stitch at first, but over the next few hours, it turned into a full-blown backache. You may have pain in one or both legs, in the hip or thigh area, or radiating all the way down to your heel, even your toes.

What do you do now?

You can manage this yourself, as long as you have not had trouble urinating or distinct weakness in your legs. If you *have* had such problems, get to a doctor straightaway. Why am I making such a big deal out of this rather mundane bodily function? Because if you've got a backache, and suddenly you can't urinate or hold your urine, you may have a very large herniated disc that has popped out of place. If it's displaced enough, it can hamper the nerves controlling your bladder, bowel, and legs. This situation requires immediate medical attention.

Otherwise, here it comes: "Take some aspirin, go to bed, and call me in the morning." Do not toss this book into the trash compactor yet. For reasons we will elucidate in a moment, bed rest and two aspirin every four hours as tolerated is the very best prescription at this point.

BEST BED TACTICS

What is the optimum lying-in-bed position for your sore back? Either on your back with your hips and knees bent (as in figure 5.10) or on your side, again with hips and knees bent in the fetal position. Try it: You will find that you will be more comfortable. This position relaxes the key muscles and take the burden off your spine. But if you find a more comfortable position, enjoy it, and if you will drop me a postcard describing it, I will share it with others. You can try putting two or three pillows under your knees or hanging your legs over the edge of the couch. Sometimes placing four or five blankets on the floor provides a firm surface that you may prefer to sleep on for several days. A position that's *not* apt to please your back is lying on your stomach, which causes irritating lordosis (swayback). Some patients tell me, "I'm in a real bind, because I prefer to sleep on my stomach, but my back really wipes me out when I do. If this distress applies to you, try this: Sleep on your stomach, but with your arms or a rolled towel supporting your hips, as shown in figure 5.11. This position supports the spine and may relieve just enough swayback to permit you to sleep on your abdomen.

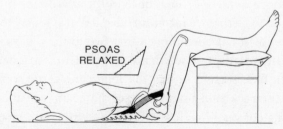

FIGURE 5.10. Comfortable Position for Aching Back

This shows an effective method for relaxing the psoas muscle and easing the stress on the low back. With the hips flexed and the weight relieved by being on the back, the spine is least likely to be irritated. Equally effective alternatives are shown in figure 8.2.

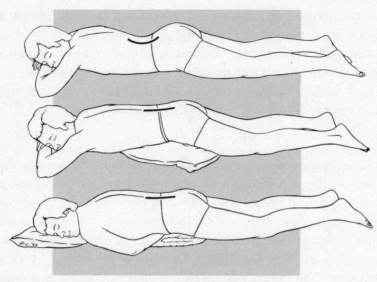

FIGURE 5.11. The Sleeping-on-the-Stomach Problem

The top illustration depicts the swayback, or slightly extended spine. Figure 8.1 shows us why that's a problem. Thus, the backache patient should avoid sleeping on the stomach. However, for variety, or if you simply must sleep on your stomach, try the tricks shown in the lower two illustrations. You can straighten out that spine a bit with a pillow or a towel and/or by sleeping with your forearms underneath your pelvic bone.

At first, you should stay in bed for two or three days. Feel free to get up to go to the bathroom and to cruise around the house two or three times a day, roughly once in the morning, once in the afternoon, and once in the evening. It used to be that we recommended bed rest for six to eight weeks. However, recently it has been proven that two to three days of bed rest is as good as many more, provided that your problem is just back pain, with no sciatica. In fact, staying in bed too long can accrue some significant negatives for the back pain sufferer: depression; stomach and bowel problems, including constipation; loss of bone and mineral tissue; blood clots in the legs; and weakening of the disc, cartilage, and ligaments. It sounds awful, I know, but that's the truth. So get out of bed as soon as you can after the first forty-eight to seventy-two hours.

On the other hand, some investigators and clinicians agree that modified bed rest (that is, up and about two to three times per day) for up to two weeks is a good idea if you happen to have severe leg pain (sciatica) along with your backache. The idea here is that the prolonged relative inactivity will allow the inflamed, irritated nerve root that is causing the sciatica to "cool down." A subsequent multicenter analysis has revealed that prolonged bed rest is less effective than staying active. They are equal if sciatica is present. The goal is to get a patient back to activities as soon as possible.

Mealtimes may be problematic, as sitting up will probably irritate your back. You *can* stay in a near-reclining position and eat from some type of tray, but make sure that you are not twisting your spine to eat from a tray at your side; you would be better off eating at the table or standing at a counter and returning promptly to bed.

MAKING LIGHT OF BED REST The banality "Forewarned is forearmed" applies here. If your back forces you to bed for a period, watch out for unwanted pounds. Inactivity plus the likelihood of boredom-inspired munching will make you less svelte than before. We have noted that weight stresses the lumbar spine. Do not fall into the vicious cycle of back pain leading to inactivity, weight gain, more back irritation, then greater immobility and so on. It may hurt, my friend, but now is the time for a little willpower. If you diet, however, follow a sensible low-calorie regimen, not a fly-by-night miracle diet. Take a generic multivitamin pill once a day.

GETTING IN AND OUT OF BED Getting in and out of bed with a backache is a sophisticated art. Consult the diagrams in figure 5.12.

To get out of bed, first lie on your side, facing the side of the bed from which you plan to arise. Then work your way over to the edge of the bed. Now, without twisting or bending your back (keep it straight), let your downside (bedside) arm push you up slowly to the sitting position. At the same time, move your legs over the side of the bed, so your feet can touch the floor. This motion is similar to that of a pregnant woman getting out of bed. Follow that example if you have ever witnessed or experienced this technique. If you perform this maneuver carefully, you will spare yourself some pain.

When getting into bed, reverse the maneuver. First, sit on the side of the bed, resting your pillow-side arm on the bed. Gradually bring your legs up as you slowly let your body down on its side by shifting your weight

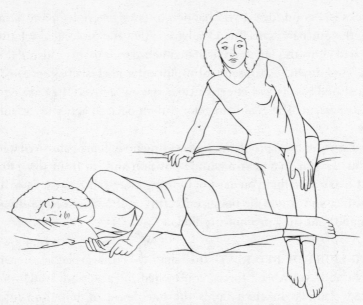

FIGURE 5.12. Proper Back Mechanics for Getting in and out of Bed

Here we see the side-lying position, with hips and knees flexed for a relaxed, pain-free back. This is also the position one should move to before getting in and out of bed. This figure also shows how to use your arm to push up when getting out of bed or to let yourself down when getting into bed.

from your palm to your forearm, then to your elbow, your shoulder, and your neck and head until you are fully reclined. Now move to your favorite position.

If your back is very painful, have someone help you by slowly lifting your legs as you let your body down.

ASPIRIN AND OTHER FRIENDS

Nonsteriodal anti-inflammory drugs have been shown to be effective for acute low back pain. However, the data on NSAID use for treating chronic low back pain are more limited.

Aspirin and buffered aspirin are two examples of NSAIDs and are usually the best for backache. Because comedians over the years have gotten a lot of mileage out of it, and because it is a cheap, over-the-counter medication, aspirin is not well respected by the layman. Once you understand how effective acetylsalicylic acid (aspirin) really is, you will probably stop sneering at the tablet. It has been estimated that 650 milligrams (two aspirin) every four hours is about as effective as 50 milligrams of Demerol (meperidine), a powerful opioid analgesic. Aspirin has also been found effective in preventing strokes and heart attacks.

When you take aspirin, you are fighting both the cause of your disease (inflammation) and its symptoms (pain). For moderate pain, two aspirin as needed are probably adequate. For more severe pain or pain that is clearly based on an inflammatory response, you should religiously swallow two aspirin every four hours (but do not wake yourself up to take it) for seven to ten days. This builds a significant blood level of the drug to fight inflammation and pain. Aspirin is a humble, homely miracle drug that is cheap, nonaddictive, purchased without a prescription, and very helpful!

However, no drug on earth is without its risks and limitations. Aspirin is an NSAID (nonsteroidal anti-inflammatory drug) and can irritate preexisting gastritis, ulcers, or just a sensitive stomach. Buffered or enteric-coated aspirin can reduce these risks, especially if taken with food or a light snack. Use of over-the-counter aid reducers such as Zantac and Prilosec may also reduce these stomach symptoms; however, you should confer with your physician. Aspirin may also be taken rectally.

Aspirin can also cause abnormal bleeding in some circumstances. Check with your physician if you think you're at risk.

If you are one of those who for one reason or another cannot tolerate aspirin, there are substitutes. Acetaminophen (Tylenol) is a similar non-prescription painkiller and very effective. Ibuprofen (Motrin) is another nonsteroidal anti-inflammatory drug. Several NSAIDs are now available over the counter, such as the brand names Aleve (naproxen) and Advil (also ibuprofen); thus, you do not need a prescription. Prescription NSAIDs (see list on page 46) are potentially helpful alternatives.

Patients with liver or kidney disease may have to avoid NSAIDs. As stated, these nonsteroidal anti-inflammatory drugs have gastrointestinal side effects, and therefore precautions must be taken. Always take these medications with a small snack. If one bothers your stomach, try a different one. Sometimes one is tolerated better than others, for no clear reason. Do not take a friend's or family member's medication. A physician should prescribe and supervise the use of all prescription medications.

The question of *muscle relaxants,* which are often prescribed with NSAIDs, almost invariably comes up. I prefer to use them selectively. The medical literature reveals that they can be effective in the management of nonspecific low back pain but, due to adverse effects, they must be used with caution. They have not been shown to be more effective than NSAIDs. In fact, muscle spasms, caused by the disease in the spine, may actually be protective. Pain prevents you from repeating activities that aggravate the affected area. When the disease wanes, the spasm should disappear.

The various relaxants seem to be similar in performance. When I do prescribe a muscle relaxant, I prefer methocarbamol (Robaxin) or metaxalone (Skelaxin), both of which tend to be less sedating. If you happen to be taking one of these drugs for low back pain and/or sciatica, remember this important point: It is possible that this medication can cause urinary retention; that is, you may have difficulty or be unable to urinate. You should report this to your doctor immediately, or, if you go to an acute-care facility, let someone know that the problem may be due to the medication you are taking. Otherwise, someone may fear that your inability to void is due to a huge disc herniation, and loss of ability to urinate based on a huge disk herniation requires immediate surgical removal of the disc.

The next chapter, on medical care for the problem back, will address these pharmacological matters in greater detail, including the side effects associated with the use of stronger painkillers (narcotic and nonnarcotic). For most backaches, however, aspirin or another nonaddictive medication is the drug of choice.

HEAT, ICE, AND MASSAGE

Heat is another ally while you are resting and recovering from your back ailment. An electric heating pad is as good as anything, although some people will prefer moist heat. Moist heating pads are generally available at any large drugstore or medical-surgical supply store. So long as it is not too hot and does not damage the skin, any form of heat will do.

What does heat or ice do for you? By soothing your aches, it can help break the cycle in which muscle spasm causes pain and so on. Refer back to the gate control theory of pain in chapter 4. The sensory input from heat or ice application (and massage too) may somehow block pain transmission, or it may cause local circulatory changes under the skin. Analysis of the evidence of efficacy from review of the medical literature, though limited, suggests that heat wrap therapy is associated with short-term improvement. There is insufficient published evidence regarding cold or ice therapy.

What is the data on massage as a therapeutic intervention? Clearly, massage, laying on of hands, tender loving care, and any sensual pleasure derived therefrom are good for the back as well as the soul. The literature indicates that massage "may be beneficial" for patients with subacute and chronic nonspecific low back pain, especially when combined with exercise and education. Overall, the reports present mixed results. Both ice and heat massage probably stimulate endorphin production and the placebo effect (see chapter 4), which can have potent benefits.

While I believe that any kind of heat application works equally well, the particular massage technique and skill of the masseur or masseuse are probably important factors. Oddly enough, ice massage—simply rubbing the back with ice cubes—comforts some sufferers. If it helps, don't worry about why. It cannot harm you.

"Which is better, heat or cold?" my patients ask. First answer: Use whatever feels best to you. Second answer: Generally, in an acute strain or with a muscle-pull injury with spasm, ice is likely to be better to reduce swelling in the first forty-eight hours, and heat thereafter.

Getting Well

HOW LONG, OH LORD, HOW LONG?

Observe yourself for signs of progress. Chart your recuperation in terms of what you can do today compared with yesterday or two or three days ago. You will no doubt find that you are improving. It may be gradual, but you will note that there are more and more things you can do without the excruciating pain that heralded your ailment. A little back diary can help you keep track.

We have indicated that bed rest should be limited to two or three days. If you are improving, even just a little bit, consider taking aspirin and reducing your activity (not bed rest) for as long as two or three weeks before consulting a doctor. (This assumes you have no problem urinating; if you do, see a doctor at once.) If you should get progressively worse over several days, even though you are doing all the right things, you may want to see a doctor about adding stronger painkillers to your regimen. Most people, however, will recover on a course of reduced activity, aspirin, *patience,* optimism, and following the advice in this book.

BYE-BYE, BACKACHE BLUES

What should you do when you start to feel better? How can you gauge how much activity your back can withstand? As soon as you can move with minimal pain, you can begin to walk around the house a little more. Then, when you have managed at-home maneuvers with little pain for two or three days, you can start pondering a more rigorous exercise program (see next chapter) and return to work. If commuting requires a long drive, have someone else do the driving during your early effort to return to work. You can either lie down in the backseat or sit in the front reclining seat, if your car has one. Sitting with your seat belt fastened is perhaps the safest choice, as required by law in forty-nine of fifty states.

Going back to work on a half-day basis at first may be wise. However, as long as your back pain does not come back to haunt you, go ahead and plunge right into a full schedule. You may need to take several breaks, getting up, walking around, or simply changing positions. Even with some residual back pain, as long as there is no major setback, you can progress to full-time work over the course of several days. Once you are almost free of pain, you can start the basic sitting and leg-stretching exercise described in the next chapter.

If your job involves heavy manual labor, however, your back-to-work scenario will be a little different. You will need a five- to ten-day essentially pain-free interval beforehand, then return to work with a *light*-duty schedule (policies permitting). That means lifting no more than twenty-five pounds and avoiding bending or twisting. If this is a problem because of your actual work situation, or if you have any questions, you should probably consult a physician about what your back is capable of handling.

Despite our keep-a-positive-attitude theme, I must warn you that sometimes patients who cautiously return to work have a setback, and their pain comes back full blast. Despair not: You will not have this severe pain forever. However, you must take it from the top, more or less, and start recuperating all over again. You will work yourself back to health sooner than you think, so try again.

CONVALESCENCE: STEP BY STEP

Let us describe the convalescent period (the time between recovering from acute back pain and returning to the workplace) in a little more detail.

First a sermonette: In the last chapter I warned you against the tribulations of compensation tragedy and the poor soul. Now I would like to address the other end of the spectrum: those individuals who think the sun will be stuck below the horizon if they do not get back to the office and make it all happen. Do not worry. The work crew, company, hospital, government, store, university, team, family, business will all still be there. Of course you are needed and missed, but do not wreck your back by playing the martyr, the hero/heroine, and "totin' them bales" prematurely. You may be as strong as an ox, but if you yield to back pain like a willow to the wind, you will bounce back sooner.

What are the risks of too much activity too soon? You may reirritate your spine and cause a setback that will prolong your overall convalescence. One signpost of recovery is the amount of time spent out of bed and moving about. You should do a bit of sitting, but not too much, as it puts a big load on the spine. When you can sit without back pain for over twenty minutes, you will know you can gradually increase your activities.

Noting the amount of pain-free time you spend each day is a good gauge of how much you can stay out of bed. Another specific milestone is how much walking you can do. You can gradually extend your distances as your back permits.

Sometimes you can do a little gentle testing of your work conditions. Try deskwork when there are other signs of recovery. Certain types of mild to moderate physical labor can also be performed as a test run.

After you return to work, stop and lie down for a few minutes if your back bothers you. This is crucial advice, as it often prevents a reinjury or setback. Let me repeat it con brio: *If your back hurts, stop and lie down for a few minutes, with your hips and knees bent!*

Here is a summary of some key back-to-work information as espoused by the late Professor Alf Nachemson of Sweden:

Back-to-Work Checklist (Reminder)

- Do not lift heavy objects.
- Whatever you lift, keep it close to your body.
- Have a lumbar support and armrest where you sit.
- Avoid bending and twisting.
- Change positions frequently.
- Do not sit in low chairs.

Exercises

Exercises are important, and they do help! Once you are able to get back to work, or even a few days before, you can start an exercise program. In my opinion, the simple, straightforward exercises below represent the best advice current medical knowledge has to offer you. A word of warning: Do not confuse complexity with efficacy. I suspect that some exercise programs may seem more compelling because they are complicated. Don't worry—sometimes simple is beautiful.

WALKING, BICYCLING, AND SWIMMING

A simple, straightforward, effective exercise program encompasses several key components: (1) regularity, (2) trunk muscle strengthening and endurance, and (3) palatability—that is, the exercises should be somewhat interesting and enjoyable. Regularity is important to stimulate endorphin secretions (our own internal pain control substances). Regular exercise is the key to building strength and endurance. There is evidence that good, functional trunk muscles support the spine and help in rehabilitation and prevention of recurrence. Finally, since we are all endowed with the inalienable right of the pursuit of happiness, among other things, we need to have fun doing the exercises. Moreover, if in this process of fighting the backache battle we can become habitual exercisers, this would be a bonus. It takes six weeks to develop a habit (a good or bad one). To develop a healthy exercise habit, tie it to a current habit—for example, your daily dental hygiene. Tell yourself, "I can't brush my teeth until I've done my back exercises." The tandem approach is a successful one. The exercises suggested, and the schedule recommended, are designed to provide aerobic fitness as well.

In our routine program, patients gradually work up to a point where they can walk, bicycle (mobile or stationary), or swim for a half hour to three-quarters of an hour at their own pace, three to five times per week. Any combination of the three activities is fabulous! The patient is advised to gradually work up to the half-hour range and to continue with mild pain as tolerated, but to stop when there is severe pain.

Walking can be done as a slow, relaxed, recreational walk, or it can be done with as much vigor as can be tolerated. A fifteen-minute mile is excellent for aerobic conditioning. Use your iPod or MP3 player to listen to music, humor, foreign-language lessons, sermons, lectures, audio novels, or unmentionables to make it fun.

Use of a stationary bike or bicycling outdoors is generally well tolerated by those with back pain. As with walking, one can gradually build up to the suggested thirty- to forty-five-minute workout and go at one's own pace. Supplementary entertainment with audio or, if stationary biking, TV, videos, or DVDs, can enhance the fun.

Swimming is often described as the best exercise for patients with low back pain, as well as the best all-around exercise. Swimming works all of our major muscle groups, provides superb aerobic conditioning, and takes a tremendous amount stress off of our backs. We ask our patients to use any stroke or any combination of strokes that they enjoy. The butterfly stroke tends to aggravate a lot of patients because of the extension component (swayback, or lordosis, of the back). However, if it does not bother you, and you enjoy the butterfly stroke, then continue without worry. The guidelines for pain are the same as stated above.

These are our recommendations. Certainly, any sport or physical activity that does not aggravate one's pain can be helpful as well as invigorating. We usually like to discuss these sports individually with the patient. Our goal, of course, is to help the patient get back to doing whatever it is he/she wants to do. Jogging or "wogging" (a combination of jogging and walking) can often be participated in successfully without pain, as can golf, tennis, sailing, softball, bowling, and many other activities, although some seem to be more likely than others to cause difficulty. The recommendation is best made after a careful and current history of tolerance and incidence. There is a lot more about sports and the back in chapter 9.

You have just been exposed to my first choices for exercises, but the following is a discussion of several other reasonable approaches that have been utilized and prescribed for patients with back problems.

SIT-UPS

Sit-ups have been considered important because they strengthen the abdomen and, in theory, relieve the spine of stress (figure 5.13).

Sit-ups should *not* be done with the leg straight, or with the feet or legs hooked under some fixed object (figure 5.14). Why? Doing them that way makes the psoas muscle work too hard, imparting high stress to your spine. And this phenomenon aggravates rather than alleviates any exist-

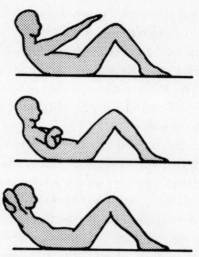

FIGURE 5.13. Exercise

These exercises are good for strengthening the stomach muscles after you've gotten over the initial sharp back pain. These sit-ups increase in difficulty from top to bottom, because you shift the center of gravity upward by moving the arms closer to the head. The top one is fine and the best for most readers.

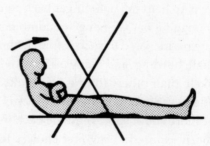

FIGURE 5.14. Exercise

This is no good for the back, even if you don't have backache. It is the best way to strain the spine, because when you do sit-ups this way, or with something holding your feet down, you use the psoas muscle and stress your back. This obviously is what you do when you lean over the side to balance a sailing craft. See Sailing, chapter 9.

ing backache. For that matter, they may even be undesirable for someone *without* back pain.

So start the exercise lying flat on your back, with your hips and knees bent. In the beginning, you won't have much strength, so you need do no more than just reach for your knees by raising your head, shoulder, and upper back off the floor (figure 5.13). If you can do this twenty to twenty-five times once or twice a day, you'll develop abdominal tone and protect your back. As you gain strength, you can increase the difficulty by putting your arms behind your head.

ISOMETRIC ABDOMINAL EXERCISE

Tighten your throat, bowel, and bladder muscles. Then press hard, as if you were trying to have a bowel movement, and concentrate on tightening all your abdominal muscles. This, my friend, is the isometric abdominal exercise. There is a minicourse on the terminology of muscle contractions in the next section, and the definitions are in the glossary. If you do not particularly enjoy studying these terms, do not worry: You can take good care of your back without memorizing all of the definitions.

The beauty of these exercises is that you can do them while riding in a car, standing, talking on the phone, or whenever. Their purpose is to tone up your abdomen, and you should do fifteen or twenty of them three or four times a day. I think that this is the best exercise of all, especially if you are only going to do one exercise. If you have heart disease, it should not be done without consulting your doctor.

BACK MUSCLE EXERCISES

Some clinical studies and a number of therapists have emphasized strengthening the back muscles, mainly the erector spinae group. There are two ways to achieve this. One is to simply lie facedown and raise your head and upper chest off the surface. The other is illustrated in figure 5.15. Start down on all fours, then lift one arm and the opposite leg to a posi-

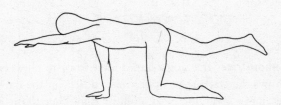

FIGURE 5.15. Exercise

An excellent (though not easy) exercise to strengthen the back muscles. *(REPRODUCED WITH PERMISSION FROM WHITE, A. A., AND PANJABI, M. M.: CLINICAL BIOMECHANICS OF THE SPINE, 2ND ED., J. B. LIPPINCOTT, 1990.)*

tion parallel to the floor; hold a second and then place them back down on the floor. Then do the same with the opposite arm and leg. This is not easy because it requires good balance and strength. If you can work up to ten or fifteen repetitions for each arm and leg daily, you will have significantly strengthened your back muscles.

KNEE-TO-CHEST EXERCISES Take a look at figure 5.16. Lying on your back with your hips and knees slightly flexed, pull one leg up to your chest, using both arms. Then return it to its original position and do the same thing with the other leg. Repeat ten times for each leg. The purpose of this exercise is to stretch the muscles and ligaments in the spine and the back

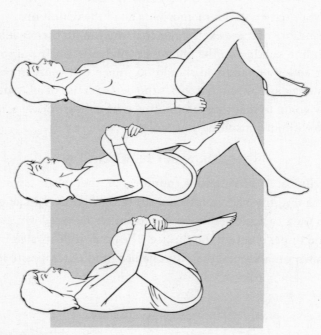

FIGURE 5.16. Exercise

This figure demonstrates the single and double knee-to-chest exercise. The top picture shows the starting position: relaxed, flat on the back, with hips flexed and feet flat on the floor. Next, pull the right knee to the chest. Complete the last few inches by pulling with the arms. Then let go, relax, and repeat with the left knee. The double knee-to-chest exercise is done as shown in the bottom drawing. If you are one of the few patients who experiences additional pain following these knee-to-chest exercises, discontinue them.

of the hip, improving posture and spine mechanics and alleviating back stresses. It can also be done by bringing both knees up simultaneously, also repeated ten times.

Twice a day is best, but even a consistent once-a-day habit should benefit you greatly.

However, be advised that some of you, especially if you are afflicted with sciatica, may find this exercise irritating. If so, don't do it. This rule applies to any activity that makes your back hurt more, for the old work-through-the-pain concept is a fallacious one.

THE PELVIC TILT If you are a dancer or a lover, or both, it may inspire you to learn that this movement is essentially the "front bump" in dancing and the pelvic motion basic to lovemaking. Back up against the wall or lie on the floor. Now put your hand behind your lower back, feeling the arch there and nothing that the back isn't touching the wall (or floor) at that point. Then try to flatten your back to eliminate the gap. When you have performed this maneuver, then you have just completed a pelvic tilt. Do fifteen to twenty of these every day, and that should suffice. This exercise strengthens the front spine structures and stretches the back ones. And it moves the lumbar spine from a lordotic (swayback) position to a straighter position that is better for your back (figure 5.17).

Some Things You Need to Know About Muscles, Exercise, and Low Back Pain

There are three important, practical questions to be discussed concerning low back pain. First, how important is trunk muscle function in the evaluation, treatment, rehabilitation, and prevention of low back pain? Second, assuming that strong erector spinae muscles are important, what is the best way to strengthen them? Third, if one decides to strengthen these back muscles, what is the importance of various types of exercise machines that are available for monitoring the muscle activity?

If you have back pain rehabilitation in the twenty-first century, you are very likely to be encounter some of the following terms. Therefore, before I discuss muscle strengthening, please allow me to share with you a brief glossary of muscle contraction terminology. Your therapist or physician may occasionally use one or more of these terms or phrases.

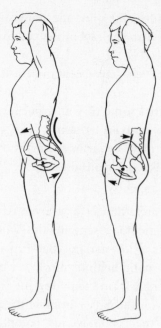

FIGURE 5.17. Exercise

The pelvic tilt exercise can be difficult to explain. However, between the text and the good work of Pat Lynch, our dedicated illustrator, you will understand the concept. On the left, we see the position of the low back and pelvis in the swayback (extended) position. I describe elsewhere (figure 8.1) the theoretical negatives of this position. The pelvic tilt shown on the right rotates the pelvis and straightens out the spine, which accentuates the positives and eliminates the negatives. The forces are better distributed with the pelvic tilt as shown.

On the left is the relaxed swayback position. On the right, the arrows show the forces that must be exerted by muscles to rotate it to the proper position. The text tells you how to get your pelvis in this more healthy position. Now you must get in the habit of keeping it there.

- **Concentric contraction:** There is tension in the muscle and it contracts, actively shortening. The load acted upon is less than the maximum tension that the muscle can generate, permitting the muscle to shorten. Lifting a weighted barbell with your hand and flexing your elbow causes the biceps muscle in your upper arm to contract (shorten).
- **Isotonic contraction:** There is tension in the muscle (contraction again); this time, it also changes its length. However, the tone or force of this concentric muscle contraction remains relatively unchanged. Take

a sip of coffee. When you lift the cup, you contract and shorten your biceps muscle. The force required to lift the cup is minimal as coffee, with its familiar, stimulating aroma, moves to your welcoming lips. That is isotonic contraction.

- **Isometric contraction:** There is tension in the muscle (it contracts), but it *does not* change its length. Consequently, there is no motion of the associated joint or limb. I discussed this type of contraction when we reviewed isometric abdominal exercises on page 125.
- **Eccentric contraction:** There is tension in the muscle (you've got it: contraction), and it changes length—but this time, rather than shortening, it lengthens! Right! It is the opposite of concentric contraction. Would *lengthening contraction* be a more descriptive term? Some people think so. You be the judge. Here is an example of eccentric contraction. You take a sip of coffee and put down your cup. The weight of the cup and its contents is resisted by the biceps muscle involved in an eccentric contraction. The muscle lengthens as it contracts to ensure a gradual, safe descent of the cup to the table.
- **Isokinetic contraction:** There is tension in the muscle (right, it contracts: the common denominator). However, this time there is a small and powerful machine that can be set to select and control the speed at which you can move your arm, leg, or trunk. The rate of muscle shortening can be held constant. Machines that do this eliminate certain variables and make possible a more standardized analysis of muscle strength and fatigue.
- **Isointernal contraction:** There is tension in the muscle and a change in length, but this time the smart machine can control and keep constant the load, or the force, that the muscle must exert.

Testing equipment is available to control resistance, rate, and range of movement (acceleration, velocity, and distance). This leaves only the torque as an independent variable, which makes it possible to compare a patient with him-/herself and with others in a standard method. The Cybex and Kin-Com are examples of computerized machines that measure the power, strength, and endurance of various muscle groups.

To briefly summarize and review, there is tension in the muscle with every contraction. It either (a) keeps the same length, (b) shortens, or (c) lengthens. Moreover, for contractions whereby there is a change in length, there are machines that can select and keep *constant* either (a) the speed that the muscle changes its length or (b) the loads that must be overcome as the length changes. Are you thoroughly confused? If not, let's move on. If so, let's move on, because understanding every aspect of muscle physiology is by no means crucial to getting rid of that backache.

Let us continue with some additional background information. Analysis of trunk muscles shows that the extensors (back muscles) are generally stronger than the flexors (abdominal and psoas). My athletic daughters were amused to find out that although men as a group are stronger than women in the absolute sense, women are stronger on a pound-for-pound basis. In addition, research shows that women demonstrate greater endurance in their trunk muscles. It seems that we are all destined to show a distinct loss of strength in the trunk muscles, beginning around age forty.

Most muscle strains and acute soft-tissue injuries of the spine and trunk recover completely in three to six weeks. Although machine-controlled muscle testing provides some quantitative assessment of functional capacity, it can be irritating if started too soon after the onset of the acute condition.

As mentioned previously, there is moderate evidence that inadequate trunk strength may predispose a person to having a backache. Studies show that sit-ups, extension exercises, and electrical stimulation of muscles enhance endurance but not strength. Trunk muscle strength can be improved with a six- to twelve-week exercise program.

In recent years, there have been some prominent studies of the use of trunk muscle exercise in the treatment of low back pain. As we have mentioned before, there are no strong, consistent ropes of evidence to support claims for their efficacy. The current literature promotes the idea that trunk therapeutic (abdominal and/or extension) exercise, in conjunction with back pain school (see page 159) and work hardening (page 161) programs, are beneficial.

Studies of the electrical response of muscles, as well as mechanical studies of the trunk muscles, show an association between trunk muscle fatigue and low back pain.

Let me now attempt to provide succinct answers to the questions posed at the beginning of this section.

Q. *How important is trunk muscle function in the evaluation, treatment, rehabilitation, and prevention of low back pain?*

A. It is very important, because patients with low back pain have decreased strength and are more likely to have less endurance. In all probability, the development of strong trunk muscles, particularly the erector spinae, is useful in the treatment, rehabilitation, and prevention of low back pain. However, the clinical evidence to prove this is not as strong as we would like.

Q. *Assuming that strong trunk muscles are desirable, what is the best way to strengthen them?*
A. Swimming, stationary bicycling, walking, back extension exercises, and the use of various exercise machines to increase muscle strength.

Q. *How important is it to use various exercise machines for monitoring muscle activity?*
A. The currently available evidence does not prove that they are essential. They are nice to have and, appropriately used, they can make a contribution. There is also an unproven but probably psychological advantage in that the patient can "see progress." This, I believe, has motivational value to the patient.

The current best available scientific evidence suggests that education in the form of a back school program, coupled with low-impact aerobic exercise, has been shown to reduce pain and improve function in the short and intermediate term. So good luck, and get to work!

WHEN *NOT* TO EXERCISE

Do not exercise right after getting out of bed in the morning. Your discs have taken in fluid while you were asleep, with no gravitational forces on them. Thus, they are tense and more prone to irritation. Wait two hours before doing your exercises.

Do not do any exercise that causes severe pain. Whenever your back gets worse, you should decrease your activity. And do not abandon hope: It is highly probable that you will gradually recover again without a relapse.

Devices for Daily Living

MATTRESS CONNOISSEURSHIP

The morning can be a stiff and painful time of day for the backache sufferer. Therefore, let us now talk about beds.

First, do not be hoodwinked by terms such as *orthopedic* or the root *ortho-* affixed to particular beds or mattresses. Words like *posture, medical, osteopathic, chiropractic*, and so on, while perhaps evocative of white uniforms, do not guarantee better sleep or a disease-free life, either. Your own preference is a good place to start; after all, you spend approximately a third of your life either recreating, procreating, or recuperating there.

Let us start with the simplest scenario. If you have a normal back and no acquaintance with backache, then in addition to being an unlikely reader of this tome, you should choose your mattress based entirely on comfort. "Sleeping around" on different mattresses in hotels or in department or furniture stores is an inevitable part of the selection process. Once you have narrowed your choice to two or three mattresses or beds, explain to the salesperson that you need to try it out for a half hour or so.

All other things being equal, a relatively firm mattress is best. Moreover, you can firm up a bed by laying down a ⅜-inch plywood board on some cinder blocks or a wood frame, then using a 3- to 6-inch piece of foam rubber as a mattress. Another alternative is to place a plywood board between your box spring and mattress.

Now, if you are a backache victim, everyone has probably told you to get a hard mattress—as hard as possible. That advice is sound. To test out how a firm mattress would treat your back, put six or eight blankets on the floor and sleep there for three to five nights. Feel better? If so, then a very firm mattress should be a good investment.

But, again, individuals are unpredictable. Some of you back pain sufferers may not sleep comfortably on a hard mattress, and something medium or even soft may suit you better. If you do prefer a softer mattress, and the sleeping-on-the-floor test does not do anything for your back, go with the soft mattress.

What about water beds? Trial and error is the best modus operandi. If you like it and it does not hurt your back, enjoy sleeping on the waves. You might first test one out in a motel. However, I do not think there is any magic to slumbering on H_2O.

Here is some useful specific information about beds that I am happy to be able to pass on to you. Drs. S. R. Garfin and S. A. Pye of the University of California at San Diego completed a very useful study. They compared the effects of four types of beds on patients with long-term low back pain. Bed number one was a hard bed (720 individually reinforced coils and a built-in bed board). Bed number two was a softer bed (500 coils, with no bed board). Bed number three was a commercially available water bed filled to a depth of 9 inches. Bed number four was a "hybrid" bed (a combination of foam and water). The results of their study revealed that the majority of patients preferred the hard bed and thought their back pain improved more after two weeks of use. The water bed came in second.

I do not mean to be inconsiderate of your partner. In any case, I had hoped that some reasonable compromise could give you both satisfactory sleeping arrangements. You probably cannot expect your mate to be happy on the floor for nights on end! One possibility is to soften a very firm mattress on one side with a foam rubber covering. There are, however, mattresses available whereby the firmness of each side can be adjusted. These are typically more expensive, but they may keep the peace in your household when it comes to sleeping arrangements. Your ingenuity may suggest other options.

CORSETS

Corsets have been around for centuries, mostly to accentuate the positives and eliminate the negatives in the female form, and occasionally the male. But our focus is on therapeutic corsets.

The rationale for use of a corset is that if the spine can be immobilized, supported, and allowed to rest, it will be irritated less and therefore more comfortable. Corsets may do so by reducing the stress on your spine. I also suspect that there is an emotional value in making your back feel more secure and supported. If it feels better for your back to wear the corset, then enjoy it and do not worry about your muscles atrophying. Remember that it is not possible for muscles that are exercised to waste away.

Next comes more sophisticated spine-immobilizing devices like braces and casts, which ought to be prescribed by a physician. We will discuss brace and cast technology in the next chapter.

A GUIDE TO SEATS

Well, you have gotten out of bed, dressed with or without a corset, and now you are about to drive or ride to work. During many parts of your day, you are going to be in a seat. The natural question is: What is the ideal seat?

That depends, in part, on what you are sitting down to accomplish. Therefore, we will break this down into categories. Much of the following information is based on experiments that measured intervertebral disc pressures as well as the sitters' subjective comfort ratings.

It appears that the more a seat is reclined, up to 120 degrees, the more comfortable it is. A distinct lumbar support in the chair is better than an indistinct or absent one. Armrests decrease the forces on the low back. Plenty of space on the seat platform is desirable, because it supports the thighs and allows for comfortable shifts of position. Readers who have compared long airplane trips in first class with those in economy class will attest to this criterion.

Another factor is the position of the entire seat in relation to the floor. That is, if the angle between the seat's back and bottom is 90 degrees in the erect position, and the entire seat is tilted 20 degrees in relation to the floor, the forces on the spine are reduced, even though the angle between back and seat has not changed. This concept (shown in figure 5.18) may seem abstract, but it can, in fact, be used by a weary driver with an adjustable power seat.

Avoid low chairs.

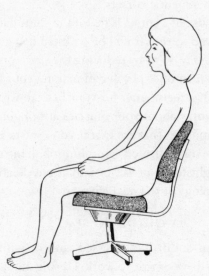

FIGURE 5.18. Ergonomic Chair

This shows the principle of fully tilting a chair to the horizontal to unweight the spine and relax the back muscles. By tilting the bottom (seat part) of the chair, it is possible to decrease considerably the stresses on the spine. This type of chair can be returned to the upright position and locked for working.

CAR SEATS Individual taste surfaces here, for we know that some people will ride in a terribly uncomfortable seat if the car satisfies the ego. But if you drive a great deal and back comfort overshadows ego gratification, then select a comfortable car seat. Why not rent several cars in order to find one or two with comfortable seats? You should drive them long enough to be certain before you make a purchase. You can also get opinions from friends in your search for the ideal seat.

It is well known that the Volvo Corporation has invested a great deal of resources in human spine research, using the information to design its automobile seats. In addition, the multiply adjustable power seat system, which allows the driver more changes of position, has its virtues.

Here are a few car-seat-enhancing tips: If there is no armrest on either side, then improvise. A pillow will serve you well, either next to the door or on the middle part of the seat. Long trips make an armrest particularly desirable. If you are driving, relax your arms by hanging them steadily on the steering wheel, which unweights the spine and relaxes the shoulders. Recline in your seat as much as you can while still being able to see the road. You may want to alternate this position with one in which the seat is more erect and pulled close to the steering wheel. You can use a towel, small blanket, or pillow between the seat and your lower back for that crucial lumbar support, if your vehicle does not have one that you can adjust. Remember to place it at the curved part of the back, the way the administrative assistant's seat fits in figure 5.1.

SEAT ACCOUTREMENTS A few devices may come in handy. An air pillow—a small 18-by-18-inch rubber pillow with a detachable hand bulb inflator—allows you to pump up your low back support to the desired bulge and stiffness. It comes with straps that attach to any car seat.

Another device, the three-way portable, adjustable orthopedic seat, can be used in the car, at home, or at work. It boasts some real advantages: The amount of recline—as well as the prominence and height of the back support—can be controlled. Therefore, the seat can be fashioned to your unique anatomy and comfort requirements. It's available through Nepsco Inc., 53 Jeffrey Avenue, Holliston, MA 01746.

Let us mention a few more car seat helpers. One is a seat-within-a-seat, usually an insert with just a bottom, a back, or both, which may have cushioned wire coils or springs. There are also wedges that fit right into the angle where the seat back meets the base in an attempt to offer lumbar support. However, these tend to be too low. Such devices can be found at large auto supply or "truck stop" stores. Nevertheless, try the towel or pillow trick first. If it helps, go to an air pillow or an adjustable orthopedic seat.

SEATS AND STANDING DESKS AT WORK Now that you have made it to work, you will probably have to spend several hours on your derriere. Sitting places more force on your spine than standing does. If you enjoy the luxury of an executive chair, have it fit the criteria of the ideal seat. Consider having all the seats under your domain come as close as possible to the ideal traits while remaining functional. While you are at it, consider arranging for all of the seats that you purchase for your company to pamper the backs of the employees.

Secretarial seats with lumbar supports, armrests, and a reclining option are available. In some cases, of course, armrests are not practical. Draftsmen and other desk workers can have appropriately designed chairs that do not interfere with their work. Improvisation can improve your work seat, as it did your car seat, if this year's budget does not allow for buying more chairs.

For several years, patients have asked me about furniture that substitutes as a chair in which people can kneel to work, read, and so on. The weight is carried partially by the buttocks, but the shins and lower legs carry a significant portion of it as well. I can now happily give an answer. Balans chairs (figure 5.19), as they are called, were studied and found to be less comfortable than more conventional chairs, and using them caused increased muscle activity in the neck and back. This implies more stress or strain occurs in the position in which this device is used. Nevertheless, some patients like them. My advice is for you to use what is most comfortable. However, there is no evidence that it is going to be helpful or therapeutic for a bad back. The price of a Balans chair ranges from $200 to more than $300. Newer versions can be equipped with wheels and/or a lumbar support.

Do not forget that just about everything you can do sitting can also be done standing up. It may be worth it to build waist-high or chest-high platforms (with bar rails) as alternative workbenches. It is not written in stone that a computer will not work if its operator is on his/her feet. You can even read—this book, for instance—standing at a high desk. In fact, a

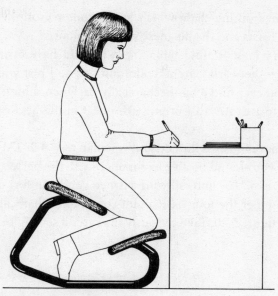

FIGURE 5.19. Ergonomic Chair

This is the Balans chair. The body weight is supported on the buttocks and the shins. While these are marketed as "more comfortable" chairs, clinical studies suggest that they are not. However, if you try it and like it, that is all that matters.

number of my patients who would usually be doing a great deal of sitting have been helped tremendously by standing desks. This is a very important point to consider. Depending on your individual preference and comfort, a standing desk should come up to your waist, at minimum, and your chest/nipple line, at maximum. It should incline up and away from you. (If you are unable to locate one, or have one built, try contacting Peabody Office Furniture, 234 Congress Street, Boston, MA 02110, (617) 542-1902, www.peabodyoffice.com, or the Comfort Store online at www.sitin comfort.com. A high stool with a backrest and a foot rail at a high desk is another option.

HOME AND HEARTH

Now you have managed to get through the working day; you have driven home in your cleverly improvised or scientifically designed comfortable car seat; and you are ready for dinner. Unhappily, I have never seen a com-

fortably designed dining chair, which may be one reason the Romans reclined at their feasts and the Japanese sit on the floor.

At the very least, dining table chairs should have armrests, and if
yours do not, forget early parental admonitions and rest your elbows on
the table. If you ever find a biomechanically designed dining chair, please
send me a picture of it, and I promise to put it in the next edition of this
book.

Now you have finished dinner, and you plan to watch TV or read a bit.
Here is where you should be able to come up with the perfect seat. Simply
shop for your own "10" until all your aesthetic and comfort qualifications
are met. Remember the four basic points of a biomechanically ideal seat,
as depicted in figure 5.20. Take seriously the careful search for a truly com-

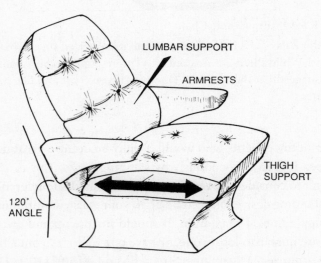

FIGURE 5.20. Ergonomic Chair

This figure depicts the important elements of the biomechanically ideal seat,
your ideal chair for maximum low back comfort. Features include (1) significant lumbar support, (2) the ability to recline at least 120 degrees, (3) armrests, and (4) ample thigh support and room to change position. As long as
you have these four basic elements, you can do anything you like with design, upholstery, and so forth, and have the best seat for relaxing your back.
*(REPRODUCED WITH PERMISSION FROM WHITE, A. A., AND PANJABI, M. M.:
CLINICAL BIOMECHANICS OF THE SPINE, 2ND ED., J. B. LIPPINCOTT, 1990.)*

fortable chair that has the biomechanical characteristics described here for you. This can be an important lifetime investment of time and money.

VIBRATING CHAIRS, BEDS, MASSAGERS

Massagers, which come with some mattresses and reclining chairs, can certainly soothe the back and relax tense muscles. A simple handheld vibrator, its honeymoon-catalogue aura aside, can also ease the painful parts of your back. The cheapest one that is safe and feels good is probably the best buy. Although these devices do not cure any basic problem, they can put you in a relaxed state, the virtues of which are laid out in chapter 4. Whether the laying on of human hands or the application of an electrical masseur works best is purely a matter of individual taste and availability.

A HELPFUL HINT

This is a tip from a patient. The severe leg pain associated with low back pain is greatly comforted by wearing substantial support stockings (support hose or long-leg supports). Just as a comfort measure, not a cure, of course.

Fellow Humans

See chapter 7 for a list of my opinions, based on the current best medical evidence, regarding how to select from the major available options for back care.

Our next chapter addresses the problem back. It is a practical guide to obtaining and profiting from the best medical care. If you suffer from chronic backache, you will want to turn the page for an inventory of all nonsurgical treatments, from acupuncture and spinal manipulation to traction and trigger point injections.

Reflecting on the various home remedies discussed here, it seems that I have painted a somewhat dismal picture of everything you must do to avoid backache. It goes something like this: Don't work too much. Don't sit too much. Don't make love too much. Don't lift too much. Don't drive too much. Don't smoke. Don't play golf. Don't get promoted or divorced. Redesign all your furniture. Don't put on weight.

And, of course, don't stress yourself.

In real life, though, just two or three minor adjustments, like a new mattress, a moderate exercise program, and making pit stops during long car trips, may do wonders in keeping your backache at bay. Now, if you *don't* have chronic or intractable pain, this is the ideal time to save your back. I believe that this chapter should be reread from time to time until it becomes second nature to you. Also, remember that most people get rid of their back pain in two to three weeks. May the "force" be with you!

CHAPTER 6

The Problem Back

Nonsurgical and Minimally Invasive Treatments

BACKACHE, ESPECIALLY THE CHRONIC OR RECURRENT KIND, is not an easy companion to live with. Back care is a field full of confusion, contradictory opinions, unanswered questions, myriad therapies—orthodox and not so orthodox—and, yes, some dubious practitioners (figure 6.1). Is it any wonder that you sometimes feel like a wanderer in a labyrinth? Alas, there are no foolproof cures. When we fully understand spine disease, we will let you know. However, we *do* know that if you follow the guidelines presented for you here and do your best to be patient, you will most likely gradually improve.

What this book can do for you is to serve as a survival manual. We will guide you through the intricacies of doctors' offices—and acupuncture clinics. The various types of spinal care available, including alternative and complementary medicine, are not all administered by MDs. This chapter will acquaint you with just about all the known nonsurgical back treatments, noting everything we presently know about their value or lack thereof. It will help you pick your way through the "bs" nonsurgical treatments. That is, through the "bold speculation." We will also review minimally invasive approaches prior to our venturing into the chapter on surgical interventions.

When to Get Help

In the last chapter, we told you how to treat your backache at home. However, sometimes you should take your back to a good doctor. Here is a list, in order of urgency, of all the circumstances that warrant medical intervention.

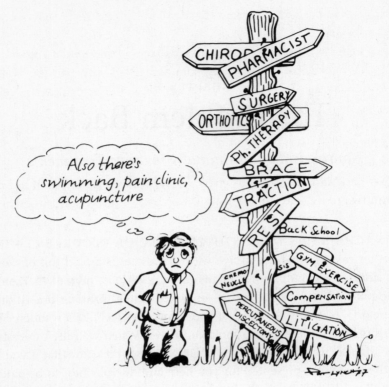

FIGURE 6.1. Decisions, Decisions

Dear Reader, I know some of you must feel like the fellow in the cartoon. He obviously does not think his situation is so funny, and you may not, either. There are many options for treating your back, and it is normal to be a bit confused at some point. We recognize that there are several paths that you may take. We have provided information here and in the next chapter to help *you* to decide which road is *best for you.* (*REPRODUCED WITH PERMISSION FROM WHITE, A. A., AND PANJABI, M. M.: CLINICAL BIOMECHANICS OF THE SPINE, 2ND ED., J. B. LIPPINCOTT, 1990.*)

Checklist for When to Call the Doctor

- You are having trouble urinating, especially getting the stream flowing or maintaining control. *Go to the emergency room right away.*
- You have weakness in one or both legs that is getting worse.
- Your severe back pain is preceded or accompanied by involuntary weight loss or pain elsewhere in the body.

- Your severe back and leg pain is accompanied by a fever that is not an obvious cold.
- Your pain is very intense and getting worse no matter what you do.
- You have a backache and/or leg pain associated with pain or swelling in other joints: fingers, wrists, elbows, hips, knees, or ankles, for instance.
- You have had moderately severe back pain for three to four weeks, or you have had several episodes of severe backache and want to find out what is going on.
- Your back and/or leg pain is constant and severe, and does not improve with two to five days' bed rest, followed by two or three weeks of home and/or self-care.
- You have done the best you can, and you just cannot stand it anymore.

These are all excellent reasons to see a doctor. I suggest that you consult a good general practitioner, board-certified family practitioner, internist, rheumatologist, orthopedic surgeon, or neurosurgeon. In chapter 7, I have provided some tips intended to help you select the best doctor for your back.

Most backaches can be well managed by your primary care physician; however, there may be situations in which you want to see a specialist even though surgery may not be in the offing. This is the case when there is long-term back pain without sciatica or neurological problems, such as weakness or numbness.

Getting Along with Your Doctor

This book should be used as a practical survival handbook as well as a reliable source of information regarding your back. Therefore, we must point out some of the potential pitfalls in your path, one of which is possible prejudice on the part of fellow humans. If you happen to be African-American, female, poor, Jewish, Catholic, Irish, Italian, Hispanic, Asian, or any other designation, you may be treated prejudicially. We in the medical profession would like to think that all of us are without prejudice, but unfortunately that just is not the case. If a doctor or some other professional treats you disdainfully for no reason, be suspicious. Consider changing doctors. I should mention that in 2003 the Institute of Medicine published a report entitled *Unequal Treatment,* which concluded that women, minorities, the elderly, gays and lesbians, the poor, the disabled, immigrants, and the obese receive disparate care due to conscious or unconscious bias on the part of some caregivers. Do not be paranoid; simply recognize the potential and consider these recommendations.

Ask around; find a doctor who has taken good care of a friend or a member of your own family. If you have a friend with a good doctor, let your friend tell his doctor about you and your problem. Then tell the doctor that you sought him/her out because of a friend's recommendation. He/she will appreciate the compliment.

Medical schools teach doctors to "humanize" our patients. This is very important. What this means is that in addition to evaluating and treating a patient, we must somehow communicate with him/her as a human being. There are infinite possibilities: How's your golf? Your wife? Your kids? Did you see the game last night? Let me suggest that you, the patient, also humanize your doctor. Most doctors are under some time pressure. You should politely acknowledge this, yet seek to obtain answers to important questions. Write them down, if necessary, to ensure that you do not forget to ask.

Working with Your Doctor

You have found a doctor that you like. How do you get the most out of your relationship with him/her? The trick is *not* to take the attitude "Okay, I hurt; now, I'll bet you can't make me stop hurting." The trick is to take the attitude "I have this disease, Doc, so let's you and I work together to defeat it." If you and your doctor can develop that type of relationship, you are way ahead of the game!

First, ask enough questions until you're satisfied that you understand what your back is doing. How serious is it? What is the prognosis? Remember that many back conditions do not have a precise diagnosis. That is okay, provided your doctor has noted your history and thoroughly examined you. You should be examined for tumors, infections, and any other specific, treatable disease such as ankylosing spondylitis, which requires special management. Ask whether other tests are necessary either to confirm the diagnosis or to search further for causes.

Once you grasp the diagnosis and the ins and outs of the disease process, you and your doctor can confer regarding your treatment. Ask for the rationale, benefits, and risks of the recommended treatment. You should know both its pitfalls and its prospects for success.

If everything makes sense to you, follow your doctor's program conscientiously. I italicize the advice because no treatment can work if you do not use it. You will never know if it *could* have worked if you do not give it an honest try. This is what is referred to as patient compliance, and *your shared decision making* in the care of *your* back is essential for a successful outcome. When you go back to your doctor, and he assumes you have tried treatment A and it did not work, he will then suggest treatment B. Generally, as you progress from A to B to C, the risks as well as the possible benefits escalate. This rule is almost as inevitable as the investment laws dictating that risks increase in proportion to profits. If you bury your money under the mattress, you probably won't lose it, but likewise you will not earn any interest. If, on the other hand, you put it into venture capital fund, you may get a 20, 30, or 50 percent return, but you risk losing your entire "bundle."

If what your doctor is telling you does not make sense and he is unable or unwilling to explain things so that they do make sense, then you deserve at least another visit, another opinion, or perhaps another doctor. You are an important human being with an important problem. You deserve to know and you deserve to understand.

Listen to Your Body

Seeing a doctor does not absolve you of your responsibility. You are still your own best physician, in that only *you* dwell inside *your* body. I inform my patients that the physician's objective is to help figure out what the problems are—that is, to make a diagnosis. You must convey the nature and severity of the symptoms.

Pay attention to what circumstances and activities seem to provoke back pain. You can do this in your head. If you are either compulsive or forgetful, jot down your observations in a little notebook. Do stress, changes in the weather, certain sports, certain chairs/beds/cars, some sexual positions, airplane trips, and a hobby or work activity seem to trigger a backache? Next, ask yourself what makes your back feel better. Some of the preceding activities might end up on the list of things that help. Things on the good list may include aspirin, a glass of wine or a cocktail, stretching, massage, and possibly certain sports, like swimming. This information will help you avoid pain and enjoy comfort. When you turn up distinct trends or correlations, tell your doctor; they could help determine your diagnosis as well as influence treatment.

Use your own mind, psyche, ego, faith, intellect, will, or whatever you call the spirit inside you. If you have mastered chapter 4, you know that a positive attitude is a potent force in your treatment program. It is something you may already possess—a philosophy of life or health, a religious or secular commitment—or something new can help sustain you. Perhaps it's some form of autopsychology, the relaxation response, biofeedback, meditation, self-hypnosis, or anything else that bolsters your will to recover. Maybe your doctor, minister, priest, rabbi, friends, or family can be of help. Utilize all the resources that are available to you. Take control of your backache situation.

The Placebo and the Natural Course of the Disease

Let us revisit our old friend the placebo. We have already introduced you to the placebo response, but further acquaintance seems fitting here.

There is a copious list of backache treatments, generating two chapters in this book, one for nonsurgical procedures and another for surgical procedures. Why such a copious list? Because, at some time in their lives, 50 percent to 70 percent of adults will suffer from an attack of low back pain. A rarer disease grants fewer opportunities to assess what different treatments are more effective, and still fewer opportunities for them to catch on.

A significant factor in the success of any treatment approach is the placebo phenomenon, which is readily built into the human psyche. When you are treated for any painful disease, a successful outcome boils down to changing your behavior from an "I hurt" mode to "I feel better; I no longer hurt." A harmless sugar pill touted as an effective medication will switch one out of every three people from "I hurt" to "I'm better." Is it all in your mind? Not exactly. There are situations in which real, measurable changes have occurred following placebo treatment.

What does all this have to do with the treatment of backache? First, when we talk about any treatment's success rate, bear in mind that one in three patients can be cured merely by *believing* that the treatment will work: the placebo effect. Furthermore, when it comes to backache, recall that by waiting and doing nothing, 70 percent of you will be well in three weeks, and 90 percent of you in two months. That is written into the natural course of the disease. Now we begin to understand that any treatment, whether traditional or exotic, acclaimed for healing 70 percent of all seekers is not necessarily the greatest boon to humanity. When we factor in the placebo effect and nature's own healing hand, the proportion of success directly attributable to the treatment drops dramatically. This is not to deprecate the placebo effect. In fact, as we discuss specific treatment, we will applaud the harnessing of your own faith and self-healing powers. Moreover, placebo treatment may also induce the body to secrete its own morphinelike drug, endorphins. Even for treatments that are deemed highly effective, I inform my patients that the role of effective treatment is to "place you on the road to recovery." After being placed on that road, you, the patient, are the most important ingredient in the formula for success. Thus, follow through on the treatment instructions and think positively.

THE PARABLE OF FROG SURGERY

There is a familiar tale in medical circles about placebo surgery.

Once upon a time, a patient complained of severe stomach pain, which he described as though it were "a frog jumping around there." Every possible test, including X-rays, ultrasound, a barium enema, gallbladder studies, CT scan, MRI, and numerous lab tests, all turned up nothing. The patient consulted a psychiatrist, who listened carefully to the description of the ailment and concluded that the patient was emotionally disturbed. Yet, several months of intense psychotherapy did not alter the man's complaint.

In desperation, the man's physicians, psychiatrists, and surgeons, after long and intensive discussion, finally decided to relieve him of his suffering with placebo surgery. They made an incision, opened the patient up, sewed him up again, and reported they'd found a large frog in this stomach. They even produced a frog preserved in a jar of formaldehyde. After a few days, the once frog-plagued patient was pain free and living a normal life.

After several weeks, however, the man felt fresh discomfort in his stomach, and its nature convinced him that it was exactly the same type of pain. When he consulted his doctors, they pointed out that they had already removed the frog from his stomach. The patient was pensive for a moment. Then he said, "I think I know what happened, gentlemen. You've done an excellent job of removing the frog. But it's clear that you left eggs behind, and now there's another frog."

The story points to some of the vicissitudes of the mind and the pitfalls of placebo treatments.

A Complete List of Nonsurgical Back Treatments

Now back to where we left off in chapter 5, which focused on the do-it-yourself mode of treatment. The current section will also include some do-it-yourself modalities. However, much of the treatment discussed here targets the longer-term back problem and is likely to be utilized by a physician or physical therapist. Many of chapter 5's lessons will also apply to those of you who have been seeing a doctor for longer periods of time and are contemplating more sophisticated remedies. So bear with a bit of recapitulation.

BED REST AND PAINKILLERS

Local inflammation in anatomic structures such as the facet joints and surrounding nerves probably produces much of your back pain. Therefore, resting in the proper position (see chapter 5) allows nature to heal most patients in two or three weeks. I recommended that you limit your actual bed rest to two or three days. Hagen coordinated a review of the best available literature on acute low back pain episodes and noted that bed rest is less effective than advice to stay active. If sciatica is present, then two days or less bed rest and staying active were similar in efficacy. Such data speak to the natural history if the disease. Prolonged bed rest has a negative effect on the rate of recovery. The goal is to get people back to activities as tolerated, with due respect to preventive measures, of course.

We also told you of the wonders of good old aspirin and itemized a few other drugs, both prescription and nonprescription, that may be useful. But what if your backache is really excruciating and the remedies have not worked?

When your pain is very severe and unrelieved by aspirin or another nonsteroidal anti-inflammatory drug, your physician may sometimes prescribe a *narcotic analgesic*. Usually this means codeine, hydrocodone (Vicodin), or meperidine (Demerol), in addition to an NSAID. Narcotics can relieve the agony of the acute phase but should not be relied upon for long-term treatment. They are addictive, and you soon build up a tolerance to them. The exception to the rule is a very serious chronic pain problem such as inoperable cancer.

What about muscle relaxants? Usually your muscle spasm will subside as the pain and inflammation wane. I repeat that I'm not an enthusiast of these drugs, which alter your central nervous system and mental processes and should be used with caution. However, the current medical evidence reveals that muscle relaxants can be effective in managing nonspecific low back pain. The different relaxants were noted to be similar in performance, although they were not shown to be more effective than analgesics or NSAIDs. Many physicians use muscle relaxants in combination with NSAIDs. They have not been proven to specifically relax muscles. However, on occasion, when a severe muscle spasm is unresponsive to rest or anti-inflammatories and other drugs, I sometimes prescribe them.

Certain relaxants tend to be more sedating, including tizanidine (Zanaflex), cyclobenzaprine (Flexeril), diazepam (Valium), carisoprodol (Soma), and chlorzoxazone (Parafon Forte). The less sedating choices include nabumetone (Relafen) and metaxalone (Skelaxin). All relaxants may cause urinary retention. The side effects may become more pronounced if used together with narcotic medications. One must use caution when taking these agents alone or in combination. As with anything else, I try to use the simplest regimen and the lowest effective dosage, prescribing medication at the earliest possible time in my patient's best interest.

HEAT AND MASSAGE

We talked about the soothing virtues of these age-old remedies in chapter 5. Their success rate is on a par with other nonsurgical treatments, and, delightfully, it is very had to harm yourself with either. Skin burns can occur in connection with heat application. Some patients have described falling asleep on the heating pad with it set at the highest setting. Try to avoid sleeping on the pad, or use a timer. The medical evidence reveals that heat rather than cold is associated with short-term improvement.

As for massage, a review of the literature noted that massage "might be beneficial" for patients with subacute and chronic nonspecific low back pain, especially when combined with exercise and education. Massage poses occasional social complications. Otherwise, I'd say massage and heat application constitute a riskless therapy that satisfies the patient's need to be treated. Who can argue against something that can make people feel better, even though it may contain no special elixir?

BRACES

In chapter 5, we said that a corset can serve as a stand-in for firm abdominal muscles. The next, more sophisticated level of abdominal support is the lumbar or lumbosacral brace. It extends from the pelvis up to the middle of the rib cage. These braces come with a variety of rigid components running down and across the body. Several common back braces are shown in figure 6.2. Some actually go down to the *trochanter,* the prominent bone on the side of the hip. Being held in a tight clasp, the wearer is reminded to restrain his/her motion.

Why use a brace? Besides giving abdominal support, the brace, with

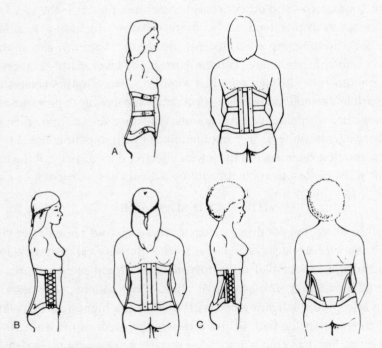

FIGURE 6.2. Lumbar Braces

Here are several braces that you might consider for low back pain. All of them can be effective. Several others are described in the text. (A) is the Mac Ausland, or chargeback, brace, (B) is the Knight brace, and (C) is the Williams brace. Note that all three have a good abdominal support. This is a key factor in their efficacy. *(REPRODUCED WITH PERMISSION FROM WHITE, A. A., AND PANJABI, M. M.: CLINICAL BIOMECHANICS OF THE SPINE, 2ND ED., J. B. LIPPINCOTT, 1990.)*

its rigid parts, further immobilizes the spine. However, by supporting the trunk muscles, some studies suggest, the brace may usurp their functions, leaving them to fade away, as inactive muscles are wont to do. Paradoxically, another experiment shows that when a patient walks in a rigid spinal brace, his erector spinae muscles are actually *more* active (as measured by their electrical response). One review of the medical literature noted that there is moderate evidence that braces are not effective for primary prevention of low back pain (LBP); however, there was limited evidence that braces are more effective than no treatment for ongoing LBP.

If you decide that maximum bracing is the treatment for you, two specific braces represent the optimum state of the art: the Boston brace and the Raney flexion jacket. Both are rigorously designed for effective abdominal compression and for a slightly flexed lumbar spine. Lumbar flexion decreases the backward bulging of the disc and reduces some of the forces on the lumbar spine's posterior elements. But these braces are not cheap. A larger variety and some less expensive braces are available. Nonetheless, like medications and surgery, they should be prescribed only after a thorough clinical exam and an adequate trial of less expensive therapy.

PLASTER CASTS

The plaster cast differs from corsets and braces only in its greater rigidity. It can be made to fit your individual contours as well as the average brace, but, of course, you do not have the option of conveniently taking it off. Because a cast is temporary and cheaper than any other bracing device, it is often used on a trial basis to predict how you would fare with a brace. It can also test to some extent the efficacy of a proposed spinal fusion.

Although the current clinical studies regarding corsets, braces, and casts are limited, there is no question that wearing them sometimes make patients feel better, and they are reasonable alternatives to more drastic therapies. Their risks come mainly in the form of nuisances. Braces may irritate the skin or bony prominences or make your back more painful. More ominously, a too-tight cast, or even a slightly snug one, can occasionally result in "cast syndrome." This is a serious problem in which one of your major abdominal arteries squeezes against the upper intestines, triggering vomiting and/or severe abdominal pain. If you develop these symptoms, take off the brace or corset and see a doctor immediately to head off major gastrointestinal upset or disease.

TRACTION (DRX9000 / VAX-D / INVERSION TABLES)

In a nutshell, traction pulls the upper and lower parts of your body in opposite directions to ease your low back and/or leg pain. It can be done either continuously for several hours or intermittently (pull—release—pull) for seconds or minutes. Traction use dates back to the time of the Greek physician Hippocrates, the "father of medicine," who used it to treat back pain, including traumatic injuries.

There have been several clinical studies on various traction techniques. Sorry, folks, but the results indicate that traction really does not seem to provide sustained relief. One team of researchers reviewed the current literature on the use of traction for low back pain with and without sciatica. They concluded that intermittent or continuous traction cannot be recommended for patients with low back pain with or without sciatica, or for sciatica alone.

Many of you may have seen the full-page advertisements in the newspapers or magazines touting the benefits of VAX-D or the DRX9000. These are "computer"-assisted *mechanical traction devices.* These devices are being marketed not as traditional traction but as nonsurgical "decompression" treatment for low back pain, disc herniations, spinal stenosis, and so forth. The early advertisements indicated that these devices were developed based on NASA research. According to recent published reports, the company Axiom Worldwide, which developed the DRX9000, was served an injunction by a federal judge for false advertising regarding its claims of NASA research and technology, FDA approval, and patent-document falsification. Some practitioners were fined for false advertising as well. The VAX-D device and several practitioners have been intertwined in similar legal wranglings surrounding fraud charges. There is no evidence to suggest that these computerized devices are more beneficial than or differ from standard traction—which itself has not been shown to be very effective, other than perhaps transiently.

Inversion therapy, using a special table, involves hanging upside down, supported by your ankles. There is also an inversion chair available. The technique is essentially gravity-facilitated traction. Although some patients have reported short-term relief, there is no scientific evidence to support long-term benefit. The concern with inversion treatment is that the resultant increased blood flow and blood pressure in your head is worrisome for patients with hypertension, heart disease, or glaucoma.

These techniques are deemed to be the same modalities approached from different angles. So let's move on.

SPINAL MANIPULATION

Yeah, I know that you have been waiting to hear what I have to say about chiropractors. Well, here it is. What I am going to say about chiropractors is what the medical literature supports. My goal is simply to present the facts as objectively as possible and let you form your own conclusions. This book is about low back pain—how to treat, survive, and live with it based on sound medical science. It is not about political, socioeconomic, and other aspects related to the various forms of practitioners in this world.

Spinal manipulative therapy is practiced by chiropractors, osteopaths, and some physical therapists. Whole books have been devoted to the numerous, complex maneuvers involved in spinal manipulation (see bibliography). Yet, whatever external technique is applied, the possible movements of the vertebrae themselves are limited by nature. You can carry out whatever body contortion you like, but your vertebrae can move only in a certain manner. All of the possible movements are indicated by the arrows provided in figure 6.3.

I have already emphasized the medical implications of a backache and provided you with my best opinions regarding how you should proceed vis-à-vis when, how, and what type of medical attention to seek for your backache. Therefore, let us proceed in a similar manner when we consider the issue of spinal-manipulative therapy. I suspect that even this disclaimer will not defuse controversy or eliminate misunderstanding, and, no doubt, chiropractic critics and devotees alike will be pleased and offended in turn by what I write here.

Now let's try to be a little more scientific and objective. In 1975 the National Institute of Neurological Disorders and Stroke (one of the National Institutes of Health) sponsored a workshop titled "Research Status of Spinal Manipulative Therapy" (see bibliography). Here is a quotation from the summary of that workshop, which drew a number of osteopaths, physicians, chiropractors, and scientists:

> The concept of chiropractic subluxation [that is, nonobservable partial dislocation in the normal position of two adjacent vertebrae] remains a hypothesis yet to be evaluated experimentally. We believe this has been one of the frustrating aspects . . . When one is correcting a

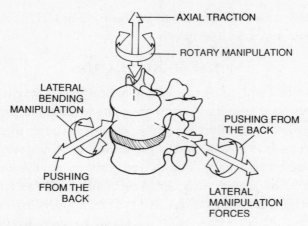

FIGURE 6.3. Spine Vertebral Motion

This is to show all the possible ways that we can cause a vertebra in the spine to move. These various movements can be achieved through spinal manipulation, traction, or exercise. No matter what you do to the spine, here are all the motions you can possibly achieve. *(REPRODUCED WITH PERMISSION FROM WHITE, A. A., AND PANJABI, M. M.: CLINICAL BIOMECHANICS OF THE SPINE, 2ND ED., J. B. LIPPINCOTT, 1990.)*

"subluxation" that cannot be perceived by independent scientific observers, it is difficult to convince those observers that the treatment
is effective . . .

In other words, the question of spinal manipulation's efficacy and mechanism of action remains in limbo, since independent clinical and scientific
observers remain skeptical of its unverified premises. Yet, spinal manipulation is one of the most popular backache treatment methods, and it deserves a detailed, fair look here.

COMMON MANIPULATION TECHNIQUES Since manipulation techniques would fill a large tome, we will confine ourselves to the best-known
methods. The simplest manipulation consists of pressure applied directly
to the spinous processes of a given vertebra. This can be performed by
pressing a finger on the vertebra or using the palm or the ball of the hand.
There is also a limited maneuver that can be performed on the front of the
neck or, in a very relaxed patient, on the front part of the lumbar spine.

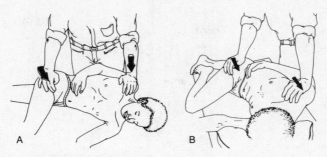

FIGURE 6.4. Spinal Manipulation

This particular technique of spinal manipulation is probably the one employed most often by practitioners. (A) This shows the technique from the front. The major force is from the therapist pushing the pelvis forward with the right hand, while with the left hand there is a moderate thrust in the opposite direction. (B) This is an axial view, which shows how the two motions impart an element of twist to the lower portion of the spine. *(REPRODUCED WITH PERMISSION FROM WHITE, A. A., AND PANJABI, M. M.: CLINICAL BIO-MECHANICS OF THE SPINE, 2ND ED., J. B. LIPPINCOTT, 1990.)*

Again, the finger is usually supplanted by another part of the hand. Most manipulations are done *indirectly*, by twisting the head, shoulders, and hips, rotating the spine, as shown in figure 6.4. A more direct manipulation is shown in figure 6.5.

DOES IT WORK? Manipulation applies certain forces and movements to the spine. Within tolerable limits, these forces and motions are considered helpful. When tolerance limits are exceeded, spinal structures run the risk of damage. Our extensive, ever-growing knowledge of spine mechanics allows us to predict what changes spinal manipulations can effect. The theory that these forces relieve nerve pressure is not compatible with our current information. Nothing suggests that manipulating a motion segment can move structures significantly into or out of the intervertebral foramen; this is the canal through which the nerve root passes as it leaves the spinal cord to go ultimately to the skin or muscle (see figure 2.6b). The fairest summation is that at present there is no compelling theory to explain the mechanism whereby spinal manipulative therapy relieves pain, if it does.

Is it therefore helpful? First, let us address the treatment of visceral

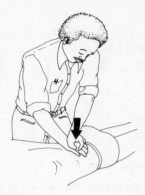

FIGURE 6.5. Spinal Manipulation

This is a simple direct thrust to the spine transmitted through the heel of the hand. These maneuvers must be done with care, as they can be irritating. *(REPRODUCED WITH PERMISSION FROM WHITE, A. A., AND PANJABI, M. M.: CLINICAL BIOMECHANICS OF THE SPINE, 2ND ED., J. B. LIPPINCOTT, 1990.)*

disease, or all diseases other than back pain. Starkly put, there is no clinical or scientific evidence to suggest that manipulation can help cure systemic diseases such as diabetes, ulcers, hypertension, and so on. Anyone who attempts to treat such diseases with manipulation renders a great disservice to his/her patients.

On the other hand, myriad studies have examined the use of spinal manipulation on back pain patients, with and without leg pain or neurological problems. The conclusions from the more recent studies are as follows: There is a brief, transient reduction of pain for patients who have back pain of short duration—that being less than three months. If you have leg pain, numbness, or weakness, or long-standing back pain (more than three months), you are likely to experience the transient pain reduction. The pain reduction is short-term and may last for several hours or a few days.

THE DANGERS OF SPINAL MANIPULATION The greatest harm comes from inappropriately performing spinal manipulation to treat an infected, fractured, osteoporotic, or cancerous spine; another disease, like diabetes or rheumatoid arthritis; or patients on anticoagulants (blood thinners). Consequences are tragic when the disease could have been cured or controlled by a mainstream medical method.

Is manipulation itself risky? Sometimes. One publication reported four cases of patients who were paralyzed in the legs or developed other major neurological problems after a trip to the chiropractor. Whenever jostling the spine, disc, and nerves makes your condition worse, it does not matter who does the jostling. Other documented, though rare, dangers include manipulation-induced herniated discs and fatal brain hemorrhages, spinal cord injuries, and nonfatal bleeding caused by neck manipulation. Forceful manipulation in the setting of acute neurological deficits should be avoided and approached with great caution.

A 1999 study published in the *New England Journal of Medicine* found that patients with low back pain without sciatica responded similarly well to treatment with either McKenzie-based (centralization) physical therapy, chiropractic manipulation, or minimal intervention with only patient education provided through a booklet. Neither treatment was superior, which suggests that we may be observing the natural history of the disease. Patient satisfaction reports following subsequent clinical trials indicates an increasing acceptance of spinal manipulative therapy for certain categories of back pain. Some insurance carriers now cover this treatment option.

CONCLUSION. Recall that to be outstanding, a treatment must outperform the placebo effect of 33 percent success, plus nature's own healing rate of 60 percent to 70 percent. Spinal manipulation, then, comes out about even with other nonsurgical treatments, but its *subjective* results run a little higher. As a bottom line, consider spinal manipulation a justified alternative, provided that you have been appropriately evaluated by a medical doctor, you have no neurological deficits, and the manipulation is not too vigorous. Forceful manipulation may be accompanied by a higher risk of injury. Prolonged, repeated, expensive manipulations that may bring only transient reduction of pain may not be the best use of your resources.

The advice I give my patients is as follows: If you do not get distinct, lasting relief after several manipulations, then do not continue them. If a patient has disc disease, I advise him/her not to have forceful spinal manipulation, because in my opinion there is a risk of potentially serious neurological complications. Your chiropractor should also screen you for any signs of an infection or tumor—two other contraindications for spinal manipulation.

EXERCISE

Exercise belongs to the pantheon of desirable states, alongside mother-hood, peace, health, and love. Furthermore, it is a bona fide back care therapy that you should not scorn. Even though exercise has been covered extensively in the preceding chapter, it seems worthwhile to return to the topic briefly here, from a slightly different perspective. Here we will divide exercises into three categories: William's exercises, miscellaneous exercises, and truncal exercises.

WILLIAM'S EXERCISES These exercises are mentioned briefly, mainly for historic interest. Their goal is to strengthen certain muscles and stretch certain ligaments in order to switch the spine's alignment from a sway-back (lordotic) position to a straightened one. The assumption is that the straighter the spine, the healthier and more comfortable it is. Our theo-retical knowledge lends some weight to this notion. A straighter position distributes the forces more evenly, reduces pressure on the sensitive facet joints, and discourages the backward bulging of the disc.

However, I have a real problem with the classic William's exercises. They're certainly not the best prescription for anyone with acute spine problems. The sit-up exercises, especially, are prone to irritating your in-tervertebral disc in the early stages of back disease, since the forces gen-erated are equal to those caused by improperly lifting forty-four pounds. Would we ask someone with fresh, severe backache and sciatica to im-properly tote around forty-four-pound weights?

MISCELLANEOUS EXERCISES Generally, these are exercises to strengthen the trunk muscles. They include back extension exercises, partial sit-ups, and range-of-motion exercises such as general bending, extension, side-ways bending and maximum twisting motions, and general calisthenics. Improvement runs in the range of 60 percent to 70 percent. Complications are minimal, but some risks are incurred by back arching and axial torque (twisting the shoulders from side to side with the hips fairly stationary). Toe-touching exercises can also irritate your back and cause leg pain, espe-cially if you have sciatica.

When your back can tolerate it, good tone in the trunk muscles and those around the spine is a healthy goal. But these exercises should be re-served for your getting-better days, not for acute backache. Most important, avoid sit-ups with the legs straight if you have low back pain. Refer to chapter 5 for a refresher.

ISOMETRIC TRUNCAL EXERCISE Remember how we compared developed abdominal muscles to an inflated football? The idea of isometric abdominal exercises is to compress your abdominal contents by tightening up your throat, holding your rectum tight, and pushing hard, as though straining to move your bowels. Do this at least ten or fifteen times, holding each contraction for about three seconds, three or four times a day. The result? Tightened abdominal and trunk muscles. Studies show that the pressure generated by compressing the fluid and air in the trunk adds considerable support to our spine, protecting it from forces imposed on it.

Any risks? If you have acute disc disease, these exercises can irritate the nerve roots. Avoid them, also, if you have either heart disease or a hernia; they can put too much pressure on your heart, interfering with its circulation, or enlarge a hernia. Otherwise, their great advantage is that you can perform them discreetly in the office, car, theater, or wherever, without equipment.

McKENZIE PROGRAM In this exercise program, a patient, under the therapist's guidance, is put through various movements. These include flexion, extension, lateral bending, and rotation. Notations are made on which of these movements best "centralize" the patient's symptoms. During "centralizing," pain initially in the back, hip, leg, and foot gradually localizes to the back and hip. The patient is then advised to repeat the movement that has centralized the pain and to do other exercises as well. Initial studies give this a favorable evaluation; however, more experience is needed to be certain of the therapeutic value of this program. The concept of centralizing pain is strictly theoretical and, to my knowledge, is without scientific basis. In its favor: It does no harm!

BACK SCHOOL

The basic back pain school was developed in Sweden by a physical therapist named Marianne Zachrisson-Forssell, who assembled the best available knowledge into a packaged lecture-and-slide program. Since then, the back school has been adopted and modified in many places. Most cities in North America have a back school of some type.

The back school course generally includes a primer on the anatomy and basic functions of the spine, drawn from recent research. We then move on to more detailed biomechanics lessons, then to an enumeration of various back problems and their causes. What follows are a series of instructions ranging from isometric abdominal exercises to practical back care tips and precautions that one can incorporate into the common activities of daily life in the home, office, factory, and playing field.

The following is how one particular school works, but it is not unlike others around the world. The YMCA, for instance, offers a back care class at many of its worldwide centers. Besides practical advice, the back school offers a form of group therapy. Such programs afford the opportunity for a healthy exchange of experiences, advice, and emotional support with individuals who have faced similar challenges. Such dialogue may be a real solace to many a frustrated patient.

As a treatment mode, the back school has proved superior to the placebo effect—and even to physical therapy alone. Volvo employees were observed in a controlled industrial study. Those who attended a Swedish back school returned to work sooner and reported sick less often than patients treated with physical therapy alone. Back schools have been effective in reducing medical expenses and industrial disability claims. Moreover, function has been increased and recurrence decreased. One review of the medical evidence regarding back school programs demonstrated reduced low back pain and improved function with the addition of this educational component to a course of physical therapy. However, back school does not work for everyone. Those who happen to be drug dependent or suffering from constant pain may not benefit. Also, one must implement what is being taught in the back school in order to reap the benefits.

Nonetheless, just in case you have not already detected it, I am a back school advocate. Not only is it more cost-effective than most conservative therapies, it is complication free. In addition, it can head off more expensive treatment, such as hospitalization and surgery, down the road. It is also a productive way to share information in an ambience of professional expertise and human understanding. In the ideal world, there would be a back school program for chronic pain sufferers as well as those with acute pain, plus a follow-up refresher course after several months for all students.

> ## Representative Outline of a Back School Course
>
> 1. Anatomy
>   Function
>   Cause of back pain
>   Who gets it
>   Treatment results
>
> 2. Biomechanics of the spine
>   Effects of activities on disc pressure
>   Importance of controlling loads on low back
>
> 3. Ergonomics (how to use your back safely)
>   Individual advice about work and recreational activities
>   Effective back exercises
>
> 4. Review and summary
>   Instilling self-confidence
>   Encouraging sports, activity, ingenuity, common sense, and having fun

WORK HARDENING, FUNCTIONAL INTERVENTION PROGRAMS, AND PAIN CLINICS

In work hardening programs recommended by your doctor and physical therapist, there is intensive goal-oriented physical training to improve strength and endurance. The patient/worker is also rehabilitated and re-educated to be able to perform tasks at a capacity similar to his/her actual work. Specific advice on how to best use the body in these tasks is provided.

Functional training, or work conditioning, is somewhat similar. The patient is reeducated and taught exercises, activities, and postures that will allow him/her to return to work. There is a rigorous selection process that eliminates all but the well motivated and psychologically able. Group dynamics are involved to facilitate and sustain progress. We have discussed low back school; some of these programs may be considered low back *boot camp*. The strong survive and become successful "combat" personnel in the workplace. A multidisciplinary approach is utilized, with a physical therapist, an occupational therapist, psychologists, and a vocational specialist often being involved. In a well-controlled clinical study, this type of program was shown to be effective.

Pain clinics are designed primarily to teach patients coping mechanisms for dealing with their pain and to supervise the use of various medications. The cause of the pain, although it may be known, traditionally has not been treated specifically. The goal is to reduce the pain so that the other modalities can be used more effectively. However, some pain clinics that are run by anesthesiologists and physiatrists have pursued various interventions to address low back pain. These interventions will be discussed in the next section.

Conservative Treatment: Passive and Minimally Invasive

To complete our nonsurgical-treatment list, we need to consider those approaches that "invade" the body in some way. Do not be put off by the word *invasive;* most of the following treatments are actually pretty mild. The needles used in acupuncture, for example, hurt no more than a pinprick and pose no danger. I should point out that invasive procedures used repeatedly and without proper indications may foster patient dependency and tend to prolong the pain. This is a kind of psychological dependency on the treatment and development of a "pain habit"—something we want to avoid at all cost, because it *will* cost.

ACUPUNCTURE

This procedure evolved out of thousands of years of Chinese history, culture, and tradition. Lately it has entered the West, charged with controversy and confusion stemming from our Western attempt to make it fit our own scientific models and biases. As two worlds mix and mingle, certain things are happening for the first time. Recently, experts from all over the world met in a congress to launch research studies to bridge some of our East-West gaps through collaborative research on the use of acupuncture.

Acupuncture is used in several contexts. One application is as an anesthetic. In China, in the fall of 1979, I witnessed a cesarean section performed entirely under acupuncture anesthesia, accompanied by a low-voltage electrical current delivered through the needles to the acupuncture points. This is called electroacupuncture (EA). In my opinion, there was not a trace of hoax involved. It does work. Clinical studies have shown an increase in spinal fluid beta-endorphin levels (our own internal pain-killers) after EA.

Acupuncture's other use is as a treatment for pain. Over thousands of years, Chinese doctors have mapped out a complex system of meridians—pathways of energy—running up, down, and around the human body. We have not found any equivalent in our anatomy system. During acupuncture, thin needles are placed at specific points along the meridians in order to dull pain in the back, elbow, or another anatomic location. Acupuncture is a common Chinese treatment for low back pain, with low-voltage electrical current often supplementing the needles. Even here in the United States and in other Western countries, acupuncture is being used to ease back pain.

Does it work? While I have not had acupuncture myself, several of my patients have. As you would expect, some felt that they were helped, while others found only transient or negligible relief. Complications are relatively nonexistent, save for the final word of caution outlined below. The fine sterilized needles that are stuck in the skin carry no more risk of infection than a routine blood test.

The placebo recovery range is 25 percent to 35 percent; most studies show that acupuncture's success rate is not significantly better than this. The point is that although it may provide temporary relief for some, acupuncture probably does not have very much of a specific effect on back pain to cure or change the condition. In one study, researchers reviewed the current medical evidence on acupuncture and dry needling for low back pain. They noted that for acute low back pain, the data did not allow firm conclusions regarding effectiveness. For chronic low back pain, there was a trend toward limited effectiveness. A more recent (2009) study yielded similar results, with a small analgesic effect being observed.

If you would care to hear a traditional explanation of acupuncture's effects, refer back to chapter 4's discussion of the gate control theory of pain. Presumably, the moving or electrically stimulated needles affect the central nervous system, blocking or dulling pain. It is also possible that acupuncture works through our system of internal opiates. In fact, some studies have shown acupuncture to be capable of stimulating endorphin production.

If you have decided, after reading this section, that acupuncture is the thing for you, then heed this note of caution: Acupuncture should be avoided if you are taking blood thinners or have a bleeding disorder. Discuss the treatment with the acupuncture specialist and, above all, follow these three steps: (1) make sure the needles are sterile, (2) make sure the needles are sterile, and (3) make sure the needles are sterile. There are several potentially fatal diseases that can be transmitted through contaminated needles!

TENS (TRANSCUTANEOUS ELECTRICAL NERVE STIMULATION)

This can be viewed as a kind of Western medicine answer to acupuncture. Transcutaneous electrical nerve stimulation units are portable devices that have electrode patches that are placed on the skin over or around the painful area. Low-voltage electrical current, set at a low or high frequency, can be adjusted by the user. Studies suggest that TENS works by stimulating the body's endorphins, thus blocking perception of pain. The theory and explanation are similar for both treatments. It does appear to help control pain for some patients. There is no clinical risk except that patients with pacemakers should avoid TENS due to potential interference with the function of the pacemaker. Transcutaneous electrical nerve stimulation is not effective for everyone. If it doesn't seem to be helping, discontinue its use.

TRIGGER POINT INJECTIONS

Sometimes patients point to a particular painful spot on their backs that, when touched, triggers pain even in distant sites in the back, hips, thighs, or legs. Some of these patients probably have myofascial syndromes, such as fibromyalgia or fibrositis. Some practitioners believe that injections of a local anesthetic, perhaps with cortisone or saline, relieves the pain. Supposedly the trigger point injections break up the pain cycle somewhat.

There is little solid evidence for this notion. If it works for you and keeps your pain at bay, be happy. As long as the needles are sterile and you are not allergic to Novocain, there are no risks. Multiple cortisone shots are not advised. If it does not work after one or two tries, you are probably wasting your time and money.

DEEPER INJECTIONS OF CORTISONE AND NOVOCAIN

The assumption is that a long-acting local anesthetic agent will interrupt any pain cycle existing between the local pain and a secondary muscle spasm. Locally acting cortisone is also injected in the hopes of minimizing local inflammation.

Under the same theory, cortisone has actually been injected into the intervertebral disc in an effort to stop inflammation. And the same approach has been launched on the facet joints. Most rheumatologists and orthopedists advise against injecting cortisone into joints; this should also apply to the joints of the spine.

Unfortunately, I do not think that any of these is a very good treatment for low back pain. Deep injections constitute an invasive and painful technique that, according to the evidence, is no more effective than milder therapies. In fact, cortisone may occasionally irritate structures with which it comes into contact, and we know that repeated cortisone injections into other joints can accelerate arthritis.

Sometimes an injection may be used for diagnostic purposes. For example, in an effort to assess whether a pars defect or a facet joint (see figures 3.5a and 3.5b) is the source of the pain, an injection may be helpful. The relief, though temporary, may provide useful information.

PROLOTHERAPY

Prolotherapy is a technique used to treat pain by injecting a sugar solution into affected ligaments and tendons with the intent of stimulating proliferation of connective tissue, thereby restoring the strength and stability of these structures. A 2007 review of several well-designed studies concluded that prolotherapy was ineffective in treating chronic low back pain.

RADIOFREQUENCY NEUROTOMY (RHIZOTOMY)

This is a technique whereby a small electrode, threaded through a needle, is placed adjacent to the nerve of interest around the facet joints. A pulsed electrical current interrupts, or ablates, the nerve, impairing its ability to transmit pain signals. The reports that tout the efficacy of neurotomy state that the relief is only temporary, while others report no benefit at all. There is redundancy or overlap in certain nerve pathways (innervations). Some reports have suggested that the transient relief is short-lived because the adjacent nerve pathways assume the roles of those that have been ablated. One published review of the current literature concluded that there is conflicting evidence regarding the effectiveness of this modality and that additional studies are required.

LUMBAR EPIDURAL STEROID INJECTION (LESI)

It is not at all rare that one of our patients with low back pain and sciatica due to disc disease, spinal stenosis, or some other cause will ask our opinion about *lumbar epidural steroid injections (LESI)*. This procedure performed by anesthesiologists, surgeons, interventional radiologists, and physiatrists, entails injecting a liquid corticosteroid plus a local anesthetic into the epidural space, using a needle or small catheter tube. The epidural space is the area around the sheath (dura) that contains the nerves, cauda equina, and spinal fluid (see figure 2.6b). The goal is to reduce inflammation around the nerve roots due to mechanical, chemical, and immunological irritants and thereby diminish pain. Use of this procedure, performed with fluoroscopic guidance, has been increasing in the United States.

I rarely suggest epidural steroids, because most of the evidence indicates that it is not particularly helpful, particularly to patients suffering from sciatica. Moreover, although complications are not frequent, they can and do occur. Some, such as headaches, and dizziness that may result from a spinal fluid leak, are not very serious. The latter is usually resolved with bed rest; however, surgical treatment is occasionally required to repair or seal the leak. Some patients may experience an increase in back and leg pain after the injection. Others complications are *very serious;* this includes infectious and noninfectious inflammation of the nerves.

A 2007 scientific position paper from the American Academy of Neurology that assessed available data concluded that epidural steroid injections used to treat radicular and lumbosacral were ineffective. A multicenter, randomized controlled trial of epidural steroid injections used to treat sciatica published in 2005 revealed that at three weeks there was a transient benefit over the placebo; however, no benefit was demonstrated from six to fifty-two weeks. However, in addition to initial symptomatic relief, these injections can be of diagnostic benefit. Transient relief following an epidural steroid injection has been reported to be a predictor of successful surgical decompression of the affected neural structures in patients whose symptoms persist.

Some practitioners have recommended a series of injections. Because there is no data to support the routine use of this approach, repeat injections should be considered only after an assessment of the response to this treatment method.

Anyone with signs of an infection should not receive an injection until the infection has been resolved completely. Blood thinners, including NSAIDs, heparin, Coumadin, and Plavix, must be discontinued an appropriate amount of time prior to an injection to minimize the risk of bleeding into the spinal canal (epidural hematoma). Consult your physician. Those with an allergy to iodine or contrast agents (medical dyes) should inform their physicians so that these agents are not used.

Individuals exposed to steroids may also have systemic or generalized effects, because taking steroids suppresses your body's ability to make its own steroids in the adrenal glands. Common side effects include fluid retention, elevated blood sugar (diabetics must monitor closely), nausea, facial flushing, insomnia, elevated blood pressure, and menstrual irregularities.

You should not consider such an intervention unless you have been properly evaluated by your physician and the appropriate imaging studies have been performed (for example, X-rays and MRI or CT-myelogram). These will allow an understanding of the diagnosis and rationale for treatment.

In summary, LESIs are being used as a diagnostic and therapeutic tool with greater frequency in the United States despite evidence that they do not provide sustained relief. The temporary response may be of benefit while awaiting the natural resolution versus that of predicting the outcome of subsequent surgical treatment. Although serious adverse side effects are exceedingly rare, utilize the appropriate precautions prior to considering this choice.

CHEMONUCLEOLYSIS

In the 1950s, a prominent researcher, writer, and physician named Lewis Thomas was involved in an experiment in which meat tenderizer, injected into the bloodstream of rabbits, caused their ears to collapse. Why? Because the meat tenderizer contains chymopapain, an enzyme that dissolves mucopolysaccharides. These chemicals constitute a major component of the cartilage in rabbits' ears and the nucleus pulposus of the intervertebral disc. Recognizing that backache and sciatica may be caused by a herniated disc, Professor Carl Hirsch of Sweden suggested that chymopapain, injected into the disc, could dissolve some of it. Dr. Lyman Smith, of Chicago, popularized the idea in the United States, and chemonucleolysis was born.

Chemonucleolysis was very popular in the early and mid-1970s. As

the patient lies under an X-ray machine, a needle placed into the intervertebral disc is used to inject chymopapain. The results? Patients with a distinct clinical picture of disc herniation, including back pain and sciatica,
got the greatest benefit. Most studies computed the success rate at 60 percent to 70 percent. Chemonucleolysis was, at that time, on a par with other
treatments. There were a few reports with more glowing results. In one
interesting experiment, chemonucleolysis was compared with surgery for
lumbar disc disease—and came out on top. But I am not convinced that
the study was properly designed.

The major risk of chemonucleolysis, although it's rare, is a severe, even
fatal hypersensitivity reaction. The material can also inflame the disc and
cause scarring and inflammation around the lumbar dura and nerves if
it comes into contact with them. Some studies show that the substance is
toxic to nerve tissue; others maintain that it is safe.

The concern with chymopapain is that it be used appropriately and not
indiscriminately. How, you might ask, can patients determine this? Here
are two specific guidelines that should help: (1) Your condition should
have all the indications that would make disc surgery the primary procedure (described in chapter 6); and (2) you should have confidence in the
advice of a well-qualified spine surgeon (neurological or orthopedic) in
the form of a second opinion.

When considering injection with chymopapain as an alternative to
surgery, bear in mind that its success rate is about 70 percent to 75 percent,
comparable to many other nonsurgical treatments. In addition, following
injection, about half of those treated with chymopapain will have moderately severe to very severe back pain for three to twelve weeks.

Another potential difficulty is allergic reactions. If you are allergic to
iodine or to any meat tenderizer, you should not be treated with chymopapain. You should not have a second injection of chymopapain, as the first
injection will sensitize you to it and a second is likely to cause a more pronounced allergic reaction. An allergic reaction that does develop can range
from a simple rash, with or without itching and edema, to anaphylactic
shock, the most severe kind of allergic reaction. In fact, anaphylactic shock
is a big-league problem. Many events occur in the body during this kind of
reaction, the most deadly being a rapid drop in blood pressure that must
be controlled if the patient is to survive. The chance of this kind of reaction
is one in one hundred. Anaphylactic shock is ten times more common in
women than in men.

In summary, then, this treatment did have a place in the management of herniated discs. Overall, it was shown to be safer than surgery, and it will not cause scarring if it does not come into contact with the neural structures. However, it is not a risk-free therapy, and you should acknowledge that fact. Chymopapain was removed from the U.S. market in 2003 after several adverse reactions—including a few fatalities from anaphylactic shock. Therefore, it is no longer readily available in the United States. A few centers still offer this technique. It is available in Europe, Canada, and several other countries.

Discuss with your doctor some of the problems presented here, and if you decide to go ahead with it, maintain a positive attitude. You may want to confer with an allergist/immunologist to test whether or not you would react adversely if exposed. These specialists can perform a skin test with a small amount of the compound to assess how you would respond. Such testing may prevent an anaphylactic reaction, should you go on to have the procedure.

If it turns out not to help, you have not burned any bridges. Surgery is still an option. If it does help, you will have allowed our hopes for this treatment to rise incrementally. Minimally invasive procedures may offer virtually all the benefits of chemonucleolysis, without the risk of an anaphylactic reaction. There are reports that over time the benefits may not be sustained.

INTRADISCAL ELECTROTHERMAL THERAPY (IDET)

Intradiscal electrothermal therapy (IDET) is a technique developed as a treatment alternative to spinal fusion surgery for patients with chronic discogenic low back pain. Unless your doctor has identified disc disease as the source of the pain using lumbar discography (see figure 3.1b), it is unlikely that he will recommend IDET. The procedure, performed through the skin (percutaneously), involves fluoroscopy-guided placement of a heat probe into the affected disc. Thermal ablation destruction of the nerve fibers along the periphery of the disc is thought to relieve pain by blocking the nerves' ability to convey pain signals. Another theory is that heating and cooling may affect the biomechanical properties of the disc.

Early physician enthusiasm over this technique has faded, perhaps because of inconsistent results in clinical studies.

PERCUTANEOUS, ENDOSCOPIC, ARTHROSCOPIC, AND LASER DISCECTOMY

Percutaneous discectomy is the removal of a portion of the nucleus and annulus of the intervertebral disc by placing a probe in the disc using fluoroscopic X-ray control. Dr. Gary Onik and associates in the United States invented a 2.5-millimeter-diameter probe with a reciprocating suction cutter for dividing the disc material into small pieces and aspirating it from the disc space. This approach allows for an indirect decompression of a herniation from the center of the disc (figure 6.6).

Percutaneous discectomy was first performed in 1975 by Dr. Sadahisa

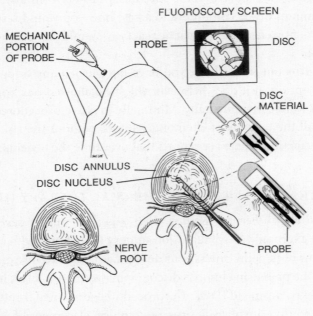

FIGURE 6.6. Percutaneous Discectomy Technique

The patient lies on his/her side. A small probe, 2.5 millimeters in diameter, is inserted through the skin, muscle sheath, and muscles and into the central portion of the disc. With the use of an automated cutting-irrigating-suctioning device, some of the nucleus pulposus and annulus fibrosus is removed from the central and posterior-lateral portion of the disc. The relationship of the protruded disc and the nerve root before and after percutaneous discectomy is shown. As a result, there is a reduction in both pressure and volume within the disc. Treatment is successful in about 70 percent of patients.

Hijikata in Tokyo. He used long surgical instruments and worked through a cannula tube that he placed into the center of the disc. Several other surgeons in Europe and the United States have developed variations of this methodology. The 2002 *Clinical Orthopaedics and Related Research* and *Journal of the American Academy of Orthopaedic Surgeons,* referenced in the bibliography, provides a synopsis of the current status along with the various modifications and advancements in the techniques. These modifications include the same basic approach to gaining access to the disc, but either an endoscope, an arthroscope, or tissue dilation tubes/expandable retractors are utilized to minimize the size of the incision required to perform the procedure. Advanced fiber-optic visualization has been important in improving such techniques.

Laser disc decompression is likewise an indirect decompression of a disc herniation using laser probe vaporization rather than a nucleotome (mechanical disc shaver) to remove a portion of the disc material. Patients appropriate for *laser discectomy* are the same as those for the percutaneous procedure. Essentially, the same precautions and complications have been observed: for instance, infection and nerve and organ irritation. Concerns regarding potential injury to the adjacent nerve and vascular structures from the heat generated by the laser may be minimized by the use of cool holmium-YAG lasers in conjunction with endoscopic visualization. Further study is needed.

Microscopic discectomy (discussed further in the next chapter) is basically the standard open procedure performed through a much smaller incision afforded by the use of a microscope. The size of the patient will have an impact on the size of the incision(s) in most cases. This approach is considered the gold standard to which other techniques are compared with respect to success rates and complications. The important factors to consider are adequate visualization to ensure that the objectives of the procedure are achieved (such as decompression while protecting the important anatomic structures). The other minimally invasive procedures to date have been associated with a higher complication rate and incomplete decompression of the nerve.

These procedures can often be performed under local anesthesia, and you may go home the same day or the next. General anesthesia may be required and is individualized based on the patient's medical history. You are probably thinking, "Sounds good, so am I a candidate?" There are some specific factors to consider. You should have clinical evidence of a disc herniation, sciatica, physical exam findings to go with the sciatica, and imaging evidence that confirms the abnormality. The abnormal disc should be at a level and on a side that fits with your symptoms and physical examination. The imaging study, preferably an MRI, should show that the herniation is likely to be still connected to the disc and is not a "free fragment." In such a case, the herniated disc material is separated from the central portion of the disc and in this setting, the percutaneous/endoscopic/laser/arthroscopic discectomy will fail to completely decompress the nerve. If you have multilevel disease, the same rule applies. A history of previous surgery may prevent such an approach, due to the presence of scar tissue. If you are pregnant, then discuss the matter with your doctor. Moreover, if you are sexually active, take steps to prevent conception from the time of your last menstrual period up to the time of the procedure. The reason for this is that the fetus would be exposed to fluoroscopic radiation at the time of the procedure. Ample precautions are routinely taken to prevent problems from occurring, but if you are pregnant, you may want to forgo this course of treatment. You also should not consider the procedure until you have given your back problem four to six weeks to heal under appropriate nonoperative care—something that you are an expert on if you have read this far.

Now, you may ask, "What is the chance of this thing working?" The current evidence is variable and the studies are evolving; however, the success rate can reasonably be put in the range of 60 percent to 85 percent. As for the risks, there is significantly less than 0.5 percent chance of getting a disc space infection. There is a *small* chance that in the process of placing the probe, the inflamed nerve root could be irritated or damaged. If only irritated, this would be enough to cause some pain, numbness, or a tingling sensation for several hours or days afterward. If damaged, a patient could have leg weakness, persistent pain, and/or numbness. The risk of a spinal fluid leak is higher. Also, there's the extremely low risk that an internal organ could be irritated or injured. The complication rates are higher than that of a standard open procedure (discussed in the next chapter), due to the fact that the exposure or room for maneuvering is limited by the tools that allow for this minimally invasive approach. Conditions during minimally invasive surgery may occur that necessitate conversion to an open procedure in order to effectively complete the surgery or repair important anatomic structures. As a result, some surgeons pursue an ap-

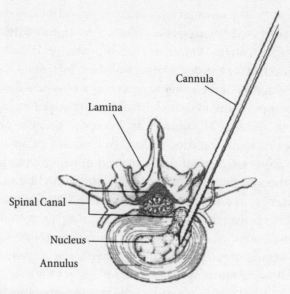

Cannula

Lamina

Spinal Canal

Nucleus

Annulus

FIGURE 6.7. Minimally Invasive Spine Surgery

This is one example of a technique whereby a cannula or endoscope is placed in the disc to facilitate removal of the herniated fragment. The approach to inserting the cannula is identical to the percutaneous discectomy technique.

proach that allows for a more direct visualization of the pathology, such as the microdiscectomy.

Review of the current randomized controlled trials reveals no difference in the long-term outcomes between minimally invasive and open treatment of lumbar disc herniations. Finally, as with any new procedure, there may be some complications that have not yet been documented or recognized. For example, is there any long-range liability to removing a portion of the disc in this manner? On balance, however, when used with appropriate indications, these techniques merit a place among with the armamentaria available to attack the ache in your back and/or leg.

INTERSPINOUS PROCESS SPACERS

This new class of devices was designed to be used as a treatment alternative for patients with symptomatic mild to moderate spinal stenosis at one or two levels of the spinal column and have not responded to nonsurgical measures. We reviewed the anatomy of spinal stenosis in chapter 3 (see figures 3.6 and 3.7). Its symptoms—back pain and neurogenic claudication—are exacerbated by extension of the spine. That is why many people with lumbar spinal stenosis have an altered posture and walk leaning forward. The rationale for the development of these *interspinous process spacers* is that distraction of the spinous processes and yellow ligament (figure 3.7) will decompress the neural elements in the spinal canal and neural foramen by increasing the volume, or space, for these important structures. The device keeps the affected level in modest flexion and limits extension. The anticipated result is a reduction in pain and improved blood supply. It is thought that pain may also be diminished by reducing stress across the facet joints and pressure in the disc and posterior ligaments.

These devices can be placed between adjacent spinous processes through a small incision, often with just a local anesthetic. General anesthesia is sometimes required, with most patients able to go home the same day or the following morning. This technique is not for every patient with spinal stenosis. Contraindications include severe osteoporosis, lumbar instability, history of a fracture, scoliosis, and obesity. Patients with severe spinal stenosis are not candidates and may require a laminectomy.

Examples of such implants include the X-STOP spacer (figure 6.8), which is the only FDA-approved device for use in patients with neurogenic claudication due to spinal stenosis at one or two levels between L1 and L5. Early reports indicated a success rate of 60 percent to 80 percent. However, follow-up studies at two years reveal that this figure can drop—in some series, as low as 33 percent. Additional study is being pursued.

There are theoretical and practical concerns regarding these types of devices. Will they cause pain or instability through the distraction or forced flexion of the involved segment? Will they exacerbate or produce spondylolisthesis? Will a fracture of the spinous process occur with repetitive extension against the implant? We patiently await the results of further clinical study.

PERCUTANEOUS TREATMENT OF VERTEBRAL BODY (SPINAL COMPRESSION) FRACTURES (VERTEBROPLASTY, KYPHOPLASTY)

Spinal compression fractures are a common problem in patients with osteoporosis. When there is no associated compromise of the neural structures, these injuries have traditionally been treated conservatively. Medication and the use of a brace, or orthosis, are utilized to support the spine and

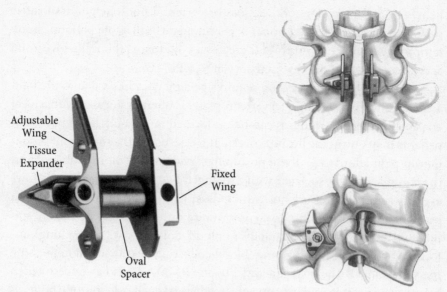

Adjustable
Wing

Tissue
Expander

Fixed
Wing

Oval
Spacer

FIGURE 6.8. The X-STOP Interspinous Process Decompression System
This device is outlined above. The figures on the right reveal the position of
the X-STOP after it has been implanted. *(REPRODUCED WITH PERMISSION*
FROM KYPHON.)

control pain. Detection of these fractures also presents an opportunity to
begin treatment for the osteoporosis. Pain can at times become so severe
that it limits function. However, in the absence of nerve compression by
a fracture fragment, patients usually fare well if they can endure the pain.
Miacalcin (calcitonin) is a hormone that improves absorption of calcium,
which is important for healing these fractures. When given to patients
with compression fractures in the setting of osteoporosis, it has the dual
benefit of substantially diminishing pain.

Vertebroplasty and kyphoplasty are minimally invasive methods that
can treat severe pain and provide structural support in the setting of spinal
compression fractures and metastatic lesions. Metastatic disease, in this
instance, refers to cancer that arises elsewhere in the body and has trav-
eled to the vertebrae. Cancer in the spine can weaken the bone and subsequently lead to what's called a pathologic fracture.

Often referred to as augmentation, vertebroplasty and kyphoplasty involve percutaneously injecting the fractured vertebral body with a liquid
acrylic cement, which then hardens. Kyphoplasty has the added potential

benefit of reversing some of the loss of vertebral body height associated with fractured or diseased bone. A percutaneous inflatable balloon (bone tamp) is used for this purpose. It creates a void that is then filled with the acrylic cement (polymethylmethacrylate, or PMMA).

The kyphoplasty procedure requires general anesthesia due to the pain associated with the technique; vertebroplasty is often performed with a local anesthetic. These procedures can be performed on an outpatient basis, but patients may stay in the hospital overnight. Because of the significant reduction in pain afforded by these procedures, patients are more mobile. Thus, the complications associated with prolonged bed rest are prevented. However, these procedures are not without risk. Complications include cement leakage that can result in nerve compromise or blood vessel occlusion, spinal fluid leak, pulmonary embolus (a blood clot that goes to the lung), infection, and epidural hematoma (blood collecting next to and compressing the spinal cord). The heat generated by the PMMA is also a concern when considering healing in the setting of already weakened osteoporotic bone, in addition to the potential threat to the neurovascular structures if the cement leaks. The firm cement in the fractured vertebrae adjacent to neighboring osteoporotic bone may alter the mechanics of the spine such that there is an increased risk of fracture at the next vertebral level. Efforts to develop a cement that is bioactive and can be metabolized into new bone are ongoing.

These percutaneous cement injection techniques have been shown to be useful aids in reducing pain and providing some stability in the setting

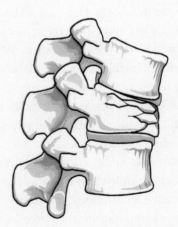

FIGURE 6.9. Vertebral Compression Fracture can cause prolonged, severe pain and create deformity.

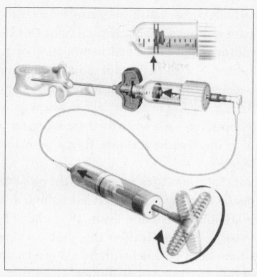

FIGURE 6.11. Vertebroplasty generally relieves pain with injection of acrylic cement into the fractured vertebral body. *(PHOTO COURTESY OF DEPUY SPINE, RAYNHAM, MA.)*

of vertebral compression fractures and metastatic cancer. Remember, although the procedure may bring pain relief and make the patient more mobile, the fracture has not healed. I recommend wearing a brace until it does. Diligent follow-up with the treating physician is very important.

Patients who have associated spinal stenosis, disc herniation, or a fracture fragment that compresses a nerve should not undergo such a procedure; they may require a more direct surgical approach.

SPINAL CORD STIMULATION (SCS), OR DORSAL COLUMN STIMULATION (DCS)

This technology has been around for approximately thirty years. Although the mechanism of action is not completely understood, the goal is to reduce chronic nerve-related pain. The method involves use of an implantable device that delivers pulsed electrical energy to the dorsal surface of the spinal cord through leads placed in the epidural space. Recall our discussion of the gate control theory of pain in chapter 4. This approach is thought to "close the gate" via L fiber activation (see figures 4.1a and 4.1b) and promote the release of inhibitory neurotransmitters that reduce the response to a painful stimulus.

Patients for whom conservative measures have failed, such as those with nerve root pain without a clear structural cause (for example, chronic regional pain syndrome and peripheral neuropathy) or failed back syndrome, are candidates. Not all patients respond to this technique; therefore, prior to placement of a permanent stimulator, temporary leads are placed, on a trial basis, for five to seven days to assess patient response. A successful trial is considered one whereby there is greater than 50 percent reduction in pain. If this threshold is met, then a permanent implant can be placed.

It is important that candidates for permanent placement understand that relief may not be sustained. The effect seems to fade when the body learns where the stimulus is coming from. Thus, the SCS may not provide long-term relief. Efforts to address this problem through modulating the stimulus have been pursued with mixed results. In addition, you should know that these techniques are minimally invasive surgical procedures (percutaneous or via laminectomy) that carry the risk of infection, epidural hematoma, paralysis, spinal fluid leak, and implant migration. Patients who have these implants cannot undergo an MRI scan due to the risk of migration and heating of the implanted electrodes in the presence of the large magnet. Spinal cord stimulation is not for everyone; however, for those with neuropathic pain who have exhausted other treatment options, it may be reasonable to consider.

Summary: Nonsurgical and Minimally Invasive Treatments

For a listing of my respectful opinion regarding how to select from the major treatment options for back care, see the table at the end of chapter 7.

We have listed an awesome variety of treatments in this chapter. The objective was to provide accurate and practical information with respect to how their success rates and risks compare. We found that many treatments fall into the success range of 60 percent to 70 percent—some higher, some lower.

Caregivers will assess each patient and make treatment recommendations. Individual physicians and therapists may choose among a variety of treatments, for complex reasons. One factor, of course, is their own familiarity with particular therapies.

How do *you* navigate the treatment maze?

The chart at the end of chapter 7 summarizes the relative risks and benefits associated with the various treatments we have discussed. It will give you an idea of the likelihood of success from selected treatment modalities, balanced against my considered opinion and their relative risks for the patient.

It makes sense to try two or three different conservative therapies first. If one fails, it is possible that another will succeed, as the odds work in your favor. On the other hand, do not seek out every backache therapy on the planet, or you will dissipate your time and resources. If, after giving two or three kinds of conservative treatment your best shot and you are still stuck with intractable pain, then you should consider one or two basic alternatives.

One alternative is surgery, discussed in the next chapter. However, an operation is the answer only when you have a clear-cut diagnosis that can be helped by a specific surgical procedure. Your doctor can explain your diagnosis and the proposed surgery so that you understand your situation and the treatment. If you are still in doubt, obtain a second opinion.

The other alternative is a well-conceived and organized program for managing chronic back pain. I hate to see patients struggle along with an unsuccessful treatment after it has proven to be unsuccessful. There are no magic cures. Rely on a comprehensive, conservative back pain management program, which includes a psychological and/or psychiatric assessment. I am not saying that the pain is all in your head. But when you have had severe pain for a long time, you may need emotional as well as medical or physical help to make yourself better.

CHAPTER 7

To Operate or Not to Operate?

The Risk-Versus-Benefit Equation

My task is a moral and legal one: to provide my patient with the opportunity to give informed consent. The gist of what we do for the patient is to give an idea of the *risks* associated with treatment choices, and the *benefits* that are likely to be gained from these choices.

The concept is expressed symbolically in figure 7.1. This means looking some cold statistics squarely in the eye. We talk about the one or two patients out of forty-four thousand who do not wake up from their anesthesia; not bad odds, but nonetheless . . . We mention the possibility of pneumonia following anesthesia, and the remote chance that a blood clot in the leg will travel to the lungs as a dangerous pulmonary embolism. In addition, I must point out that one or two out of every hundred patients develop an infection at the surgical site.

I tell them that during surgery, the nerve root may be irritated, damaged, or lost, causing numbness or weakness in a part of the leg after the operation. Some patients ask, "Could I be paralyzed by the operation?" This is asked when the patient fears the "helpless" situation where he/she cannot move arms or legs, or simply cannot walk at all. It is fair to say that none of the operations discussed here is likely to result in such a tragedy. There is the risk of significant weakness, numbness, or tingling in one or both legs that is associated with some of the operations. I will explain those as we come to them.

There is also a tiny risk of severe bleeding in the small vessels around the disc or in the major ones in front of the spine. Although the latter com-

RISK/BENEFIT

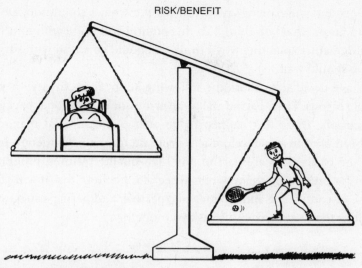

FIGURE 7.1. Risk and Benefit

Every operation has an associated risk but offers the possibility of benefit. The patient and surgeon must evaluate the situation and determine that the benefits outweigh the risks.

plication is rare, it may require a separate lifesaving operation through the abdomen to control bleeding.

Now, on the other hand, I reassure my patient. I review the probabilities of a good to excellent result. I point out that these major complications rarely occur. What I have given you is the most rigorous inventory of possible risks, and if I were talking to an extremely anxious patient, I would try to transmit the essence without dwelling on rare tragic possibilities.

Then I explain to my patient how his/her uniqueness bears on these concrete statistics. That is, if you are a vigorous, assertive, positive, healthy person, then you have a significantly lower risk profile than someone who is just the opposite. Likewise, there may be aspects of your particular diagnosis and condition that warrant more optimism. Whatever the diagnosis and treatment, a patient without a sincere, realistic desire to get well is not a good surgical candidate.

With all of this under our belts, I ask the patient whether he/she prefers surgery or continued attempts at nonsurgical treatment. In most cases, the patient has a clear-cut opinion. But sometimes the ball is returned to my court and the patient says, "You tell me what I should do, Doctor; I want to know what you think." At this point, I will share with him/her my best judgment, explaining why I think we should go ahead with surgery or why we should wait.

I have decided to share the following surgical maxims with you for several reasons. First, permit me to give you some additional background information. These just happen to be orthopedic surgical maxims that have been used in our development program for young surgeons. In principle, the basic ideas are part of any high-quality training program. My reason for presenting them here is threefold: I believe that it will give you a sense of confidence and a better perspective, and perhaps suggest some questions that you may wish to ask your doctor.

A Doctor's Surgical Maxims

- Do the least amount of surgery that is necessary to solve the patient's problem(s).
- Each additional risk to the patient must be justified by substantial evidence of incremental benefit for the patient.

To Operate or Not?

In medical textbooks, the terms of this dilemma are deemed *indications* and *contraindications* of surgery, and the question has been the focus of many a journal article, conference, and informal talk. Doctors, in fact, spend a good part of their careers figuring out how to select from among all the possible treatments the one that is best for a particular patient.

Indications for surgery? First, a specific abnormal process in the spine should be identified and documented. And it should have been present long enough to assume that nature alone is not going to cure it. Finally, before anyone gets wheeled into the operating room, there should be reasonable evidence that surgery will correct, eliminate, or substantially improve the problem. Surgery is the controlled disruption of tissue performed for the purpose of removing, augmenting, or repairing an injured, malfunctioning, cancerous, or infected anatomic structure.

When surgery is not beneficial, or is likely to be harmful, it should not be performed. Of course, there is not always a crisp, clean yes-or-no judgment.

In this chapter, we will list the common low back operations, with the indications and contraindications of each. Although reading this chapter is no substitute for a thorough discussion with your surgeon, it will equip you with the information you need to engage substantively in that conversation.

How to Choose a Surgeon

Things are getting serious. You need a spine specialist to evaluate and possibly treat you. Here is a checklist to help you identify that person. The key questions are: Is this person qualified? Does he/she care about me? Will this doctor explain what's wrong with me and answer my questions?

That's essentially it. The checklist will help you to find a qualified, caring, explaining, and good question-answerer.

Who should operate? Simple: someone well trained and experienced in low back surgery. Your surgeon should understand patients as people and be thoroughly knowledgeable about the diagnosis and management of lumbar spine pain. How do you know if a given surgeon is qualified? I would recommend seeking one who is a spine surgeon, fellowship trained and board certified in either orthopedic surgery or neurosurgery. The hospital where a surgeon admits patients will generally provide board-certification information. Perhaps even more useful references are the

---

Checklist for Finding a Good Spine Care Surgeon

- Ask your internist or primary care physician.
- Try a doctor referral service in your hospital or clinic.
- If one or more of the major hospitals in your city has a physician referral service, try that.
- Do you have a friend in the health care profession—a doctor, a nurse, or an administrator? Ask him/her.
- Make sure your doctor is board certified.
- While there are good doctors outside university-affiliated hospitals, if in doubt, go with teaching centers.

websites of the American Board of Medical Specialties (www.abms.org), the American Academy of Orthopaedic Surgeons (www.aaos.org), the American Board of Orthopaedic Surgery (www.abos.org), and the American Board of Neurological Surgery (www.abns.org), where you can obtain this information electronically. Sometimes you may see advertisements in various commercial magazines highlighting some of the "best" doctors. These may display good doctors, but the ads do not tell you much regarding their credentials, quality of care, or bedside manner. Ask fellow back sufferers, listening for the kinds of traits that we have mentioned. Do not hesitate to query your surgeon about how comfortable and experienced he/she is with your contemplated procedure if his/her training in a certain technique is not evident. Nowadays, this is perfectly acceptable patient-doctor etiquette. After all, it is *your* back. Finally, heed your gut feelings of confidence and rapport.

Which should you choose: an orthopedic surgeon or a neurosurgeon? If a spinal fusion is called for, I would advise you to have an orthopedic surgeon perform the procedure. This is a procedure at which he/she is generally more experienced. But otherwise, either is fine. An Australian study compared a large group of patients with low back pain and sciatica. Half were treated by orthopedic surgeons and half by neurosurgeons, and the success rates were nearly identical. In addition, several training programs combined the efforts of both orthopedic and neurosurgery department faculty with respect to educating young doctors in residency and fellowship postresidency training.

If a surgeon seems to be rushing you into surgery, beware, unless you have the bladder problems we previously described. Also, shun any self-proclaimed miracle worker. On the subject of doctors, let me tell you a little story. (My apologies are extended to any doctors who may be reading this book, as they may have heard this story at least three times.)

After bidding farewell to this good life, a woman finds herself outside the pearly gates. She is about to have her credentials checked by Saint Peter. There is a long line of prospective applicants in front of her. Of course, everyone is on his/her best behavior. Suddenly, along strolls a tall, stately person in a white coat with a stethoscope around his neck. Without any timidity whatsoever, this self-possessed individual walks past everyone to the front of the line and enters heaven. "Who was that?" the people in line whisper to one another. "That was God." The word filters back. "But why the white coat and stetho-scope?" the people ask. The answer comes back: "Oh, He likes to play doctor sometimes."

Sometimes in our zeal to help, or laboring under an unrealistic belief in our own powers, we doctors can do *too much* surgery on backache patients. This is a consideration especially in the case of salvage back surgery, which we will discuss later.

Surgery for Disc Disease

(DISCECTOMY)

Let's start with what is probably the most common operation for backache. The rationale for removing the intervertebral disc is that it's presumed to be the offending body part and has become abnormal. This was one of the first surgical principles, and it still holds.

What does disc surgery consist of? Operating through the back, the surgeon dissects down the back of the vertebrae, making an entrance into the vertebral canal. He then carefully moves the dura and the bundle of nerves called the cauda equina aside, exposing the disc itself. The important, somewhat sticky part of the procedure is to expose and protect the nerve elements and control the bleeding from the network of veins in this area (figure 7.2).

Now the disc can be clearly identified. At this point, one of three things happens:

1. If a portion of the disc has separated from the main part and moved out into the nerve canal, it is called a free fragment (figure 7.3). It can simply be plucked out or dissected from the scar tissue and ligaments in the canal.

2. The disc may be incompletely displaced, with the fragment still partially within the space between the two vertebrae (figure 7.4).

3. The disc isn't fragmented at all but is bulging extensively (figure 7.5).

In either of the second two cases, the surgeon removes the bulging or displaced part and a part of the disc that lies in the interspace between the vertebrae.

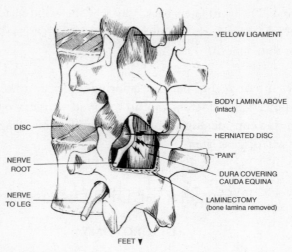

Labels on figure:
YELLOW LIGAMENT
BODY LAMINA ABOVE (intact)
DISC
HERNIATED DISC
"PAIN"
NERVE ROOT
DURA COVERING CAUDA EQUINA
NERVE TO LEG
LAMINECTOMY (bone lamina removed)
FEET ▼

FIGURE 7.2. Laminectomy

A lumbar laminectomy is an operative procedure in which part or all of the lamina (a portion of bone on the back of the vertebra) is removed. In addition, a part of the yellow ligament is removed, as shown here. The purpose, in this example, is to get to the herniated disc. The herniated portion of the disc is then removed in order to decompress, or relieve, the irritation of the nerve root.

What shape the disc is found in at the time of surgery has much to do with whether or not the operation relieves your leg pain from sciatica. The best prognosis—a 90 percent success rate—comes with complete disc herniation. When the disc fragment is not completely separated from the rest of the disc and the space between the vertebrae, the success rate drops to 80 percent. When only a bulging disc is found, success is in the range of 60 percent. It may interest you to know that when the disc is not abnormal at all, surgery still cures 30 percent of patients—an example of the placebo effect. The mind is a puzzling machine!

Patients often ask, "What happens when you remove the disc? Do you just leave nothing there? Nature must have put it there for some reason." That is a reasonable question, and the reply is that the patient is better off without the disc than with an abnormal one. Most surgeons are aware that, for good reasons, the patient is best served by removing just the herniated part and a small portion of the remaining disc. And while the back is not restored to its original perfection, it's improved enough to be only very

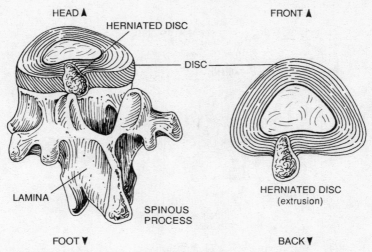

FIGURE 7.3. Disc Herniation with Extrusion

A portion of the nucleus has isolated itself from the rest of the disc and all or part of it is displaced well out into the canal. This situation is the one that responds best to surgery. It may not respond to conservative therapy, including manipulation. *(REPRODUCED WITH PERMISSION FROM WHITE, A. A., AND PANJABI, M. M.: CLINICAL BIOMECHANICS OF THE SPINE, 2ND ED., J. B. LIPPINCOTT, 1990.)*

subtly different from a normal one. In most instances, of course, the patient has residual reminders that his/her back isn't quite its old self: When the weather is bad, a heavy item is lifted improperly, or he/she goes for a long drive, there may be mild or moderate pain similar to what the patient felt before surgery.

The question frequently arises as to whether there is too much disc surgery done in the United States. Here are some statistics. In Great Britain, ten in one hundred thousand patients with a disc herniation will have surgery. In Finland, the number is between thirty-one and forty-one. In the United States? About seventy out of one hundred thousand men and women with disc herniation will have surgery. Rates of surgical treatment in the United States have been observed to vary by region. The reason for is unclear. These statistics, of course, *do not* answer the question of whether too much disc surgery is performed in the United States. There could be other explanations for these figures. The diagnoses could be different, or patient demands and expectations could be a factor. Nevertheless, there may, in fact, be too much disc surgery performed in the United States.

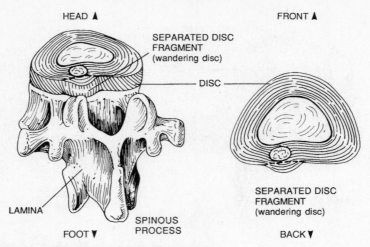

FIGURE 7.4. "Wandering" Disc Herniation

This one I like to call the "wandering disc." Some annulus fibers have iso-lated themselves and wander about due to movement of the spine. In some positions, they cause pain; in others, they don't. Traction, or manipula-tion, may help. The problem may come on suddenly following just a slight twist or bend, and it may go away almost as rapidly following a fall, twist, or cough. Surgery is sometimes required when severe pain and disability persist for three to twelve weeks or more. *(REPRODUCED WITH PERMISSION FROM WHITE, A. A., AND PANJABI, M. M.: CLINICAL BIOMECHANICS OF THE SPINE, 2ND ED., J. B. LIPPINCOTT, 1990.)*

The goal of this chapter is to provide the necessary information for you to make a wise decision about surgery.

WHO SHOULD HAVE DISC SURGERY?

For openers, consider a history of back pain that has lasted for at least six weeks. Now, much hinges on certain diagnostic tests, and this brings us to the matter of a thorough preoperative exam. If you are being evaluated for disc disease, several tests will clarify your condition.

First, your history and a few neurologic findings tell your doctor some-thing about the state of your disc. One part of the physical exam, called the straight leg raising test, is especially critical. If positive, this results in pain radiating down your leg, which indicates nerve root compression. Your doctor may recommend an electromyographic/nerve conduction study (EMG/NCS) to help identify abnormal electrical activity in the muscles

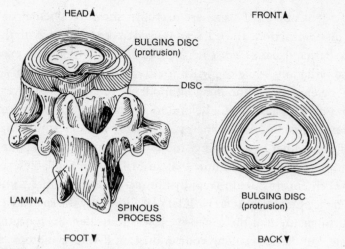

FIGURE 7.5. The "Bulging" Disc

Here the disc is herniated but bulges just enough to cause nerve root irritation and sciatica. These patients may be helped with traction, manipulation, and medication/observation. Surgery is sometimes needed if there is a positive MRI or CT-myelogram and the back pain and sciatica do not subside in three to twelve weeks. The results are good with surgery, but not as good as when there is a significant fragment of disc out in the canal. *(REPRODUCED WITH PERMISSION FROM WHITE, A. A., AND PANJABI, M. M.:* CLINICAL BIO-MECHANICS OF THE SPINE, *2ND ED., J. B. LIPPINCOTT, 1990.)*

supplied by the sciatic nerve. This test is not usually bad at all, particularly if you can manage to relax. Very fine needles may be inserted into several muscles to pick up and record their electrical patterns.

Let me suggest a little mental trick that can make this test a breeze for you. Think of it as a little mosquito bite, followed by an itch or tickle. I'm serious—the sensations are amazingly similar. You must faithfully convince yourself of that. People have trouble with these tests because they build up anxiety over the words *needle* and *electrical.*

Abnormal activity suggests nerve root damage caused by an encroaching disc. There is something called a *water-soluble myelogram,* a technique that's more accurate than the older fat-soluble myelograms in visualizing a herniated disc. The difference between the two is the solubility of the contrast medium, or dye. (See chapter 3 for a discussion of the myelograms.) Happily, the water-soluble dye does not have to be removed after the test. This simplifies the procedure.

CT scans and MRI scans are useful in showing whether or not you have a disc herniation. The CT scan is used in conjunction with the myelogram to better visualize a disc herniation. The CT-myelogram exposes you to some radiation, while the MRI does not. The MRI has nearly replaced the CT-myelogram as the imaging modality of choice. However, the CT scan and myelogram are still helpful tools that need to be used in certain situations. There are times when your doctor will determine that one or both of these other two imaging studies are best to evaluate your particular condition. You should know that an MRI is not available everywhere but new centers are opening rapidly now across the country. Some Health Maintenance Organizations (HMOs) will allow only the specialist to order an MRI to ensure that the expensive test is indicated. Such caution is appropriate, but do not prolong your evaluation if your symptoms are escalating (see "Checklist for When to Call the Doctor" in chapter 6).

EXPECTED SUCCESS RATE OF DISC SURGERY

When your doctor can add up the evaluation of your history, the physical exam, and all the test results, then he/she can gauge your odds of successful surgery. Bear in mind the correlation between disc herniation and pain relief. If you have a three-month history of back pain with sciatica and clear neurologic problems, an abnormal straight leg raising test, an abnormal EMG/NCS, and positive imaging studies, your odds of being helped by disc surgery are around 90 percent to 95 percent. If the diagnosis of a herniated disc is based on your history and neurologic exam alone, it may be only 60 percent accurate. Add the abnormal straight leg raising test, and we go up to 70 percent; with an abnormal EMG/NCS, to 80 percent.

Good news for senior citizens: You, too, can expect a favorable outcome from disc surgery when the proper indications are present. The data show that 87 percent of patients over sixty will enjoy a good-to-excellent result.

PROS AND CONS OF DISC SURGERY

Major complications of disc removal include damaged nerves in the lumbar area, damaged major blood vessels in front of the disc, and wound infections. Most of these complications are quite rare, although wound infections occur at a 1 percent to 2 percent rate.

Now, you may ask, "What will happen to me if I *don't* have the surgery?" A Swedish study addressed this question, dividing a group of patients with a clear diagnosis of herniated disc for six months into two groups. One group underwent disc removal and laminectomy (see figure 7.2), while the others were treated nonsurgically, with immobilization. How did they fare?

Well, those with definite disc prolapse or herniation who were operated on enjoyed quicker relief of their sciatica and returned to work sooner than the nonsurgical patients. But the experiment did show that nature can cure sciatica, too. Six months after treatment, there was little difference between the two groups. But the patients' subjective self-evaluation differed. The surgical patients rated their condition as more improved and took less sick leave than those who'd been treated with immobilization, even though their tests of leg motor strength were identical.

Other studies from Norway show a superior outcome from surgery that lasts for two to five years. However, after ten years, nonoperated patients did about as well as those who had surgery.

A recently published multicenter randomized controlled trial called the Spine Patients Outcomes Research Trial, coordinated by surgeon Dr. James Weinstein of the Dartmouth-Hitchcock Medical Center in Lebanon, New Hampshire, examined the results of surgical versus nonsurgical treatment of lumbar disc herniation. There were patients in the surgery group who decided not to have an operation. Likewise, there were patients in the nonoperative group who decided to undergo surgery due to ongoing or worsening symptoms. Critics have suggested that such "crossover" of patients between the two groups may have affected the interpretation of the data. Nonetheless, this study revealed that sciatica and associated nerve-related symptoms from the disc herniation has an excellent prognosis. There was an advantage to surgery, with the surgical patients improving faster and doing significantly better out to two years. There was a significant treatment effect of surgery on low back pain, with leg pain improving significantly more at each follow-up period. The back pain improved more with discectomy than in the nonoperative group. In other words, if you can endure the pain, you will do fairly well without surgery. If you want to improve faster, surgery can be quite helpful. This highlights the importance of being involved in the decision-making process regarding treatment options. In fact, Dr. Weinstein has started the Center for Shared Decision Making at Dartmouth-Hitchcock Medical Center, with educational materials and aids to help patients make informed choices regarding their care. He states, "We see patients as part of the solution, not as part of the problem."

As a result of this new center, he has observed that the rates of surgery for disc herniations fell by 30 percent, while operations for spinal stenosis increased by 10 percent, noting that the patients felt better informed and more knowledgeable.

Once your symptoms are severe, and you have low back pain, sciatica, and a diagnosis of a herniated disc, how long should you wait before considering an operation? At this point, remember that 90 percent of patients recover in about six to ten weeks with no treatment, because that is the natural course of the disease. If you are going to have elective disc surgery, consider the information discussed above. Previous data have indicated that the ideal time is at about forty to fifty days (six weeks) after the onset of leg pain. Timely and appropriate surgical intervention has the advantages of minimizing pain and psychological distress. Furthermore, patients who undergo disc removal after having persistent pain for a year are only half as likely to get pain relief as patients who have surgery earlier.

Even motor weaknesses, such as foot drop, can improve without surgery. Assuming that we are still within the six- to ten-week interval, and the pain is improving or tolerated, the presence of continued weakness alone does not necessarily force our hand in surgery. If, however, one watches a *foot drop* (motor weakness in the ankle and foot) too long—more than three to nine months—it may not recover for one or two years after surgery, if at all.

Permanent damage may be the result of chronic nerve root compression, inflammation, and scarring. Over the years, I have detected scarring and other evidence of nerve damage in discs that have presumably been herniated for a year or more. There may be a curious psychological reason, too. We know that pain that has hung around for more than a year is not usually completely banished when you correct the disease that caused it. It is as though the pain acquired a life of its own—and some psychological or emotional support may be necessary, in addition to removing the physical cause of the pain.

However, when it comes to you, the individual, do not interpret these statistics to mean that you must have the disc out by 11:59 p.m. on the fifty-ninth day of your illness. There are many intertwined considerations and few absolutes. If you cannot spare too much time away from work, you should seriously consider surgery around two to three months into your illness. However, your particular surgical risks, your anxiety about or confidence in the scalpel, and the extent of your pain, disability, and life disruption must all be taken into consideration.

There are two noteworthy exceptions to the two- to three-month principle. The first is the professional athlete who performs or participates in heavy lifting or high-risk sports, and workers with strenuous lifting tasks. These individuals should wait to see if time will heal them spontaneously. During this time, they will be out of work, out of competition, and eventually out of shape. We have developed a program for the well-trained athlete with acute low back pain (see bibliography). Here we focus on the highly competitive athlete with low back pain and significant sciatica—more precisely, with a herniated disc. We think that if these competitors are not rapidly improving after six to eight weeks (in general), they should have a minimally invasive discectomy, if appropriate. The best results and the lowest complication rate are achieved following *microdiscectomy*. It is simply the standard open procedure performed through a much smaller incision with the assistance of a surgical microscope. The disc herniation is removed under direct visualization and the athlete can begin rehabilitation and perhaps return to competition sooner. If there are any doubters as to the wisdom of this recommendation, consider the spectacular Joe Montana, who recovered from disc surgery and was rehabilitated to come back as a superstar quarterback of the National Football League. The great Major League Baseball pitcher Randy Johnson also recovered from this procedure and returned to a Cy Young Award–winning career.

The second exception is that of patients with severe sciatica who suddenly cannot control their bladders. This suggests that a large herniated disc fragment may have popped out. Sometimes there will be severe leg weakness, numbness, and/or loss of the ability to control the bowel and bladder. In these instances, so much of the disc has been displaced that the nerves involved cannot provide the usual control of the bladder, bowels, and legs. In this situation, I view surgery not as elective but, rather, *urgent*, and I would urge my patient to report to the emergency room to be evaluated by me for surgery as soon as possible, provided that the disc can be seen on an MRI.

There has been some gratifying feedback on our first endeavor to write a helpful low back book. The following vignette exemplifies a situation in which a reader converted herself into a heroine by applying this information about bladder control. Apparently our patient, who was reading the book, had a friend who had low back pain with sciatica. It was mild pain, but with some slight weakness in the leg. She had been to see several doctors and was being treated conservatively and appropriately. However, she began to develop some difficulty getting her urination started and had mentioned this to her doctor, who was not particularly alarmed. The reader of the book suggested that she contact her doctor again and reemphasize this particular symptom. This was done, and although the response was one of concern, it was not apparently one of recognition of the importance of this symptom. Our conscientious reader then insisted that her friend see another physician and again emphasize the problem. This was done, the physician ordered the appropriate imaging studies, and a large herniated disc was diagnosed and subsequently removed by a surgeon. The patient improved, and her bladder function returned to normal.

Surgery for Spinal Stenosis

Before we discuss surgery for spinal stenosis, I would like to emphasize a couple of points. First, this is a pretty important disease. The most common form is degenerative and it affects primarily our senior citizens. There are happily quite a few of them, and a lot more coming with the baby boomer wave of retirees already upon us. The disease is fairly common among those sixty-five years of age or older. The exact prevalence in the U.S. is unknown; however, it is estimated that those with symptomatic stenosis may range from one-quarter to one-half million individuals. As the population ages, the figures may increase. Now, the other point that is important to consider, before discussing surgery, is nonsurgical treatment. For the sake of emphasis, I have provided a conservative treatment checklist in chapter 3.

As we outlined in chapter 3, spinal stenosis is a condition in which there is too little space in the spinal canal. The typical symptoms include leg pain and difficulty walking. The leg symptoms may include numbness and weakness. The symptoms are usually relieved with rest and/or sitting. Sometimes a person is simply born with an abnormally narrow spinal canal. In the degenerative form, bony changes in the back of the vertebral bodies or in the posterior vertebral joints (the facet joints) may crowd the canal. A herniated disc or a bulging and/or thickened yellow ligament can contribute to stenosis as well. Please refer to figures 3.6 and 3.7 to refresh your memory. Finally, several diseases can compromise that space.

An individual with poor circulation in the legs secondary to peripheral arterial disease (PAD) will also experience difficulty walking, or claudication. Our senior members of society are also at risk for developing PAD. It is possible for both conditions to exist in the same individual. Assessment of which condition predominates will allow treatment to be prioritized.

What does surgery accomplish? Any and all structures impinging on the nerves within the canal—and causing pain, weakness, or discomfort—can be removed surgically. The prognosis for patients having surgery for spinal stenosis is quite good: About 85 percent of patients have a good or excellent result.

Beforehand, radiographic studies, including X-rays, an MRI, and possibly a CT scan and myelogram, can generally unmask the identity of the encroaching structure(s). During surgery, the surgeon opens the spine from the back, usually removing the lamina, spinous process, yellow ligament, and sometimes a part (but rarely all) of the paired facet joints at the affected levels of the spine (L2–L3, L3–L4, and so on). Please refer to figure 7.5a, which will give you a good sense of what is removed. Here the lamina on just one side has been removed. For spinal stenosis, the spinous process would be removed as well as the lamina on the other side. This would then be done at as many levels as the imaging studies showed to be constricted, taking as much as needed of the facet joints to relieve encroachment. Sometimes part of the disc is excised, too. Depending on the patient's age, the extent to which important structures have been dismantled, and the surgeon's judgment, a fusion (see page 196) may be performed to lock the spine in one position and prevent it from displacing. The likelihood of displacement is proportional to the amount of bone and other anatomic structures that had to be removed to relieve the stenosis. As we discussed in chapter 6, an interspinous process spacer may be an option for those with mild to moderate stenosis.

If you are an elderly person with a documented case of lumbar spinal stenosis and you have tried conservative treatment without success, here is my suggestion to you. If your pain and difficulty in walking are such that you are losing your independence and not able to socialize and otherwise enjoy life, consider the following: Unless you have some major illness that your physician thinks will make you an inordinate anesthesia risk, I suggest you explore the idea of surgery, which offers you about an 80 percent chance of improvement and perhaps as good or better a chance of keep-

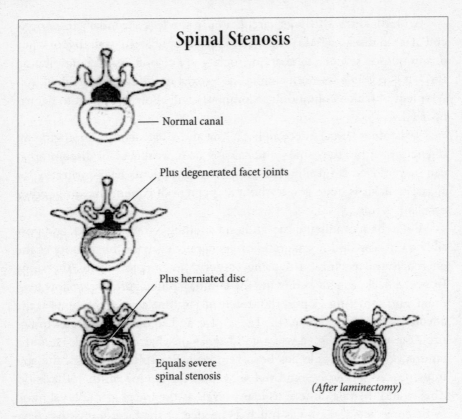

Spinal Stenosis

Normal canal

Plus degenerated facet joints

Plus herniated disc

Equals severe
spinal stenosis

(After laminectomy)

FIGURE 7.5A. Spinal Stenosis and Laminectomy

This figure highlights the nature of degenerative changes that lead to lumbar spinal stenosis and the reexpansion of the neural elements in the spinal canal following a laminectomy.

ing you from getting even worse. My point is that, barring major illness, your age alone is no reason not to give yourself a good chance to improve and/or preserve good quality of life. A reasonably healthy elderly person with lumbar spinal stenosis should not wait around to get worse and worse while assuming that he/she is too old to have surgery.

SPINAL FUSION

This is an operation in which bone from somewhere else in your body, or from a donor's body, is grafted onto regions of living bone in the back. After a period of usually four to nine months, a natural process known as *creeping substitution* transpires. Although it may evoke scenes from *Inva-*

sion of the Body Snatchers, all it means is that the bone graft is gradually replaced by living bone produced by the patient's own body. The result is a bony connection between two or more adjacent vertebrae. The graft serves as a scaffold and stimulus for the formation of new bone: usually a strong, solid, stable union between the bones selected for fusion.

Why fuse bone, anyway? The idea is that fusing the bone reduces motion at an abnormal segment of the spine. The anticipated result is that the pain produced by irritating and unstable excessive motion will fade. Normal motion of a diseased spinal segment, abnormal motion of a normal or near-normal segment, or an abnormal positioning between two segments can cause backache.

Your bone or someone else's may be used. Most evidence suggests that they are almost equally effective. Not infrequently, using your own (autograft) will require a second incision. Because the bone comes from your own body, there is no chance of your immune system rejecting the graft. What's more growth factors from your own bone cells will facilitate healing. It is considered to be the gold standard for spinal fusion surgery. Most often the bone graft is harvested from the iliac crest (the top of the pelvis). There is postoperative pain associated with taking your own bone. Additional risks include possible complications of infection or a hematoma. Antibiotics are given at the time of surgery to minimize the risk of infection.

Banked bone (someone else's) carries an *infinitesimally small* risk of transmitting a blood-borne disease such as hepatitis or AIDS. There have been documented cases whereby patients contracted acquired immunodeficiency syndrome (AIDS) and hepatitis as a result of bone transplantation (allograft) used in spinal fusion and other types of surgery requiring a bone graft. The bone in one case was unwittingly donated by a patient with AIDS, and the patient who received the bone developed the disease and symptoms within three weeks from the time of the surgery. There have been reports of errors in the manner in which the allograft donor bone had been harvested, with a subsequent FDA-ordered recall of the specimens. There were several cases where the tainted bone had been implanted in patients. These cases were traced, and there were a handful of hepatitis and HIV virus conversions reported. Other potential infectious organisms include clostridium, enterococcus, and staphylococcus. While there are risks associated with the use of banked bone, if the allograft is obtained and managed according to standards for surgical tissue banking established by the Musculoskeletal Transplant Foundation and the American Association of Tissue Banks, the risk is virtually eliminated. The most reasonable and balanced estimate is a 1 in 250,000 risk. Estimates by experts range from 1 in 75,000 to 1 in 500,000.

Processed human bone for spinal fusion is available for purchase from American Red Cross Transplantation Services. Its graft material is appropriately prepared and sterilized. There are no living cells in such prepared grafts, which minimizes the possibility of an immune response. Most important, the donors are very carefully screened for AIDS, hepatitis, syphilis, and other diseases that might be transmitted through bone grafts. This and other commercial sources are considered safe, but consult with your surgeon. The healing time may be longer when compared to that of your own bone, but you do not have the discomfort associated with the surgery site where the graft is harvested.

We advise our patients of the risks and benefits of both of these bone graft options, and engage them in the decision-making process.

Another commercially available option is that of specially treated animal bone, or xenografts. This type of bone graft is thought to be almost as effective, if not as effective, as banked human bone. These graft materials are typically obtained from cow or pig sources. Many xenograft types have been used successfully in humans. You may have heard of a friend, relative, or neighbor having had a pig valve utilized to replace an abnormal heart valve. There are many examples where bone or collagen xenografts have been used safely in orthopedic surgery. Concerns have been raised regarding the risk of an immune response, disease transmission, and the possibility of recombination/mutation with typically nonpathogenic organisms (i.e., bacteria that do not usually infect) in humans to form new infectious organisms. Additional study is required to further evaluate this graft option, define universal guidelines, and assess the long-term efficacy and risks associated with xenograft implantation in patients.

Modern technology and genetic engineering have produced yet another alternative to bone grafting. Study of the cellular and chemical stimuli for bone healing and regeneration has lead to the discovery and synthesis of bone morphogenetic proteins (BMPs). These naturally occurring proteins have been discovered to induce new bone formation, even in tissues where bone is not usually present. Further analysis has led to the isolation of the responsible compounds. Recombinant cloning techniques, also known as genetic engineering, have made BMPs available for clinical use. Potential clinical applications abound, but our interest here is in the promotion of spinal fusion. The delivery mechanism and the proper dose for specific applications are still under investigation—too much compound may promote an excessive amount of bone formation, while too little may not allow for an adequate stimulus—but studies have shown BMPs to be quite effective in promoting successful spinal fusion. Earlier studies suggested that BMPs were equal to or better than an iliac crest bone graft. This data led some clinicians to assume that BMPs could replace autograft and allograft as the gold standard, but the costs associated with BMPs have been somewhat prohibitive.

Reports that BMPs used in conjunction with donor bone can result in a rapid resorption (dissolving) of the graft suggest that these two procedures should not be combined. On the contrary, if BMPs are combined with your own bone, more abundant bone formation is observed.

Some patients respond to BMPs with a pronounced inflammatory reaction. Such a reaction suggests an allergic reaction to these proteins. The manufacturer has recommended that with patients for whom such a reaction has been observed, future exposure to BMPs should be avoided.

The FDA has approved the use of two forms of BMP: (1) rhBMP-2 (Infuse Bone Graft, Medtronic, Minneapolis, Minn.), and (2) rhBMP-7 (OP-1, Stryker Biotech, Hopkinton, Mass. RhBMP-2 has been approved for use in the treatment of acute open tibial shaft fractures in adults treated with an intramedullary rod fixation, following appropriate wound management. It has also been approved for spinal fusion surgery used together with the LP-CAGE fusion device. RhBMP-7 is approved only for humanitarian use when all other options have failed in the effort to promote bone healing in long bones (nonunions/pseudoarthrosis).

Concerns over the potential cancer risk associated with BMPs have been raised. RhBMP-2, or Infuse Bone Graft, the FDA's preferred BMP, has been shown to suppress certain types of tumor cells, but rhBMP-7, approved by the FDA only when all other options have failed, is associated with increased cancer cell growth in animal studies. There is a report from human trials where 5 of 570 patients who received rhBMP-7 developed cancer, and one patient with a previously treated cancer suffered a recurrence. The cause-and-effect relation has not been proven.

The FDA therefore requires the manufacturers of all BMPs to include the following contraindications:

- Pregnant women or those attempting to become pregnant.
- Children or skeletally immature (still growing) patients.
- Patients with a history of malignancy (rhBMP-7) or undergoing treatment for malignancy (rhBMP-2).
- Women of childbearing age should be advised to prevent pregnancy for one year after treatment with BMPs.

An additional bone graft option is synthetic or naturally occurring calcium-based ceramics that serve as a scaffold onto which bone can grow. These substances include calcium phosphates (calcium hydroxyapatite and tricalcium phosphate) and calcium sulfate and can be fashioned into porous forms that are structurally similar to bone. The healing process takes longer when this approach is used, but ceramics have the advantage of being readily available and typically lower in cost than other bone graft substitutes. In addition to serving as bone graft substitutes, these substances are often used as bone graft extenders. Some studies suggest that this is the most effective manner in which to use these compounds.

As we can see, technological advancements may be associated with certain risks. BMPs require additional study, but the concerns are legitimate. As we have previously discussed, the objective is to provide you with the most up-to-date information so that *you* can be engaged in the decision-making process regarding what treatment options are chosen for your specific condition.

The spinal fusion procedures can be performed either *anteriorly*—that is, from the front, between the vertebral bodies—or *posteriorly*—from the back, between the posterior elements of two or more adjacent vertebrae (figures 7.6 and 7.11). A combination of these techniques can be utilized. This will effectively result in fusion along the front and back of the spine, often referred to as a *360-degree fusion*. As discussed, the bone used for the graft is often taken from the top of the ilium, the portion of the pelvic bone that defines how your clothing drapes across your waistline and hip area. The top of the ilium is referred to as the iliac crest. This is where bone marrow is harvested if you were to make a donation for a cancer patient. The bone marrow cells within your own bone graft help stimulate the healing of the spinal fusion. The iliac crest bone graft is the gold standard to which all the other graft options must be compared.

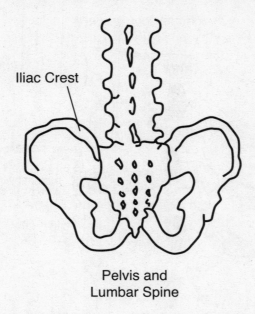

Iliac Crest

Pelvis and
Lumbar Spine

FIGURE 7.5B. Location of Iliac Crest Bone Graft Harvest Site

WHO SHOULD HAVE A SPINAL FUSION?

First of all, should spinal fusion be a routine fellow traveler on a disc-removal trip? The answer is *no.* In simple disc surgery, fusion is neither desirable nor necessary, unless there is some other abnormality. Where previous surgery has caused extensive damage to the anatomic elements of the spine, or definite arthritis exists, spinal fusion may accompany disc surgery. Spinal stenosis may also call for fusion, but this will be discussed under a separate heading.

Otherwise, when is spinal fusion a good idea? Sometimes considerable arthritis or damage from a fracture results in definite spinal instability requiring a fusion. But these conditions are not run-of-the-mill. A more straightforward case for spinal fusion is spondylolisthesis, or slippage of the vertebrae (see figure 3.5a). When spondylolisthesis causes severe back pain with or without leg pain, a spinal fusion may spell substantial relief, especially for younger patients.

But now we come to our main topic here: fusion of the lumbar spine as treatment for pain due to degenerative disc disease. Unfortunately, the success rate is not overwhelming. Many patients have some disc degeneration that is not painful. The first line of treatment is always conserva-

ANTERIOR INTERBODY FUSION

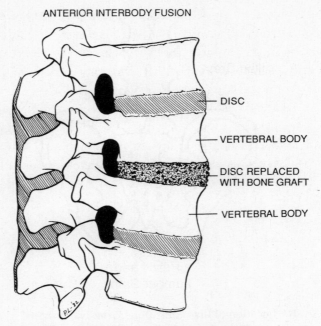

— DISC

— VERTEBRAL BODY

— DISC REPLACED
WITH BONE GRAFT

— VERTEBRAL BODY

FIGURE 7.6. Anterior Lumbar Interbody Fusion (ALIF)

In an ALIF, the disc is surgically removed through the front of the spine, and bone graft is substituted in the disc space. There are a number of variations on this basic theme, having to do with the shape of the bone graft, how much if any of the vertebra is removed, and whether metal fixation or a spine replacement is used.

tive. For most, the tincture of time, exercise, and perhaps medication will suffice. A few patients may require a spinal fusion for degenerative disc disease. Results in the 60 percent to 70 percent range barely lift lumbar fusion above the host of undistinguished nonoperative therapies discussed in chapter 6. Patients with spondylolisthesis, scoliosis, fractures, or a well-documented clinical instability of the spine enjoy much rosier odds. Surgery for tumors, infections, or extensive decompression of neural elements that require removal of part of the spine's major support structures may dictate a spinal fusion.

SPINE FUSIONS WITH IMPLANTS

Spinal instrumentation, or internal fixation, has matured from a time period when there was considerable interest to a clearly defined benefit with regard to stabilizing the spine, correcting deformity, and improving fusion rates. The rationale behind instrumentation is that it decreases movement of the spine–bone graft complex and thus helps it to heal and mature. Prior to spinal instrumentation, long bed rest and body casts were often utilized to immobilize the spine until the fusion matured. With the advent of spinal instrumentation, the inherent stability has allowed for early mobilization postoperatively. A brace or corset is still often required. Since it is quite possible that your surgeon may mention one of these implants or a similar type, I have provided some illustrations. Examples of four classic types are presented in figures 7.7 through 7.10, with modern versions outlined in 7.11 and 7.12.

In figure 7.7, the vertebra is attached to a rod by wires that must pass under the lamina into the spinal canal and loops back around the rod. The second (figure 7.8), called *Harrington rods* and hooks, is an instrumentation system that was initially used for scoliosis and later in lumbar spine fusions, especially for trauma. In figure 7.9, an internal fixator is demonstrated, whereby a screw is placed into the pedicle and the body of the vertebra and attached to a rod or plate. The fourth (figure 7.10), the *Cotrel-Dubousset apparatus,* also used for scoliosis, combines concepts of

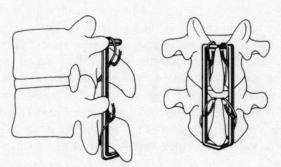

FIGURE 7.7. Spinal Instrumentation

This is a technique for internal fixation of the lumbar spine. On the left is a side view of the heavy metal rectangle, which firmly holds vertebrae in place by connecting them through wires attached to the rectangular rod structure. The wires are passed around the lamina (the back part of the vertebra) and the metal rectangle and twisted tightly. On the right is a view of the surgical construction from a posterior perspective. Bone graft is added to this construction.

(REPRODUCED WITH PERMISSION FROM WHITE, A. A., AND PANJABI, M. M.: CLINICAL BIOMECHANICS OF THE SPINE, 2ND ED., J. B. LIPPINCOTT, 1990.)

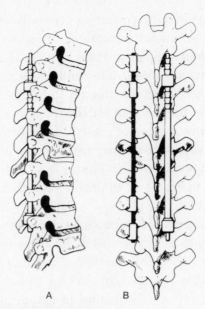

A   B

FIGURE 7.8. Spinal Instrumentation

On the left we see a lateral view of the stainless steel rod with hooks applied to the back portion of the spine. These hooks go underneath the lamina of the vertebrae and are designed not to irritate the spinal cord. The rod is designed so that it can be cranked up (somewhat analogous to a jack on a car) to correct curvature of the spine, or to fix the spine by applying pressure through the tension created by the ligaments as they are stretched. On the right-hand side of this picture, we see a posterior view of the rod that we see on the left; we also see a Harrington compression rod on the left-hand side of the spine, and the distraction rod with the jacks on it on the right-hand side. The mechanics of these rods are somewhat complex, but it is important only that the patient understand that these are useful implants. They provide some immobilizing capacity of the spine while a spinal fusion heals and takes over the loads and forces from these instruments.

the preceding two methods—that is, laminar hooks and pedicle screws— to provide a very rigid fixation system.

There are more modern versions of spinal instrumentation that are based on what we have learned from the earlier systems. In addition, there are implants that can be combined with bone graft and placed into the disc space to promote stability, improve spinal alignment, and increase the surface area for the fusion to take place (figure 7.11). These systems

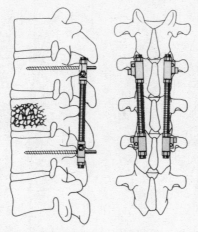

FIGURE 7.9. Spinal Instrumentation

This is a specific device; however, it is a prototype of a transpedicular fixation device. The screw goes through the pedicle and into the vertebral body and is attached to some kind of plate or rod, which connects to one or more additional vertebrae. This is shown on the left as a side view. The pedicle shown here from the side is well seen anatomically in figure 2.6a. To the right the system is seen from behind the vertebrae. The pedicle screw is shown, but the heavy longitudinal screws (which are replaced by a plate in some systems) are seen here. These surgical constructs are augmented with bone and are thought to provide the most rigid immobilization. Note also the fracture (broken area) of the vertebral body. This particular form of fixation is sometimes used to treat fractures of the vertebrae. (REPRODUCED WITH PERMISSION FROM WHITE, A. A., AND PANJABI, M. M.: CLINICAL BIOMECHANICS OF THE SPINE, 2ND ED., J. B. LIPPINCOTT, 1990.)

can be used to hold together two or more vertebrae if needed. Evidence indicates that using instrumentation improves fusion rates, and there are some circumstances, such as surgery for spinal fractures, deformity, or tumors, whereby the use of surgical instrumentation is essential to achieve the objectives and enhance the probability of a successful outcome.

COMPLICATIONS OF FUSION Besides routine anesthesia complications, we must list wound infections and chronic mild to moderate pain at the site where the bone graft was removed. Sometimes, too, the graft does not take (nonunion) and the operation must be repeated.

Bone healing requires stability and a good blood supply. Proper nu-

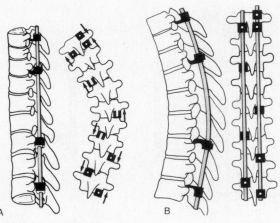

A   B

FIGURE 7.10. Spinal Instrumentation

This is a Cotrel-Dubousset apparatus. This shows two views of the spine on the left (a lateral view and a posterior view), and then two views of the spine on the right (a lateral view and a posterior view). These rods are used primarily for correcting scoliosis, or severe curvature of the spine; they are also used in some cases following trauma to the spine, and for other elective spine fusions.

First, on the left we show a lateral spine that is very straight. When the rods are applied on the right, the lateral view of the spine shows some curvature. This curvature is a more normal situation for the lateral view, so it is being corrected. Viewing again the posterior views of the spine, on the left we see a posterior view with the hooks placed in it, and on the right we see the posterior view after two rods have been applied and the correction has been made. The posterior view on the right shows correction of the scoliosis and correction of the lordosis—that is, too much extension of the spine. It is now flexed a bit, which is a normal position for the thoracic spine. Again, this is a bit complex, but it is important for the layperson to understand that these mechanical implants can sometimes be helpful in the correction and maintenance of the spine. Ultimately, though, the long-term correction always depends on a satisfactory fusion of the spine.

trition is very important for your recovery. I advise taking supplemental calcium, vitamin D, and vitamin C along with a multivitamin. Exposure to tobacco in any form (smoking, chewing tobacco, secondhand smoke, and nicotine patches) significantly inhibits bone healing, possibly leading to a nonunion (often called a *pseudoarthrosis*). Therefore, if you use tobacco, it is in your best interest to stop!

Osteoporosis, advanced age, severe anemia, diabetes, obesity, and infection are also risk factors. Your physician may suggest the use of an electrical bone stimulator, an implantable or external device that is reported to promote bone healing. The data regarding the implantable electrical bone stimulator are more compelling, but the device is associated with risk if infection or pain develops at the site of the generator under the skin. In such a case, the device would be removed. The diminished efficacy of the external stimulator is thought by some to be due to a lack of compliance—patients forget to use it. More research is required. Not everyone needs these devices. Your physician will aid in determining whether an electrical bone stimulator is a good choice for your unique condition.

Of course, you must also follow your doctor's advice and protect your spine during the healing phase. Excessive physical activity too soon after spinal surgery can put you at risk.

WHICH WAY IN? ANTERIOR? POSTERIOR?

Now, as discussed, there are two basic types of fusion. Most lumbar fusions are done from the back and are called posterior fusions, as we noted. (See figure 7.11, which shows the technique.) In an anterior fusion, the bone

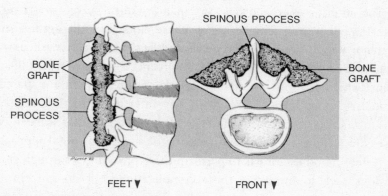

POSTERIOR SPINAL FUSION

SPINOUS PROCESS

BONE GRAFT

SPINOUS PROCESS

BONE GRAFT

FEET ▼   FRONT ▼

FIGURE 7.11. Posterior Spinal Fusion

This shows two views of a posterior spinal fusion. Three segments have been fused here, with the bone graft traversing four vertebrae. The picture on the right shows an axial, or horizontal, plane view of the fusion; this is the typical view a doctor studies when a CT scan is utilized to evaluate the spine. There are several variations of this surgical technique, but this is the basic idea.

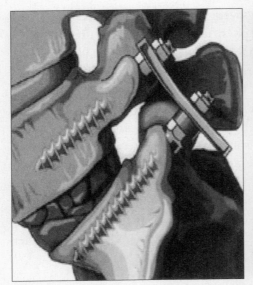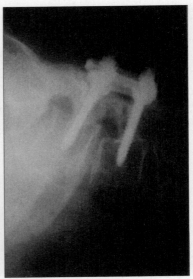

FIGURE 7.11A. Anterior and Posterior Instrumented Spinal Fusion
Posterior pedicle screw and plate instrumentation with an anterior lumbar interbody fusion demonstrated by the X-ray on the left. *(THE IMAGE ON THE RIGHT IS COURTESY OF DEPUY SPINE, RAYNHAM, MA.)*

graft is placed either between the vertebral bodies or across the vertebral body. The incision is made in either the front or side of the abdomen.

The anterior approach has certain mechanical advantages over the posterior, but it carries higher risks. Blood clots are more apt to form in the major vessels supplying the pelvis and legs. Males run a very low risk of impotence or sterility (roughly 0.4 percent) if the nerves in the sacral plexus, which governs ejaculation, are damaged. Women are spared reproductive complications. Finally, gastrointestinal function (constipation) may suffer transient interference for several days after surgery. All of these complications seem to hark back to the surgeon's frontal approach to the vertebral bodies. Efforts to perform these procedures through smaller incisions seek to minimize these complications but do not eliminate them.

By the way, there are two techniques for performing an interbody fusion from the back. A PLIF (posterior lumbar interbody fusion) and a TLIF (transforminal lumbar interbody fusion) effectively allow a posterior and anterior fusion to be performed through one incision. This combined approach has been associated with higher fusion rates. The TLIF technique

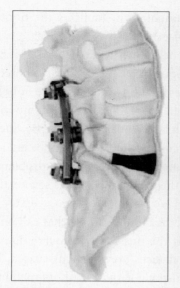 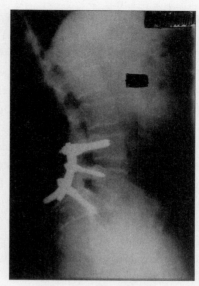

FIGURE 7.11B. Posterior Instrumented Lumbar Fusion with Fusion Cage

This is an example of an all-posterior procedure whereby placement of the pedicle screws and posterolateral and interbody fusion are performed through one incision. The figure on the left is an example of a lordotic fusion cage used to promote the interbody fusion and maintain alignment (balance) of the spine. *(PHOTO COURTESY OF DEPUY SPINE, RAYNHAM, MA.)*

has gained favor because it requires less retraction of the nerves. In my opinion, patients with risk factors for developing a nonunion (pseudoarthrosis) should be considered for a combined posterior and anterior fusion. If you are a spinal fusion candidate, discuss all the options with your surgeon.

Recently, a host of minimally invasive spinal fusion techniques have been introduced. The goal of performing spinal stabilization procedures through a small incision deserves much consideration, but the efficacy has not been proven by long-term follow-up data: It is not tried-and-true, and may not for everyone. Also, it may be associated with a higher complication rate. The key to any successful spinal fusion is adequate surgical visualization to protect the important neural structures, to control any bleeding, and to prepare the spinal segments for and placement of the bone graft as well as safe introduction of the instrumentation. In other words, the soil must be properly tilled before planting the seeds. Although we have discussed the potential benefits of spinal instrumentation, these implants are not the fusion. The instrumentation stabilizes the bone to promote healing. Fusion has not taken place until the bone heals!

Although spinal fusion can be quite helpful with respect to stabilizing the diseased or unstable segment of the spine, the mechanics are altered to achieve such stability. Over the years, the mobile segments above or below the fused vertebrae will develop degenerative changes. A component of these degenerative changes are age related, but some may be due in part to the altered mechanics and stress concentration at the adjacent segments. There is therefore a greater likelihood of developing a problem at the spinal level adjacent to the fusion. If the problem becomes severe, then surgical intervention may be required.

You deserve to know about some of the complications that can ensue from the use of metal implants. There is the possibility of nerve damage or irritation associated with each of the devices previously discussed. The probability of infection is greater than in spinal surgery without metal implants. Finally, for a variety of reasons, it may be necessary to have an operation to remove the device. If spinal instrumentation is recommended, it may be appropriate; you should understand why the incremental risks are justified by sufficient benefits.

SUMMARY: SURGERY FOR LOW BACK PAIN AND SCIATICA

The discussion that you have just waded through is extremely complex, so let's review the main points briefly.

Key Indications for the Most Common Low Back Operations

- The surgery is elective. Its purpose is to improve the quality of life, not save your life. You do not *have* to do it. Your big question: Is the reasonable expectation of pain relief worth the risks?
- If you are losing control of your bladder and have increasing leg weakness, we are no longer talking about elective surgery. You need urgent surgery.
- If you think you want surgery, the longer you wait after two or three months of properly treated backache, the more you may dim your surgical prospects. We are speaking only of selected, thoroughly diagnosed conditions that call for surgery.
- If you are having disc surgery, know that it can help both your back and your leg pain; however, you can expect most pain reduction to be in your leg.

- You generally do not want to automatically have a fusion with disc surgery. If there is a good, clear reason to do so, your surgeon will explain it so that you can *understand* and *agree*.
- In properly evaluated patients with disc disease, surgery is successful 90 percent to 95 percent of the time.
- When there is spondylolisthesis or some other cause of significant painful motion between vertebrae, spinal fusion should be considered.

Surgery for Infections

Infections of the spine can cause considerable back pain. Sometimes antibiotics alone can wipe them out, but surgery may be necessary. For example, there may be an abscess (a pocket of pus) or an area of chronic osteomyelitis (a region of infected bone, some of which is dead and some alive, with bacteria or fungus growing in it).

Surgery is performed to evacuate the abscess, remove the infected bone, and wash out many of the germs with sterile solutions containing antibiotics.

According to the circumstances, the surgeon may elect to perform some kind of fusion during this operation. Or he/she may clean out the infection first and carry out the fusion later. Each patient's problem is highly individual from the perspective of surgery and reconstruction. But the basic surgical principles are (1) to decompress or drain the abscess, (2) to remove enough bone to cure the infection while preserving as many of the spine elements as possible, and (3) to use bone graft to fuse and reconstruct the spine. Spinal instrumentation may be required to stabilize the spine in extreme cases.

Surgery for Tumors

To recapitulate chapter 2, when low back pain is caused by a bone tumor, its treatment depends on whether or not the tumor originated there (a primary tumor) or migrated from elsewhere (a metastatic tumor). When the tumor is primary, much will hinge on whether it's benign or malignant. Sometimes, metastatic tumors are better treated with radiation or chemotherapy, but surgery also sometimes offers benefits. This is particularly true when the tumor is very painful and aggravated by movement of the spine, or if the tumor is growing close to the nerves.

A tumor originating in the spine, with or without nerve involvement, is the most likely candidate for surgery. Here the principles governing infection apply again, except that the surgical challenge and risks are raised a notch or two. That is because the surgeon's mission is to eradicate *all* of the tumor, plus an appropriate margin of normal spine. Many of the spinal structures may need to be removed, and a radical procedure employed.

SPINAL RECONSTRUCTION

In this case, the spine may be rebuilt with bone graft, metal, or sometimes a prosthetic replacement. The latter may be developed with polymethyl-methacrylate (PMMA), a bone cement that we reviewed in our discussion of vertebroplasty and kyphoplasty. This sort of extensive spinal operation should be performed at centers with special expertise in spinal surgery (figure 7.11b).

I would like to reiterate here that malignant tumors that originate in the spine are extremely uncommon, so please do not start attributing every backache to cancer.

Surgery for Injuries

Most mild to moderate spinal fractures can heal without very serious pain. In the absence of nerve root or spinal cord compromise, nonoperative treatment is pursued. Simple fractures usually heal within twelve weeks, often with the support of a brace. For a review of vertebral compression fracture treatment options, please see chapter 6's discussion of vertebroplasty and kyphoplasty. Surgery for old fractures is considered only if the fracture has not healed and there is associated severe pain. Diagnostic studies may be performed that include X-rays, an MRI, a CT scan, and possibly a bone scan. Many surgeons first immobilize the patient in a brace as a trial. If the pain lessens, spinal fusion can be expected to help. A posterior fusion is usually adequate, affording considerable relief.

What about recent injury? This can be a very complex area. If you were involved in a major traumatic injury, such as a fall from an elevation or a high-speed motor vehicle collision, you may be taken to the emergency room or a trauma center. You would then consult with your surgeon about your individual needs and condition. Unless the vertebrae are extensively damaged, and the spine is unstable, surgery is not generally advisable. But

if there *is* severe vertebral damage, especially in the lower spine, and associated neurologic problems (with fragments of bone in the spinal canal),
surgery may be required to remove the bone from the spinal canal, stabilize the spine with the assistance of spinal instrumentation, and perform a
spinal fusion. These rods are attached to the normal spine above and below
the injury. They help to hold the spine in place while it heals (figure 7.11).

Motion Preservation Surgery

Over the past few years, there has been a great surge of interest in what we
now categorize as motion preservation surgery. This new heading was assigned to capture the broad spectrum of approaches that have been or are
being developed to address various spinal pathologies with the objective of
preserving or restoring the normal physiologic functional motion of a diseased or damaged segment of the spine, thereby doing away with the need
to perform a spinal fusion.

ARTIFICIAL DISC

This is a topic that has fascinated both patients and biomedical researchers for over forty years. Patients ask, "Well, if the disc is the problem, isn't
there something that can be put in there to replace it?" Surgeons and other
researchers have experimented in the laboratory with a variety of materials and devices.

The technology that has received the greatest amount of attention is
that of the *artificial disc* (disc replacement, or *arthroplasty*). The desire to
develop an effective disc replacement is not a new idea. The first effort was
developed in the mid-1950s by a trio of doctors who injected an acrylic
into the evacuated disc space after discectomy. The idea was abandoned
after observing no clear advantage. Dr. Alf Nachemson of Sweden developed a silicone rubber insert in 1962; it performed so poorly in laboratory
mechanical testing that he abandoned the idea proceeding to human trials. The first clinical series of disc replacements was presented in the early
1960s by another Swede, Dr. Ulf Fernström. He placed a stainless-steel ball
into the disc space following discectomy. This approach realized early success but later failed as a result of collapsing or settling of the bone around
the steel balls.

With the success realized from total hip and total knee replacements,
interest in an artificial disc has resurfaced. The first lumbar disc replace-

ment approved by the U.S. Food and Drug Administration (FDA) was the SB Charité III, in 2004, followed two years later by the Prodisc-I. Several other designs are under investigation (see figure 7.12).

The rationale for this technology is sound: in addition to the merit of motion preservation discussed above, the primary goal is to eradicate or diminish pain while restoring functionality of the diseased segment of the spine. There is also the theoretical benefit of a faster recovery; no need for bone healing, which eliminates the nonunion risk; and prevention of the development of adjacent segment disease that we have observed in a percentage of spinal fusion patients. Early enthusiasm surrounding this technology led some to claim that "total disc arthroplasty will make spinal fusion a thing of the past." Such has not been the case. Patient selection is of great importance with respect to a successful outcome. Of note, Medicare and several insurance companies will not pay for disc replacement surgery.

The indications for lumbar disc replacement:

- Adult patients younger than sixty years of age.
- Degenerative disc disease (DDD) at one level from L3 to S1.
- DDD is defined as discogenic back pain confirmed by patient history, radiographics, and discography.
- Patients must have failed a minimum of six months of conservative treatment prior to being considered candidates for an artificial disc.

Contraindications to lumbar disc replacement:

- Spinal stenosis
- Facet arthritis
- Pars defect (spondylolysis)
- Spondylolisthesis (slippage of the vertebrae)
- Herniated disc
- Multilevel degenerative disc disease
- Scoliosis
- Osteoporosis
- Chronic steroid use
- Previous infection
- Fracture

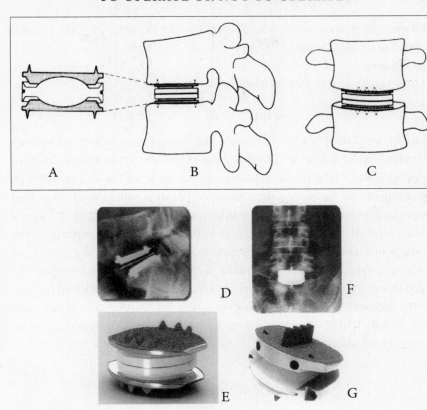

FIGURE 7.12. Artificial Disc Replacement

(A) shows a prosthetic intervertebral disc. This device is made up of a plastic biconvex disc (ultrahigh molecular weight polyethylene) that articulates with two concave metal (cobalt chromium alloy) components on each side of the plastic disc. The metal components on either side of the plastic disc are embedded into the vertebral bone above and below the disc space. (B) shows a view from the lateral perspective. (C) shows a view from a frontal perspective. *(REPRODUCED WITH PERMISSION FROM WHITE, A. A., AND PANJABI, M. M.: CLINICAL BIOMECHANICS OF THE SPINE, 2ND ED., J. B. LIPPINCOTT, 1990.)* (D) shows an X-ray following disc replacement with the SB Charité III. (E) shows the SB Charité III. *(COURTESY OF DEPUY SPINE.)* (F) shows an X-ray of an implanted Prodisc-L, and (G) shows Prodisc-L *(COURTESY OF SYNTHES.)*

- Obesity (a body mass index greater than 35 or weighing 100 pounds above your ideal weight)
- Pregnancy
- Long-term narcotic dependency

COMPLICATIONS

The risks associated with disc replacement surgery include those associated with anesthesia, as well as bleeding, infection, nerve injury, fracture of the vertebral body, impotence, and failure/wear of the components or migration of the implant. The surgical revision (reoperation) rates that have been reported range from 7 percent to 17 percent. Despite the use of the disc replacement, some patients have been noted to have spinal fusion occur spontaneously around the implant. In addition, there are reports of the development of adjacent segment disease at rates similar to that observed following fusion. If the disc replacement has to be removed for any reason, the options include putting in a new implant or conversion to a spinal fusion. These observations suggest that this technology has room for further advancement.

Salvage Low Back Surgery

The term sounds like something the sanitation man picks up. Nevertheless, it refers to surgery performed on a patient who has had two or more operations for spinal pain and is back for another. If you detect a subtle note of pessimism, you are correct. There's nothing sadder than the all-too-common multiple-scar collector who suffers the dolorous cycle of spinal pain, spinal surgery, more spinal surgery, more spinal pain, more surgery, and so on, racking up *twenty* or more operations.

The statistics are disheartening. After one operation, the chance of success from a second is diminished. However, if there is a clear, surgically correctable abnormality that correlates with your symptoms and physical findings during your examination by the treating physician, then the outcome can be quite successful. The associated risks are greater, however. The odds of success following subsequent procedures are further reduced with each effort to address the same problem. I might add that the fourth operation's odds of success are equal to its prospects of exacerbating your condition. Some studies suggest that even the third operation has a reasonable chance of making you worse.

Only in *extremely rare* circumstances is salvage surgery a reasonable option; for example, in cases where spinal stenosis recurs, a disc herniates, or there is a well-diagnosed painful pseudoarthritis of the spine (when all or part of a fusion fails to take, leaving the spine painful and unstable). Perhaps I should add that a highly motivated patient who has had several back operations without fusion may benefit from a spinal fusion if the proper indications are present. Otherwise, additional surgery leads to a dismal outcome. For those with chronic pain in the absence of a clear *etiology*, spinal cord stimulation may be a consideration.

I recommend that any salvage surgery be carried out in a center that has spinal care specialists. It should be performed after a thorough psychiatric evaluation, as neurotic patients and poor souls have extremely depressing success rates from salvage operations. A second opinion is a must before undergoing that third incision.

On the Horizon

DYNAMIC STABILIZATION

Dynamic, or elastic, stabilization is a concept that is currently being investigated. It is another motion-preservation technology that seeks to stabilize the affected segment of the spine without performing a fusion. Two studies to date have examined the effectiveness of such implants (the Graf system and the Dynesys system) in patients with spinal stenosis and spondylolisthesis. Once the nerve tissue has been freed, the device is placed in an effort to stabilize the spine and prevent progression of the spondylolisthesis, while still allowing motion. In these small preliminary studies, no significant progression of the spondylolisthesis was noted, but there were a significant number of patients with recurrent leg pain as well as a smaller number that required revision surgery. In the Dynesys series, the implant failure rate was 17 percent. Another potential application involves the use of this device to supplement a fusion procedure to minimize the risk of adjacent segment disease. Further investigation is required.

BIOABSORBABLE IMPLANTS

Bioabsorbable implants have been utilized in a variety of clinical settings. With the advent of newer polymers with improved biomechanical proper-

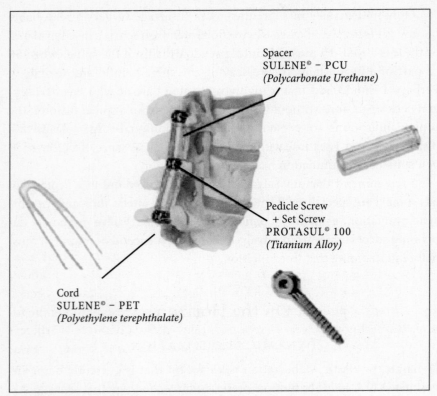

FIGURE 7.13. The Dynesys System

(COURTESY OF ZIMMER SPINE.)

ties, interest has risen regarding their use in spinal surgery. Several investigators are examining the use of such polymers as interbody fusion cages and pedicle screws to support the spine as the fusion heals. The idea is that the polymer implants, used together with bone graft or BMPs to perform spinal fusions, have the theoretical benefit of dissolving slowly after the fusion has had time to heal. In addition, these nonmetallic implants would allow for an easier assessment of the fusion's success.

NUCLEUS REPLACEMENT (NUCLEUS ARTHROPLASTY)

The basic objective of nucleus replacement is to replace the nucleus of a diseased disc with a prosthesis made of polymers or polymer combinations. Here are two examples of compounds that are currently being assessed:

- PDN-Solo and HydraFlex. These implants are polymers encased in a woven polyethylene jacket that expands in the presence of water. Their purpose is to diminish pain from a degenerated disc by replacing the nucleus and restoring disc space height while preserving motion of the affected spinal segment.
- DASCOR. This product is a curable polyurethane and expandable balloon that can be inserted into the disc after discectomy. When filled with the injectable polymer, the balloon conforms to the shape of the nucleus.

We patiently await the results of the ongoing studies.

GENE THERAPY / STEM CELL THERAPY

With the great advances in our understanding of the human genome, coupled with an expansion of our knowledge of the biochemical and cellular mechanisms through which degeneration of the intervertebral disc occurs, gene therapy and/or stem cell therapy may become a real option in the future. This technology seeks to restore or rejuvenate damaged cells, whereas many of the current treatment options remove, replace, or augment our anatomy. As with all advances in technology, there will be moral, ethical, and political issues that must be addressed as this story unfolds.

These are intriguing new prospects. If you've read this and the preceding chapter, you can surely anticipate my closing suggestion on the advisability of having a new surgical procedure. Make certain that there is ample evidence that the added risks are fully justified by good evidence of significant benefits—in other words, that your condition will be improved in a major fashion.

Some Suggestions for Postsurgical Rehabilitation

Comments from patients who read an earlier edition of *Your Aching Back* have been very helpful. This section was written in direct response to a request by a patient who observed, "One thing that you don't have any advice about is how to look after yourself following surgery." My theme for you after surgery is the same as it was before surgery: Do what you're supposed to do, be patient, and you will gradually get better.

Postoperative care really begins when you and your surgeon form a partnership. Set as your goal your ability to get back to work on your pre-back-pain life and to have some fun.

I will offer some general comments, but if in doubt or in conflict, follow *your doctor's* advice. No matter how we consider it, your surgeon knows *you* and *your* back infinitely better than I do. Just so you will be certain to have some guidelines, I will provide some general points about postoperative rehabilitation.

We believe in the liberal use of pain medications to keep patients comfortable during the first few days after surgery. Especially during the first forty-eight hours, sometimes doctors and nurses may underutilize painkillers, for fear of addicting patients. We don't worry about this right after surgery. When someone is having postsurgical pain, we provide whatever it takes to control the pain, and we know that this will not cause addiction. We even offer a system that allows patients to control the painkillers—yes, they medicate themselves as needed (PCA, or patient-controlled analgesia). We like to see the patients sitting up, standing, or walking a few yards, if possible, within the first forty-eight hours after surgery. (Of course, there are some patients who, for a variety of reasons, should not or cannot be up that soon.)

Patients who have general anesthesia are strongly encouraged not to smoke. This is to cut down on developing problems with the lungs, such as pneumonia. Smoking and tobacco in any form can slow or prevent the healing process from maturing after surgery. If your condition is such that you require surgery, you then want to do all that you can to heal properly. We also encourage patients to try and drop the habit completely, as this can add several years to one's life.

It's also important that the patient use an incentive spirometer. It looks like a toy, but it is good friend that should stay at your side after surgery. This device has a mouthpiece, a tube, and a vertical volume indicator. The patient inserts the mouthpiece and breathes in as vigorously as possible. The volume of air inspired is measured on the indicator. Use is strongly encouraged for the first three or four days after surgery to minimize the risk of contracting pneumonia. We tell our patients that this is one of the more important things they can do for themselves after surgery.

We'll divide patients into three broad groups and discuss each. The three groups are (1) routine laminectomy or microdiscectomy/percutaneous discectomy, (2) routine lumbar spinal fusion with or without fixation, and (3) miscellaneous complex and reconstructive procedures.

Routine disc procedure patients are handled in the following manner: The percutaneous and microdiscectomy patients will go home either the day of the procedure or the next day. I find that most want to stay overnight. The patients with surgical laminectomy usually leave the hospital on the second or fifth day after their operation, depending on how many levels were addressed. This group is advised as follows: Avoid prolonged sitting—that is, more than fifteen to twenty minutes. When sitting, the use of a reclined chair is preferable. Avoid bending, twisting, and lifting. Begin gentle walking inside or outside and gradually increase that as tolerated. After two weeks, you can begin stationary bicycling or gentle swimming as tolerated. For the next four weeks, patients are encouraged to continue any combination of gradually increasing amounts of walking, bicycling, or swimming. If more than minor pain in the back or leg occurs and persists, the activity should be reduced to a better-tolerated level. Six weeks after surgery, management is more individualized, according to progress, occupation, motivation, sports, hobbies, and so forth. Consult with your physician if you have questions.

The patients who have spine fusions with internal fixation may get out of bed on the first or second postoperative day, depending upon the fixation and the surgeon's opinion. The rest of the routine is similar to the discectomy patient's except that the progress is slower, extended for a much longer time (three to six months), and may call for wearing a corset or brace.

If, however, there is no internal fixation, this is what we do. (Please understand: There are several different programs here that are acceptable, although they're quite different.) For patients with low back fusion operations in which no internal fixation is used, I think it is best to keep patients in bed until a custom-made rigid brace is applied. This brace goes from the nipples down to the hip, and includes one thigh (the patient usually decides, without help), down to but not including the knee. This "extra length," or immobilization of one hip, is required in order to control the spine. The goal is to hold the spine and fusion mass (bone graft) still for early healing. The brace is worn for three months, which is the minimum amount of time required for early healing. The patient returns for a follow-up appointment. If the X-rays reveal that the fusion is healing, the brace is removed and the exercise program begins. This involves gradually increasing some combination of walking, biking, and swimming. It generally takes six months to a year for a lumbar spine fusion to heal.

Two questions may be on your mind. First: "What about removing the stitches?" Either your surgeon uses absorbable sutures (we do), so they don't have to be removed, *or* the stitches are removed about two weeks after surgery. Second: "What about physical therapy rehabilitation and the like?" Again, lots of legitimately varied opinions here. A patient who is cooperative and understands what's going on needs little in the way of special programs. For a variety of other reasons, some such program may be necessary. If you have an area of muscle weakness, for instance, the therapist can help with exercises that focus on that area. Other useful examples include a back school and work hardening program. (See chapter 6.)

Summary of Major Treatment Options for Associated Back and Leg Pain

The various treatment modalities have been discussed in this and the two preceding chapters. The chart on the next page summarizes their risks and benefits. It will give you an idea of the likelihood of success to be had from several treatments, balanced against my opinion of their relative risks for the patient.

Comment

Just a word about the risk-versus-benefit chart on the following page. It is provided as a framework for thinking about what kind of treatment you wish to pursue. There is a tendency for the higher-benefit procedures to carry a higher risk. (The McKenzie exercise therapy program is an exception.) To some degree, you will be offered only treatment that is appropriate for your individual medical condition while considering the risks and benefits. Obviously, you should not be offered surgery unless the time is right. Also, this chart is not based on a common diagnosis. Note, too, that "liberal" selection for surgery carries the same high risks but low benefits when compared with "conservative" selection. Conservative selection is where the patient has imaging evidence of a distinct disc herniation, confirmed by a physical exam, and a comprehensive trial of nonsurgical treatment. Liberal selection is when one or more of these criteria are not present.

If you do not understand things regarding your back condition and you want to know what to do next, then I will tell you. It is very simple:

Get a second opinion. You need to listen to your body and communicate effectively with your physician. We will delve deeply into the important judgment calls about surgery in the next chapter.

Risk Versus Benefit Chart

RISK	BENEFIT (RATE OF SUCCESS)			
	Outstanding (90 Percent or Better)	**Good** (70 Percent to 80 Percent)	**Average** (60 Percent to 70 Percent)	**Less Than Average** (50 Percent or Less)
Serious	• Discectomy • Microdiscectomy • Laminectomy	• Spinal Fusion	• Percutaneous, Endoscopic, and Laser Discectomy • Disc Replacement • Vertebroplasty/ Kyphoplasty	• IDET • Spinal Cord Stimulation
Moderate			• Bed Rest • NSAIDs • Muscle Relaxants • Analgesics	• Epidural Steroid Injection • Trigger Point Injection • Prolotherapy • Radiofrequency Rhizotomy
Minor	• Prayer • Psychotherapy • Meditation • Conflict Resolution/ Stress Reduction	• McKenzie Exercises • Patient Education	• William's Exercise • Heat and Massage • Back Brace/Corset	• Acupuncture • TENS Unit • Traction, VAX-D, DRX9000, Inversion Table

— CHAPTER 8 —

Sex and the Aching Back

IF YOU HAVE BACKACHE BUT NO SEXUAL PROBLEMS, DON'T read this chapter at all. I'm serious: If you are not aware of any problems in this area, then I don't want you to read this chapter and start thinking up problems for yourself. However, if you do have some problems, you have plenty of company, and a careful study of this chapter will give you some help.

I've done clinical work with spinal problems for many years, and only a handful of patients have ever asked about guidelines for sex during episodes of low back pain or sciatica. How odd. I've included in my patient questionnaires the question "Do your back and legs hurt when you have sexual intercourse?" A significant number of people have answered yes. I now take more initiative in discussing sex with patients. Obviously, many low back patients who are experiencing difficulties with this rewarding form of human activity don't feel comfortable querying their doctors about it. And despite all the lovemaking manuals on display everywhere, little literature has been devoted to making love with a bad back. And so this chapter was born.

For starters, I'd like to share with you a patient's letter. Although I've abridged it somewhat and changed certain names and identifying details, it speaks eloquently for many a low back pain sufferer.

Dear Dr. White:

I used to have an antidote for being under the weather: Get up, get moving, get busy, and everything will be all right. This worked for colds, pregnancy, nausea, sore throat, menstrual cramps, the flu, etc., but not for low back pain. I'd trade a month of the flu for relief of my back problems.

As I lie here, I hear a crash and ensuing tears. I know one of the babies has fallen in the tub and I cannot move to soothe her, hold her, and wipe away the tears. Incidents such as these occur all day. Demands are placed on me continuously, and I cannot respond. My mind responds, my body cannot. Arlene no longer comes to me when she falls. She knows I cannot pick her up. In her feverish state this week, she ran to Marian, our babysitter, for comfort. Marian brought her to my bed, but she didn't want to be with me. She knew I could not walk with her and hold her.

Susan smiles on me all day, comes to the bottom of the stairs, and calls "Momma" if I'm up here. When I'm on the sofa, she comes over and nuzzles me, filling my face with kisses. But Susan does not come to me when she is thirsty, hungry, or tired. Babies know who meets their needs and who doesn't.

Jane demands to see my incision to check my progress. It's visible evidence to a four-year-old that something tangible has been accomplished. She verbalizes, "*When* will you be better? *When* will you drive me to school?"

My husband expresses his aggravation with his short temper. This is a man who has always relied on me, and now our roles are reversed. He's always trying to encourage me to get well, be happy, etc., but finds life pretty tough right now. Every now and then there is an outburst: "I'm tired this weekend, but how would you know what it's like to be tired? You're always in bed."

I guess it's all I can expect from a man who has lost an exciting sex life, has given up his social life (he won't go without me), has been under financial strain, has had his privacy taken away . . . and does not have the haven of a well-kept, well-organized home and family life after a long and arduous workweek.

People—neighbors, family, "friends"—are tired of seeing me in a helpless, supine position. So am I. I tell everyone what a wonderful job they're doing so they will keep coming, tell my husband and children everything will be all right, and then, because I'm so helplessly frustrated and angry and distressed, I drown myself in music, books, and writing, and cry myself to sleep so that I can sanely face the next day with a smile.

I always faced each day with a smile. I love the morning, to walk, go out, play with the children. I was so happy with my life, with myself and my accomplishments . . . but somehow I don't feel quite so good about myself now.

I cannot care for my family and my home. I cannot shake this damn disability and related pain no matter how many weeks (God, it's really been months now) go by. I've had to give up my job counseling new mothers, and my consultations for the Lexington schools. How can one be terribly happy when all outlets are taken away?

Sex is really a painful loss. We used to have an active, innovative, and exciting sex relationship. Amazing—after living with one man for ten years. What a great way to share feelings and release tensions.

The most aggravating part of sexual deprivation is knowing how long it took to reach the stage of being free and passionate, [having spent] too many innocent years and the first ignorant years of marriage . . . To be deprived of it now is really unfair.

I need and want sex, but I'm afraid of hurting myself. Prior to surgery, really active sex aggravated my condition terribly. Passive sex ("Let me know when it's over" sex) is very possible. So are alternative, less direct ways of being close, but really active sex (with lots of muscle involvement and orgasm) was terribly difficult prior to surgery, rendering me unable to walk for several days. Positioning is crucial (whatever is comfortable is fine), and the level of involvement is also a major problem—I'm too afraid of being hurt.

We have become awfully good friends. I have always cherished this thought: A helpmate surpasses a lover, and loving kindness surpasses love, even passion . . .

I am usually reliable, emotionally stable, and basically positive, but not having control over my life pains me. My body won't do what I want it to. I'm at everyone's mercy for help and care. My independence has been taken away and my positive self-esteem lowered . . .

Dr. White, this excerpt is rather personal and verbose, but I have decided to share it with you because I feel you are discreet and humane. I trust you, and perhaps it might provide some useful insights for your ongoing study of spinal disorders and their effects . . .

Sincerely,
C.D.

This letter from a normal, intelligent, well-adjusted wife and mother depicts the devastating side effects of a chronic back problem. C.D. was spiritually, intellectually, and materially wealthy, in my opinion, yet only marginally able to cope with her shattered life. Finally, she did conquer her bad back, largely because of her own determination. Surgical removal of a lumbar disc helped. So did mastery of the principles for lovemaking with a bad back.

In conversation, C.D. confided that the fear of hurting her back distracted her during lovemaking and interfered with her orgasmic response. This was a patient who had many things going for her, including sexual openness, a positive attitude, a happy marriage, and considerable resources, both material and intellectual. How do you think a neurotic, repressed, or unhappily mated person would fare?

Sex is only one of the activities that may be cramped by chronic back pain, but because it's right up there on the list of trouble spots, it deserves its own chapter. So here we'll take what we know about the pathology and biomechanics of back pain and translate it into guidelines for lovemaking. We'll start by setting out the general principles, then follow them up with specific recommendations for men and women with low back pain and/or sciatica.

Pain, Emotions, and Sexual Gratification

I would submit to the reader that a fully satisfactory sex life is no small achievement even *without* backache. One study of "normal," well-educated, happily married couples runs counter to the presumed happily-ever-after sequels to classic Cary Grant–Ingrid Bergman movies (and to our own dreams). Even though 80 percent of these people considered their marital and sexual relations happy, there were manifold problems. Two-fifths of the men had problems with either erection or ejaculation, and 63 percent of the women expressed difficulty in "turning on" or climaxing. Among another group of family practice patients, 56 percent had at least one lovemaking impasse. The real world rarely meets our romantic expectations.

The reason I'm presuming to add a couple of paragraphs to the thousands of pages already written about sex is to make the point that sex problems are by no means simple. I don't have to tell you that back disease isn't easy. As we grapple with the compound problem of sex and backache, we do indeed have a challenge.

Although I'd prefer to extol the beauty of sex and lovemaking, that is not the purpose of this chapter. In order to be helpful, I must focus on the problem. So let me offer a simple categorization of two types of sexual problems.

One category is exemplified by the person who tends to avoid sex—but doesn't *want* to avoid it. This is usually a virile, sensual person who loves sex but feels frustrated both for himself/herself and his/her partner. An element of guilt often rounds out the mental anguish.

The other category includes the person who tends not to avoid sex but doesn't enjoy it. The lack of pleasure is based on some combination of mental and physical pain. While back pain could be preventing enjoyable lovemaking, a person may also feel used or "locked in" by sex and therefore fail to get pleasure from it. One can readily appreciate the complexity of the mental or physical problems when we consider that the characteristic avoider occasionally participates in lovemaking and the traditional participant sometimes avoids it.

Emotional problems such as stress or depression and/or medications involved with pain management may result in male impotence or premature ejaculation. A patient may be handicapped by an inability to enjoy sex because of *fear* of pain as well as *actual* pain. Our patient C.D. springs to mind.

There's an oft-circulated story about a patient who asked his distinguished hand surgeon just before his operation, "Doc, will I be able to play my piano after you operate on my hand?" The confident surgeon reassured him, "Why, of course you will." "That's great!" replied the patient. "Because so far I haven't been able to play the piano for the life of me!" The same principle holds here. This advice doesn't speak to any preexisting sexual problems, not even those that get channeled into the backache. On the other hand, if you follow the suggestions for open, honest discussion about sex as it relates to your back, helpful communication about other sexual problems may surface and add to your overall satisfaction.

Sex and the Bad Back

Here we'll analyze the sexual problems that stem directly from backache.

A sexually well-adjusted person with a short-term, nonchronic backache is obviously the most easily treated. You need use only proper body mechanics so as not to irritate your back during sex. When your back is acting up, follow this chapter's recommendations closely. If you fit into this category, I must warn you against falling into an enduring sexual-avoidance pattern as a backache side effect. Once set in motion, our habits have a way of sticking with us.

Most of us want to please and be pleased by our lovers. When sex is very painful or impossible because of a back condition, several kinds of emotional turmoil eventually affect both partners. Without clear communication, misunderstandings build. For example, the pain-free partner may become less physically affectionate out of consideration for his/her lover's backache, but the disabled mate may interpret this as rejection, punishment, or loss of love. The disabled person may then react with guilt, depression, or hostility—which, in turn, may provoke rejection or hostility on the part of the "considerate" nondisabled lover. A vicious cycle starts, which candid communication could have avoided from the beginning.

Or the sexually disabled person can sink into depression, anxiety, guilt, or hostility, irrespective of the mate's behavior. Here a more profound adjustment problem may be rearing its head, and specific medical or psychiatric therapy may be what is needed.

SEXUAL MALADJUSTMENT AND BACKACHE

Then there's the situation in which a preexisting sexual problem is worsened or revived by backache. Obviously, an already marginal relationship will be significantly penalized by a sore back. And it's also possible that the disabled person will consciously or unconsciously use the backache to escape from or manipulate his/her lover, as in the "Sorry, I have a backache tonight, dear" syndrome. This behavior pattern can lead you down the dismal path of guilt, anxiety, hostility, and depression.

SHORT-TERM VERSUS CHRONIC DISABILITY

Of course, it makes a world of difference whether your backache is short- or long-term. Short-term, in the medical universe, means six weeks to six months. Long-term, or chronic, means longer than six months. A short-term back patient can think in terms of carefully following this chapter's guidelines on a temporary basis, while a chronically disabled patient must consider revamping his/her sex life indefinitely.

The sexually active couple facing a long-term sexual disability must cope with a potentially very serious problem. Over the course of my practice, I've been made aware of two divorces caused by prolonged sexual disability—on the part of the man in one case, the woman in the other. The pain-free lover simply couldn't stand the deprivation for months on end. In both cases, emotional strain, distrust, and hostility culminated in a definite split. How can you avoid such a drastic state of affairs?

STAYING SEXY WITH A BACK PROBLEM

Let's now lay down a step-by-step plan for a more satisfying sex life for the backache sufferer and his/her lover.

PELVIC POWER: USE IT OR LOSE IT Step 1: The pelvis and its dynamic muscles are an integral source of sexual satisfaction. The woman's pubococcygeus (PC) muscles, stretching from front to back, form the pelvic floor. It thereby helps support the rectum, uterus, and bladder, controlling urine flow and vaginal contraction. Isometric exercises can strengthen and create voluntary control of the PC, intensifying the enjoyment for both partners.

Exercise First, locate the muscle. Simply practice tightening the muscle you would use to stop the flow during urination. Now you've found it.

While sitting or standing, contract the PC twenty-five to fifty times twice a day. It shouldn't hurt your back. You can do it standing at the checkout counter or driving in your car. (No one will know.) A variation is to contract for ten seconds, then release, continue breathing normally, and repeat several times. During intercourse, the PC will contract around the penis percussively—thus the pleasure of pelvic power!

Step 2: Begin with the doctrine that if you ever "had it good," you can have it just as good again with a back problem. Moreover, if you've never quite experienced connubial bliss, this is a good time to institute some gratifying changes. So we start with a *positive* attitude: "I know it's a challenge, but after reading this, I'm going to make it better."

Step 3: Talk to your lover. This is probably the most important advice of all. You can be subtle. Place a bookmark on this page and leave the book on your pillow or the bathroom sink. Or employ a more direct approach, placing the book on your lover's plate at the dinner table. Try to discuss the problem in a warm, clear, frank, relaxed, compassionate manner. But you must start communicating—now!

Step 4: You and your loved one must approach the problem with a sincere attitude of cooperation: a commitment to give-and-take. The goal should be the *most* pleasure (physical and emotional) and the *least* pain (physical and emotional) for both of you. Other fringe benefits may flow from a save-the-back approach to human sexuality, and we'll detail them later.

Step 5: Expand your attitudes as well as your mind and heart. Noncoital sexual activities can be mutually gratifying experiences of love. Many sexual rewards may emerge from broader attitudes and more creativity and communication about lovemaking.

Step 6: Commit yourself to understanding and following the specific practical suggestions about positions for lovemaking as well as the other recommendations provided in this chapter.

Let's face, it: There may be some rare situations in which you and your lover conscientiously follow all the advice here and have no success. Then you should go to step 7, which is to discuss the issue with a physician knowledgeable about backache and consider the advisability of a marriage or sex counselor. But take heart: It's only the very unusual "loving backache" that won't be helped by carefully following the advice on the next few pages.

HOW TO MAKE LOVE WITH A BACK PROBLEM

For starters, if what you're doing hurts, you can grin and bear it as long as there's more grinning than bearing it. If not, you shouldn't be doing it. If what you're doing doesn't conform to the guidelines given here but doesn't hurt, enjoy! Secondly, be innovative. Trying different sorts of lovemaking activities (just so they don't irritate your back!) can convert your disability into a romantic and sensual exploration.

Now you're ready for the basic mechanical principles for reducing the stress on your lower back during lovemaking.

- Don't bend forward *with the knees straight,* even if you're lying down, as this position puts tremendous forces on the lumbar spine. (A review of chapter 2 might be helpful.) It also stretches the sciatic nerve, possibly irritating it. Bending the spine slightly forward is okay, as long as you bend your knees.
- Avoid swayback (lordosis) of the low back. In the next chapter, you'll read about how extreme back arching hurts dancers' and athletes'

spines. Lovers run similar risks. Arching the back makes the disc bulge toward the back and places much stress on the posterior structures of the spine, such as the facet joints (figure 8.1). A straight or slightly flexed (forward) spine is always preferable to an extended one.

- Stay away from positions that stretch, stress, or load the psoas muscles running from the front of the lumbar spine to just below the hip joint. Examples include lying flat on your stomach or back with your hips extended straight.
- To the extent that you can flex one or both hips, you relax those muscles and take the pressure off your lower back (figure 8.2). This shows why the side-lying position and other hips-flexed positions are good.

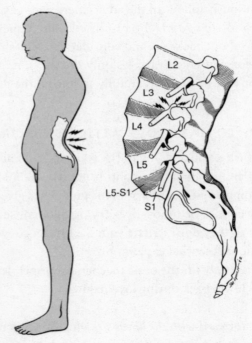

FIGURE 8.1. Swayback

This important picture shows how a swayback (extended) lumbar spine does two things that are not likely to bring pleasure to the backache sufferer during lovemaking. With this position, the disc bulges posteriorly (upper sparks) between L3 and L4, and very large forces are exerted on the facet joints (lower sparks) between L4 and L5, both of which can cause backache.

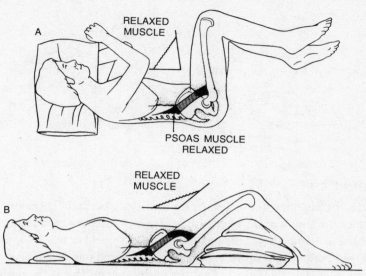

FIGURE 8.2. Comfortable Lying Positions

(A) Lying on the side with hips and knees flexed relaxes the psoas muscle.
(B) Lying on the back with pillows or some other support for the legs, with
the hips flexed, also relaxes the psoas muscle and the back. These principles are
useful to think about for general back care and especially before lovemaking.

SEXUAL BACKACHE CARE SPECIFICALLY FOR WOMEN Start by assuming that the missionary position is probably painful to the lumbar spine if the woman chooses to be active. Why? Well, lying on your back and rotating the pelvis, either back and forth or in a circular motion, extends the lumbar spine. To make matters worse, thrusting movements put demands on the abdominal and erector spinae muscles, which may be weakened and therefore uncomfortable in the acute or subacute phase of low back pain. Here, too, there is real stress on the psoas muscle and thus on the lumbar spine.

Any number of positions requiring back arching will also be irritating. But if you can get away with any of these maneuvers, go ahead. Your back will keep you informed.

In general, women with backache will do better in the positions shown in figures 8.3 through 8.6.

SEXUAL BACKACHE CARE SPECIFICALLY FOR MEN Let me begin by asking you the impossible: You must temporarily suspend your ego, or at

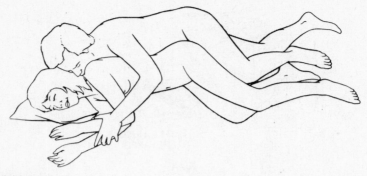

FIGURE 8.3.

This is the basic first line of defense for the "loving backache" position. It's the best for the female or the male with back pain. Both partners have their hips and knees flexed. They are lying on their sides, so neither has to support his/her own body weight or the weight of his/her loved one. The female should guard against getting into a swayback position here. This is the position of choice if you want to make love during a fairly acute stage of backache.

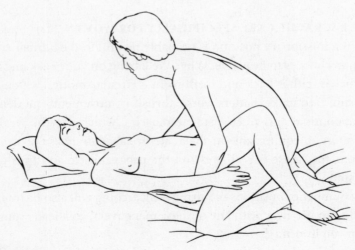

FIGURE 8.4.

This position is good for the woman with backache. It takes advantage of the principle described in figure 8.2. Care must be taken to support the woman's upper torso with pillows and her thighs with the male lover's thighs and arms.

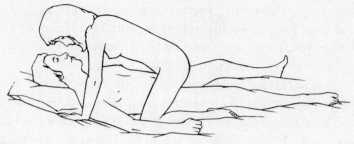

FIGURE 8.5.

This position is good for the woman with back pain. Like the male in figure 8.3, her hips are flexed. She can avoid swayback, and she can support the
weight of the upper torso on her hands. This can also be a good position for
the male shown here, should he have a backache. The upper torso should be
slightly raised with a generous number of pillows so as to slightly flex the
spine—and you must not be vigorous here, sir.

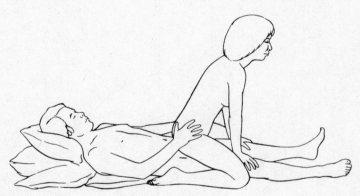

FIGURE 8.6.

This position—good for both partners—is simply a variation of figure 8.5. If
it is to be used, pressure on the man's knees from the woman's hands may irritate his back by stimulating activity in the psoas muscle.

least mix your wisdom and creativity with your lurking macho attitudes.
Bear in mind that you have a *temporary* disability to adjust to. Your bad
back not only carries biomechanical and physiologic liabilities, it also has
emotional side effects. Education and reassurance, plus the knowledge that
your sexual problems are transient, should help.

You may discover new patterns of sensuality. You may find that both you and your lover enjoy the novelty of your slightly more passive role. Remember, you're the same man you always were, but your back imposes some restrictions on your erotic athletics.

Be advised that the male's basic to-and-fro pelvic thrust is likely to aggravate a compromised spine. Sexual gymnastics (also described as "rodeo sex") are also dangerous, and sexual marathons are about as helpful to a backache as a running marathon would be. Too much, too hard, for too long can give even a healthy back some bittersweet memories the morning after.

The standard missionary position, with its thrusting movements, isn't what the doctor ordered. Instead, try kneeling or lying on your side and using less rigorous pelvic thrusts. If you have the luxury of making love in the water—a swimming pool, hot tub, deep bathtub, or anyplace where buoyancy can help—do take advantage of it. Keep your feet flat on the bottom, with your hips and knees bent as in the sitting position. Your lover faces you and, with the assistance of buoyancy, sits on your thighs. Some

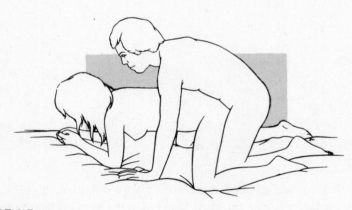

FIGURE 8.7.

This position *may* be good for the man with back pain. The reason is that the hips are flexed and the man can and should support his upper torso using one or both hands resting on the bed or on pillows. Note that his back is slightly flexed, not extended. A woman using this position may aggravate back pain if she is vigorously active or if her lover puts too much weight on her. A variation that will help the woman with backache is to have both partners with their knees on the floor and the female's upper torso fully supported by a bed, couch, or chair.

additional positions suggested for the man are shown by the male in figures 8.3 through 8.8.

There's another time-tested lover's formula that's as good for a bad back as for a robust one. I'm referring to "Slow and steady wins the race." It makes for graceful, athletic lovemaking that is good for your lover and for you. Your back will also appreciate it.

MORE SEXUAL POSITIONS THAT RESPECT THE BACK A number of recommended positions for backache patients are illustrated in figures 8.3 through 8.8. The drawings should speak for themselves, but the captions include some commentary that you should review carefully.

Use your ingenuity, as long as both partners are enjoying themselves without back pain. Admittedly, it's hard to be truly original in this ancient and profoundly expressive leisure activity, but even a minor variation may

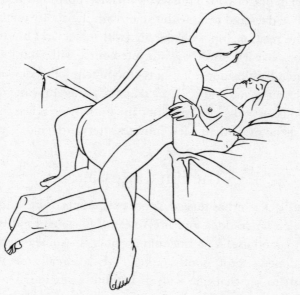

FIGURE 8.8.

This position is suggested for the male patient with backache. By resting the weight of the torso on his elbows, the stresses are taken off the erector spinae muscles in the back; also, flexing the hips reduces the stresses exerted by the psoas muscle. Of course, the position we see the woman in here is *not* for a female lover with a back problem.

please both of you. Remember, some of mankind's greatest discoveries have come about through trial and error.

In addition, you shouldn't have too much trouble finding books with sophisticated explanations of a range of sexual variations. The bibliography lists some that may prove helpful.

WHEN TO RESUME LOVEMAKING

Say that you have to abstain from intercourse because of backache. When is it safe to go back into the bridal suite? First, some negative prescriptions. *Not* when you're still on complete bed rest and taking large amounts of pain medication. *Not* the very first day or night after you go off the preceding program. One or two days after you've begun to feel better—when you can walk without much pain and require little or nothing in the way of painkillers—try a practice run. We refer to this as making love with the air, as you slowly try sexual maneuvers *without* your partner. If there's no pain, try it again, a little more vigorously. Still no pain? Then try a dry run (still with the air) in one or two of the recommended positions. If you get a sore back, wait two days and resume the affair with the air. If you have no pain, break off the relationship with the air (with grace and kindness, as you may have to revive it). Now try gentle intercourse with your lover in one of the recommended positions. If it hurts too much, wait a day or two, touch base with the air again, and if there's no pain, try again with your partner.

Once you can make love without pain, or the pain is less than the pleasure and lasts no more than a few minutes afterward, enjoy!

The Final Message

Even if your backache has turned a once exuberant sex life into infrequent, anxiety-ridden labor, don't give up. You may be able to put this chapter's guidelines to good use. A number of my patients—some of whom had virtually abandoned sex for months or years—have already met with success.

This isn't to say that life, with or without a sex life, is a picnic with backache, especially a chronic one. It's an uphill climb. But who knows? Your bad back may even translate into a rare opportunity for more sensitive, sensual, and communicative lovemaking.

How to Avoid and Relieve Backache in Sports and Dance

WHY ARE ATHLETES UNIVERSALLY ADMIRED? AFTER ALL, don't we reward our Olympic contenders, and even moderately successful Ivy League athletes, with high-paying corporate jobs? Don't professional athletes' salaries run ever more into the eight figures—not including income from selling cologne, rental cars, razors, shaving cream, cereal, candy, televisions, and alcohol? Savvy, powerful sixty-year-old men act like clumsy, excited kids in the presence of a twenty-year-old star athlete. And many people who can name all the Celtics, Patriots, Bruins, Jets, or Pirates can't identify more than three Supreme Court justices or three college presidents. How many heroes do we have, in contrast, among ministers, computer wizards, architects, and engineers?

Don't get me wrong: I, too, respect athletes. For better or worse, I probably spent as much time playing, practicing, and traveling as a member of my college football team as I did in the library. But I would trace our adulation of athletes back to our more primitive hunting-and-gathering days. The strong man brought home the bacon, literally, while the ninety-pound-weakling egghead type couldn't protect his family, village, or nation. Nowadays, of course, physical prowess doesn't count for all that much off the playing fields, and a physicist or mathematical genius can annihilate more of the enemy than all the finest warriors lumped together. Yet, we still instinctively praise the athlete.

What does all this have to do with backache? Only that a glance at our social reward system can give us insight into the athlete's consciousness and the way he or she copes with a physical problem.

First of all, athletes have hearty egos. It's not a good practice to pre-judge human beings, but allow me a few generalizations here. Athletes are highly motivated, perhaps obsessively so. Because they use and train their bodies so vigorously, they're attuned to their most subtle twinge or twitch. Furthermore, they place very high, sometimes unrealistic demands on their physical machine. So when it comes to back problems, athletes possess the *assets* of high motivation and a well-trained body, both of which would normally predispose one to "get well." However, there are the *liabilities* of heightened body sensitivity and the excessive physical demands that go with the trade.

Everything we've just said about athletes also applies to dancers, whose exquisitely trained bodies must meet equal and sometimes greater demands. As a matter of fact, when it comes to endurance, strength, and flexibility, most serious dancers rank higher than most serious athletes. Dancers (professional and social types) also rank very high in terms of the the forces they put into their lower spines.

Now, where do athletes and dancers get into trouble, specifically?

Lifting

As we've said, people who do heavy labor are more prone to back trouble than insurance underwriters, and so are athletes, for the same reasons. The lumbar spine is the workhorse of the body. Remember that bending forward and lifting imposes heavy loads on the lumbar spine, especially if you do it the wrong way—that is, by bending at the waist without bending the knees. Male dancers, for instance, are at high risk. Pity the poor male dancer! When will choreographers liberate the ballerina, allowing her to catch a male dancer after a flying leap and walk around the stage carrying him? Smile!

Football players also incur lifting damage, and not just when blocking and tackling during the game. Did you ever think about the blocking dummies, the kind the coach stands behind during practice to see how hard you're really hitting? Gymnastics, rowing, and wrestling involve heavy lifting too.

Twisting

One of this book's recurrent themes is that twisting motions are dangerous to your lumbar spine, and the deadly combo of twisting and lifting is even worse than just lifting. (Figure 9.1 explains why twisting can be a problem.) Baseball, bowling, dancing, golf, gymnastics, hockey, lacrosse, sweep rowing, tennis, racquetball, squash, figure skating, and wrestling all involve some twisting. But, of course, much depends on the circumstances. You could twist your lumbar spine at the disco, dancing the twist to one of the oldies, or you could wrench your back by releasing a heavy bowling ball a little too late. Sometimes it's *how* you play, not what, that matters.

What do the twist and break dancing have in common, besides having started in the African-American community and getting lots of play on

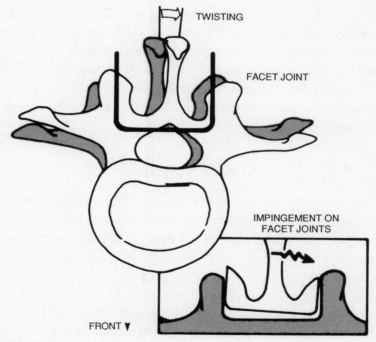

FIGURE 9.1.

Any twisting motion (axial rotation) may cause difficulty for the facet joints in the low back. After just a few degrees of axial rotation in the lumbar spine, the joints become impinged; this can result in irritation, injury, inflammation, and pain. Over time, degenerative changes will occur.

television? Answer: Both can raise havoc with the back. I've discussed the twist and how it causes stress on the back by impinging on the facet joints (figure 9.1). We should know that in break dancing, when one spins on the back, considerable bruising and painful irritation and even fracture of the spinous processes of the lumbar spine can occur. Happily, both dances are more or less out of style nowadays. But it does alert us to pay attention to potential damaging activities to the low back and recognize that even popular social dances can take their toll on this powerful yet vulnerable region of the body.

Hyperextension

Another red flag for your back is the extension lordosis (swayback) of forceful hyperextension of the lumbar spine. If you're wondering what that means, picture how gymnasts, dancers, divers, and tennis players, when serving, arch their backs. Javelin throwing, pole-vaulting, weight lifting (improperly done), swimming (butterfly or dolphin strokes), and wrestling (especially bridging) also involve a lot of back arching. So does pitching a baseball. You might be interested to know that contortionists who do lots of hyperextension suffer more spondylolysis—an anatomic gap in the back of the lumbar vertebra (see figure 3.5a)—than those who bend in the other direction.

Sports Injuries

There's no end to the variety of sports injuries. There are acute, specific injuries like fractures, and cumulative injuries resulting from repeated damage. There are self-inflicted injuries and those inflicted by competitors. By the way, one of the least health-preserving sports, boxing, more or less spares the back.

Acute injuries commonly crop up in connection with football, snowmobiling, tobogganing, and wrestling. Damage from repeated activity as well as acute injuries afflict bowlers, golfers, dancers, divers, football players, gymnasts, hockey players, rowers, weight lifters, and wrestlers. How do cumulative injuries happen? Well, usually lifting, twisting, or hyperextension is repeated until the bone breaks (it's called a fatigue fracture), a ligament or a disc fails, or you get wear-and-tear arthritis in the joint.

Now let me point out that sports can be good for you. Athletes usually have good muscle tone, or can develop it, and their bones and ligaments are stronger than those of more sedentary folk. Also, athletes' high motivation means they'll vigorously and conscientiously follow exercise programs and do everything possible to get well. But sometimes their zeal can be misdirected. We've all known jocks and jockettes who try to get back on the field (stage, court, rink, track, diving board) before their backs are ready—and reinjure themselves before adequate healing has taken place. This can lead to more serious problems.

RISKS OF DIFFERENT SPORTS

How does your favorite sport treat your back? What are its specific dangers? Is there anything you can do to protect your spine and keep on playing? Despite the high demands, the incidence of back pain in athletes (a reported 30 percent) is lower than that observed in the general population. Their excellent physical condition is thought to be the major reason. However, their stoic and competitive nature and driving desire to "get back in the game" in the face of an injury are also factors. Although the risks vary with the type of activity, a history of a previous back injury and improper conditioning and technique seem to stand out.

Baseball I'd rate it a medium- to low-risk sport. For starters, you have a straightforward twisting motion (axial rotation) as you swing the bat, and your contracting muscles exert large forces to accelerate the twist (figure 9.2). At the moment of impact, the forces required to swing the bat must be high, because they're operating well away from the pivot point (your spine). Then the twist must stop at some point, whether or not you've made contact with the ball. And this sudden stop applies pressure to both the disc and the spine's facet joints. The ensuing wear and tear can result in disc disease or arthritis of the spine. Or sometimes a particular motion, usually a swing and miss, can provoke back pain. Pitchers, who arch their backs extensively, run an additional risk.

What can you do for your back if you're a baseball aficionado? First, concentrate on developing a smooth, even swing. Come out of it by decelerating gradually and twisting your hips and knees to absorb some of the twist. Don't use a bat that's too heavy for you. If you pitch, smooth out your technique to avoid extreme arching.

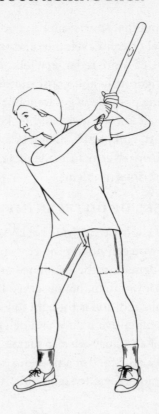

FIGURE 9.2.

In going from this position to a full swing of the bat, the spine goes through considerable axial rotation (twist), which can be irritating or damaging to the disc or the facet joints.

Basketball How can you write about sports and not mention the big round ball? Well, simply put, basketball players get backache, but the sport seems not to be one that particularly puts the back at risk. Thus, a medium- to low-risk sport.

Bowling Another medium- to low-risk sport. The twisting motion in bowling is similar to batting in baseball. The bowler's shoulders and upper torso twist in one direction while his/her hips and legs twist in the opposite way. He/she is also bent slightly forward with a heavy ball at arm's length (figure 9.3). This motion provides an efficient mechanical advantage—exerting very high loads on the spine and stressing the disc and facet joints.

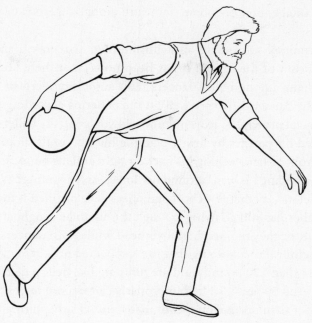

FIGURE 9.3.

From this flexed starting position to the twisted release position, consider-able forces are exerted on the spine. The forces are compression and shear, both of which can be irritating or damaging to the spine.

You can protect your back by developing a good technique. Try for a smoothly accelerated delivery and avoid releasing the ball late, which transmits heavy stress to the spine and results in injury or excessive wear. Don't use a ball that doesn't fit your fingers or is too heavy. The former problem can cause a jerky delivery, a delayed release, and a sore back.

Cycling This sport is generally not devastating to the back-pain-prone athlete. In fact, it's a good option for the jogger. It provides the leg exercise, the cardiopulmonary stimulation, and the change of scenery of jogging, but without the repeated impact loading. It also has the advantage of being a bedroom sport, if you use a stationary bike. Thus, it is considered a low-risk sport.

Dance Medium risk, depending on the kind of dancing. I won't attempt to separately classify classical ballet, modern dance, jazz ballet, slow dancing, and folk dancing, but, of course, some are more dangerous to your spine than others.

The women's movement notwithstanding, the male dancer's back bears the brunt of the action. It has been noted that there are more low back problems among ballet dancers than among modern or jazz ballet dancers. The dancer can't very well lift the ballerina according to the best biomechanical principles. How often would you go to the ballet if the male dancer lifted his partner by firmly planting his feet on the floor, squatting slowly in front of her, keeping his back straight and his buttocks placed on his heels, wrapping his arms around her knees, and grunting? While you're deciding, let me say that few choreographers have planned it that way.

The ballerinas still go flying through the air, to be caught at chest level by the male, or they're lifted high overhead while both dancers arch their backs gracefully. I'm assuming that the lovely creatures being lifted rarely weigh more than 120 pounds and are jumping like hell to help their partners. Still, even 50 pounds lifted improperly can impose forces four or five times heavier than normal on the lumbar spine, clearly putting the back at risk.

The dancer's risks relate to back arching and various pelvic motions that impart twisting and flexion to the lumbar spine. Naturally, these pelvic movements account for much of the dance's sensual and aesthetic appeal, and I wouldn't want to tamper with them. But dancers pay a price in wear on the disc and other structures, and in injuries from the muscle forces required to start, stop, or modulate movements to fast, complex rhythms. You'd have to do a lot of bowling, golfing, or baseball playing to swing your hips as forcefully and frequently as a performing dancer.

How can you save your back if you dance? Good conditioning, pacing yourself in rehearsals, and cutting down on routines that obviously hurt your back can help. If a particular routine is causing a lot of backache in the troupe, perhaps the dance master or dance mistress could be persuaded to drop or change it. This advice won't win me a place on the board of trustees at the Juilliard School, but it's good preventive medicine. I'm assuming a well-trained dancer has already developed optimum muscle control, strength, and suppleness. There's nothing more I can suggest to help your body do what it *wasn't designed to do*. We appreciate and enjoy your contribution to the arts—just be careful.

A precautionary note: Beware of new social-fad dances. Think about them, apply the principles, and decide for yourself whether or not the dance may aggravate your back. Remember the twist and break dancing? Well, neither was a friend of the low back.

Diving Medium risk. The main danger in diving comes from arching the lumbar spine as the diver snaps in and out of the dive's various maneuvers (figure 9.4). Hitting the water wrong—jackknifing the lower torso into a hyperextended position as the upper torso is being decelerated by the water—can also hurt your back. Acute injury or progressive wear of the spine's posterior elements can result. Repeated wear can cause spondylolisthesis (see figure 3.5a). Good conditioning and careful attention to technique are your best allies.

Forgive me, but I can't resist this opportunity to practice a bit of preventive medicine for the neck, as opposed to the back. One of the more common causes of broken necks and paralysis of the arms and legs is diving in unknown waters. Folks, it's preventable if you follow this simple rule: *Never!*—I repeat: *never!*—dive into unfamiliar waters, and don't let your friends do it, either, no matter how many or how few cocktails they may have had. If we would all follow this safety rule, so much sadness could be avoided. End of sermon.

Football (U.S., Canada, and others) A high-risk sport. Besides the United States and Canada, only one other country on earth has adopted football,

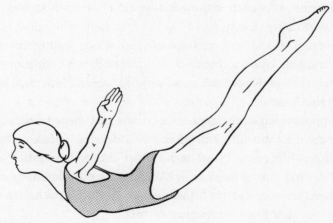

FIGURE 9.4.

The forceful hyperextension as the diver goes through various maneuvers can irritate the low back.

and that is the nation known for hara-kiri and kamikaze pilots. I enjoy and respect football, but I believe you ought to know its dangers.

Football players engage in frequent heavy lifting in less-than-ideal ergonomic circumstances. Linemen are especially burdened, both in games and in practice; up to *half* report back pain. You may notice that blocking and tackling are usually done with the back in a position of forty-five degrees or more of flexion (bending forward), followed by hyperextension as the "hit and lift" to push away an opponent. Weights being lifted are the 200- to 300-pound bodies of competing linemen. The lift is usually performed with an extended spine, using the back and leg muscles, which places forces several times one's body weight on the lumbar spine.

The result? Severe damage to the back part of the vertebrae, for instance. Is it surprising that spondylolisthesis—in which the destroyed back elements of the vertebrae cause the lumbar vertebrae to slip forward—runs four times higher in football players than in the general population? It's probably the number one cause of severe, persistent backache in the active teenage football lineman. (See figures 3.5a and 3.5b.)

To the list of football woes we must add acute injuries, for the impact to the spine in this contact sport may result in spinal fracture. When there's severe back pain immediately after an impact injury, fracture is the prime suspect. Quarterbacks, running backs, and pass receivers are vulnerable to a semipassive twisting injury. It occurs when the upper part of the torso is being twisted in one or more directions by tacklers while the lower torso is being held fast or twisted in the opposite direction by other tacklers. The resulting twist injures the spine.

And we're just talking about back injuries, which account for only one in twenty football injuries. The neck and the knee are even more vulnerable on the gridiron. Knee injuries account for about 25 percent of all the injuries in this sport.

What precautions can you take? Get in the best shape possible, not neglecting a good weight-lifting program. This develops blocking and tackling techniques that respect your back a little. This is easier said than done, I know. But while lifting helps with blocking, it's not absolutely essential. It's not altogether necessary to lift while tackling, either, although it is one of the lineman's few plays for the grandstand.

If you have a persistent, severe lower backache for fourteen days with no improvement, have it checked for spondylolysis or spondylolisthesis, either of which should be treated before it gets worse. (Spondylolysis is the result of two defects, or cracks, in the back part of the vertebra.) Herniated discs are also common in football players. When you have a sore back, remember that you may be awkward, weak, and prone to a more severe injury if you insist on playing. Sometimes your doctor may let you resume playing in an appropriately prescribed brace.

Golf Low to medium risk. Those who've been around golf much at all know that back pain goes with the divot (figure 9.5).

The twisting motion accompanying the drive is the dangerous part of golf, as it can damage the intervertebral discs and the intervertebral (facet) joints.

I had the occasion to meet an avid golfer who for twenty years after a disc removal and spinal fusion had done very well, playing golf regularly.

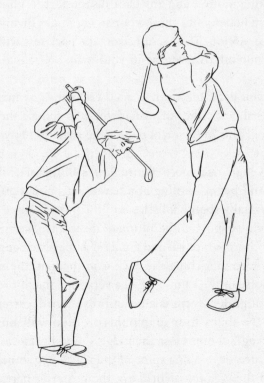

FIGURE 9.5.

This shows quite clearly how a full golf swing can result in a considerable axial rotation (twist) to the lower back. This can irritate not only the facet joints but also the disc. Smooth out the swing and rotate the hips to reduce the stress on the back.

Then one day he completed a long driving swing with a number two club and fell to the ground with excruciating back and leg pain. At the hospital, a myelogram revealed a large disc extruding just above the fused area of his spine. He underwent immediate surgical removal of the disc. After his recovery, he was advised to stay away from the green.

What probably happened was that his very efficient twisting swing was accentuated by the stable fusion beneath his normal disc. Over the years, the efficient, progressive wear and tear on the disc *adjacent* to the fusion had damaged it. The final swing was enough to cause disc herniation and the golfer's drastic symptoms.

This case, with its clear-cut dramatic cause and effect, is unusual, but if you do have back trouble, you should know that golf may expose you to further difficulties. To pamper your back, develop a swing that minimizes the twisting motion and any back discomfort. A good pro could no doubt guide you better, but I think your swing might involve more hip rotation and knee motion. This would stress the back less without introducing too many potential variations in your swing. Gradual warm-ups are also helpful.

Finally, if you used spiked or cleated golf shoes, switch to nonspiked shoes or tennis shoes, either of which will help reduce the impact at the end of the swing. This in turn will reduce the irritation to your back.

Gymnastics A high-risk sport (figure 9.6). In Bulgaria, where gymnasts are identified and begin training at a tender age, about 50 percent suffer back damage, usually spondylolisthesis of the lumbar spine.

This marvelous sport is the ultimate in balance, strength, coordination, courage, choreography—and forceful hyperextension of the spine. The forces involved in arching the back—on the mat, the uneven parallel bars, and the horse or the vault—are of a very high magnitude. Indeed, one of the criteria of perfect form is a beautifully arched, extremely extended lumbar spine. The ability to snap into this position with almost imperceptible speed and agility impresses the judges—and hurts the back, particularly the immature, developing spine of the youthful gymnast.

Fracture of the *pars interarticularis,* the posterior part of the vertebra where one finds the cracks of spondylolysis, can result in severe back pain. Due to the vigorous extension of the spine, the gymnast's risk of spondylolysis is four times higher than average. These athletes also have more disc disease and facet joint arthritis. Until the rules are changed to de-

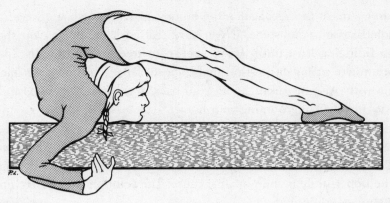

FIGURE 9.6.

If golf is the prototype for the twisting problem, gymnastics is the prototype for the *hyperextension* problem. This position causes large forces on the facet joints, the posterior part of the vertebra, and the disc.

emphasize the importance of hyperextending the spine, there is little the competitive gymnast can do other than to be careful and minimize the hyperextension—at least in practice. If you have prolonged, severe, and unimproved backache, seek appropriate medical care.

Hockey High risk. The sidearm shot, which requires twisting with a very high torque combined with leaning forward, is hockey's main backbreaker. The arms and shoulders are twisted in one direction as the hips and legs either hold steady or twist in the opposite direction. This shot hurts the back the same way that a golf swing may, except that in hockey you also hang out in a bending forward stance and put considerable pressure on your spine by contracting the erector spinae muscles. I should mention to the careful reader that the reason I rated golf low to medium risk and hockey high risk is because the twist is frequently associated with collisions with other players or, in the men's game, being "checked" against the wall. Hockey players have an increased risk of traumatic spine injuries. Precautions include good conditioning, good technique, and adequate warm-up.

Horseback Riding The risk is inversely related to the cumulative skills of horse and rider. Through alphabetical positioning, this sport almost appears next to jogging. The trouble with both sports is vertical impact loading—or, in the vernacular, the bumpy, up-and-down motions in the saddle that jolt your spine. If you have real back problems, you should drop riding, at least until you've been pain free for six months. In this sport, you're sitting, a position that imposes large loads on your back to begin with. Also be careful about your back in the work positions and activities involved in grooming your horse.

Javelin Throwing Medium risk. This is another sport that is believed to lead to back pain and spondylolisthesis. The twisting and hyperextension of the upper body is the probable cause. The solution is good technique and good conditioning.

Jogging Low to medium risk. Working with these athletes, one rarely encounters indifference. Joggers, in particular, often evince an enthusiasm bordering on the fanatical—which is great, in my opinion, since there's at times too much passivity in life.

However, vertical impact loading, or the *bump-bump-bump* as the road's vibrations are transmitted to your spine, can damage the discs and other structures. Fortunately, there's quite a lot you can do about it. The magnitude of the *bump-bump-bump* depends on your weight, your conditioning, your fatigue or lack of it, the smoothness of your stride, and the ability of your leg muscles and other muscles—as well as the hip and sacroiliac joints—to dampen the impact. Your shoes and the surfaces you run on also count.

Happily, few people who jog remain obese for long, but weight may handicap the beginning jogger. Start slowly, gradually adding to your distance as you shed pounds. Actually, starting with marathon distances isn't advisable for anyone, obese or svelte. The spine's bones and ligaments strengthen with practice and adapt to the rigors of this most ancient of man's sporting activities.

If you feel tired and notice that your weary muscles are allowing your legs to flop around a bit, or if you're stumbling, you're clearly in the fatigue range and susceptible to injury. This brings us to the matter of technique. The runner with smooth, excellent form is at lower risk than the clumsy runner. Read a good book on jogging, concentrate on your form, and observe well-trained runners.

Avoid running at night on anything but smooth, familiar surfaces. Irregularity in the terrain can hurt your ankles, knees, hands, and face if you should stumble—and unanticipated surface irregularities can transmit sudden shocks to your spine. Also, you should remember that unexplained knee pain without knee swelling or aggravation by knee motion can be caused by a herniated disc. Grass, wood, cinder tracks, sand, and soft ground are more forgiving surfaces than concrete and asphalt. Hard surfaces can damage your muscles and tendons, and produce stress fractures in your bones.

Hundreds of pages have been written about running shoes. In brief, a good running shoe should (1) conform to the foot's contour, (2) be made of energy-absorbing material in the heel and sole, and (3) allow the foot to breathe. It doesn't necessarily follow that the most expensive shoe is the best.

Some people think that jogging is good for the back because the forces applied to the disc contribute to the physiology of chemical exchanges and improve their nutrition. Moreover, good athletic conditioning is said to increase endorphin production (see chapter 4), and these morphinelike substances may be the physiological basis of the "runner's high." These theories are reasonable but not overriding. If you enjoy jogging and it doesn't hurt your back, continue. If you're jogging and having back trouble, try eliminating the risk factors we mentioned.

I sometimes ask joggers with back problems why they didn't consult a doctor earlier. Often they respond, "Well, I didn't go to the doctor because I knew a doctor would tell me to stop jogging, and no jogger wants to be told to stop." I can understand this sentiment. Some joggers don't want to give up their passion, and we doctors should try to help them continue jogging while reducing the stresses on their backs. If you're a jogger with a backache, know that your condition is unlikely to cripple you or threaten your life. But you do need to examine your pleasure-pain ratio. If you subtract your back pain from the pleasure of jogging, is there some net pleasure left over? If so, good luck, be careful, and if you must jog at night, use reflectors.

Before leaving this subject, I'd like to offer a bit of information to female joggers. If you're training to the point that you've developed amenorrhea—that is, your periods have stopped—you may be losing some bone mass. Female runners and athletes have sustained up to 14 percent decreases in bone density in association with the hormonal changes. Your exercise program should be complemented by a balanced diet (proper nutrition). Driven woman athletes may be at risk for developing the female athlete's triad: disordered eating, amenorrhea, and osteoporosis. The risks associated with this condition can be grave. Medical attention should be sought immediately.

Lacrosse Lacrosse was invented by the North American Indians, whose casualties, in games of eight hundred to a thousand players, included broken legs and even death. Nowadays, lacrosse, once mostly limited to private secondary schools and colleges in Canada and the Northeast, is gaining popularity, and, happily, deaths rarely or never occur. The men's game is particularly fascinating because it affords to rare opportunity to observe a situation in which it is acceptable for one player to take a stick and hit the other player on the head before they run down the field together. How strangely marvelous!

In any case, the twisting motion lacrosse requires for the side shot resembles the side shot in hockey and poses identical risks to your back. As the shoulders and arms twist vigorously in one direction to execute the shot, the hips and pelvis are stable or turned in the other direction as a stabilizing counterforce. If you stay in excellent physical condition and develop a technique that minimizes the side shot's twist, you'll protect your back.

Pole-vaulting High risk. This beautiful sport involves a maneuver that is potentially irritating to the back. During the vaulter's ascent to the bar, there are several phases: the run, the jump, the pull with the arms, and the lifting up of the legs as they are virtually snapped, kicked, and thrown over the bar. This lifting over of the legs requires tremendous action of our old friends the psoas muscles, which attach to the femurs (thighbones) just below the hip joints. And you know what that does. It's analogous to sit-ups with legs straight and feet held down. The psoas contractions needed to throw the legs up impose very large forces on the low back, the other points where they attach. Thus the back may be irritated.

Good conditioning and smooth execution of technique should reduce the risk and allow a pole vaulter with back pain to spring back, no pun intended.

Rowing High risk. There are two types of rowing: *sculling,* where a single rower uses two oars and pulls his back in the direction he's rowing, and *sweep rowing,* or team rowing. In sweep rowing, half the rowers extend oars on one side of the boat, half on the other side. The sweep rower must pull the oar with both hands, from way off to one side of his/her body onto his/her chest. This process constitutes a twisting motion as well as a forceful extension of the body. Consequently, there is a forceful twist and extension of the spine, two maneuvers that are unfriendly to the ailing back.

Both types of rowing pose risks to your back. But sweep rowing, with its characteristic twisting motion, is probably more dangerous than straight sculling, which involves only spine extension. I learned this little logical gem from a rowing coach.

What can you do about the risks? Stay in condition, concentrate on technique, and hope that your coach employs careful fatigue management and training. Some training exercises that involve simulated rowing are stressful to the back and should be kept to a minimum. When a rower's back aches, it's often hard to distinguish spinal problems from the soreness of any athlete's overworked muscles. But when there's associated leg pain, the possibility of nerve root irritation or significant damage to the spinal elements looms large. A doctor should be consulted.

Let me share a case history with you. A patient of mine, a vigorous, nineteen-year-old Olympic-class rower on the Harvard University team, started having back pain while rowing. Soon it began to crop up between rowing sessions as well, and he developed pain in his right leg. On the recommendation of an orthopedic surgeon, the young man rested and stopped rowing. First his leg pain subsided, then his back pain. When he went back to rowing after several weeks, he returned to sculling because summer vacation had arrived and his teammates were away. It caused no problems. In the fall, however, when he resumed sweep rowing, his severe back and leg pain flared up once more. Intrigued, the student did an informal survey of his rowing friends, quite a number of whom also complained of back and leg pain. Not only did he note that those who did sweep rowing had more pain than those who sculled, but the teammates who pulled oars on the right side of the boat had pain in the left leg, while those who pulled on the left side had right leg pain. This anecdote perfectly fits the mathematical model and the experimental studies of the spine as it relates to body activities and disc problems.

I learned from a rowing coach that it's good to develop *both* sides of a sweep rower. How ingenious. This provides balanced muscle development and distributes the stress on various parts of the disc and the facet joints more evenly.

Sailing Medium risk. Yes, there is risk here too. When crewing on a larger craft, there is simply the hard work of lifting that goes with the job. However, there is a more subtle problem that the small-craft sailor should be aware of. When you must hook your feet under a stable structure on the boat, extending your torso well over the side of the boat for balance, you certainly risk irritating an underlying back problem. It's the same reason why you should avoid sit-ups with your knees straight and your feet hooked under the bed. In both circumstances, considerable stress is exerted on the iliopsoas muscle (see figure 5.14) and therefore on the lumbar spine to which it attaches. This may truly cause your back to ache.

If you need this maneuver as a competitive sailor or in an emergency, you will probably have to pay the price. Otherwise you can improvise, or simply not allow yourself to get in that situation, letting a crew member with a good back do it.

Scuba Diving Low risk. There is a very rare situation in which scuba divers experience low back pain following too-rapid decompression. Unfortunately, this pain can signal the beginning of a severe neurological problem in which gases in the neural structures damage the spinal cord and nerves. This must be treated promptly by hyperbaric oxygen therapy.

Skating Medium risk. Three skating activities are potential back aggravators. First is the basic skating position with the spine slightly bent forward. The other two liabilities are related more to figure skating: The various spins are one problem, and landing after a jump is the other.

What can we do about it? The recreational skater can take it easy and skate as upright as possible if she has a back that's acting up. The figure skater must be ever so careful with the twists and ever so graceful in the jump landings. And if backache does hit, I suggest knocking it off for a few weeks until the back settles down.

Skiing Low risk overall. The main bogey here is the mogul that appears out of nowhere, or the jump where you don't land just right. Other stresses are the parallel skier's repeated twisting (figure 9.7) and the chronic back strain endured by downhill and cross-country skiers as they hold their torsos in a slightly flexed position. I suggest that if you're a skier with a back problem, avoid twisting your shoulders in the opposite direction in which

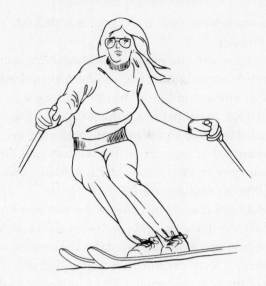

FIGURE 9.7.

Here again, axial rotation, or twisting of the spine, is a contributing factor in the skier who develops low back pain.

you're twisting your hips. Keep them as parallel as possible to avoid torque on your low back.

Another suggestion: If you ski and want to spare your back, develop your quadriceps muscles (so named for their four "heads"), the ones running from your hips to your knees, in front. They're critical shock absorbers, balancers, and controllers of the skiing body. When strengthened, they can take up much of the energy that might otherwise jolt the spine.

Here are some quadriceps strengthening exercises. Begin exercise number one by standing with your back against the wall, making sure that the floor isn't slippery and that you're wearing rubber-soled shoes. Now carefully slide down the wall, moving your feet out gradually from the wall as you go—all the way down to the point where your hips are ninety degrees flexed, your knees are bent ninety degrees, and your feet are flat on the floor. You end up in the position of a person sitting erectly in a chair—except that there's no chair and your derriere rests on air. You're supported by your feet and by your back resting against the wall. So what's the force that keeps you from sliding down the wall? The sustained contraction of your quadriceps! You'll feel it immediately. At first, you'll be able to sit there for a few seconds only, but try to gradually increase your endurance to one or two minutes.

If the wall-sitting exercise makes your knees hurt, don't do it. Do exercise number two instead. Take a ten- or fifteen-pound weight and attach it to your foot or ankle. You can improvise the weight in several ways: a sack filled with large, heavy pebbles, a pillowcase holding canned food, or a sandbag will do. Two bags or pillowcases containing weights can be tied together and draped over your ankle, one on each side. Or you can go to a sporting goods store and buy a shoe attachment that allows you to apply measured weights in various quantities.

Now sit on a high counter or table, or the side of a low bed. If you're sitting on a counter or table, rest your weighted ankles on a stool; if you're sitting on a low bed, rest it on the floor. Start the exercise with your knees bent about thirty or forty degrees (not ninety degrees), then slowly extend the knee of the weighted leg until it's completely straight. Gradually work up to doing this twenty-five or fifty times for each knee, once a day. After two or three weeks, your quadriceps will be strengthened for better, injury-free skiing. If both exercises cause severe knee pain, reduce the weights or the number of repetitions. If there's still pain, desist.

You can add extra protection to your back by doing the back exercises in chapter 5.

"When can I go back to the slopes?" is the question I hear most often from dedicated skiers. A quick, accurate, unfacetious answer is: when you can make love without back pain, and when you can perform regular basic back and quadriceps exercises. Then *gradually* work into skiing—sticking to the intermediate slopes for a few days if you're an advanced skier; to the beginner slopes if you're an intermediate. Though your ego may be begging for more, don't deceive yourself about how tired you really are.

There is no agreement about the status of cross-country skiing as a back-pain-risk sport. My suggestion is that if you want to do it, try it and see how your back fares. If you have a backache and you're looking for a sport, then I'd say this shouldn't be high on your list.

Snowmobiling Medium to high risk. This delightful recreation contributes to both sides of the pleasure-pain equilibrium during the winter months. The threat to your back is that of injury, pure and simple. Because snowmobiling is done at high speeds, spine fractures can result.

Commonsense precautions are advised. Don't snowmobile "under the influence" or speed in crowded or hard-to-maneuver places. Manufacturers could help greatly by designing seats that absorb the maximum impact, sparing the spine. Repeated jostlings and high vibrations that don't cause an immediate fracture can sometimes cause cumulative damage.

Squash Low to medium risk. Squash is similar to tennis as a sport and in the movements that may irritate the back. The twisting motion involved in the backhand can cause an injury that results in backache. Conditioning and the backhand technique of using the arms more than the trunk will help.

Sumo Wrestling High risk. I started to leave this one out, because it's pretty much limited to Japan. Then, thinking about global markets, patriotism, and the popularity of sumo wrestling in Japan, I decided to include it, in order to help the trade balance. But seriously, the *real* reason for including it is that this is such a marvelously fascinating sport, historically well entrenched in the finest of Japanese culture, and a brief discussion allows us to reemphasize certain points for any backache-prone athlete. Contrary to what you may have thought, these athletes are not fat, out-of-shape, over-the-hill wrestlers of the type that you may see in the ring on your late-night TV entertainment. They are exquisitely trained, powerful, lightening-quick competitors who work out early every morning almost 365 days a year. The afternoon is spent eating and sleeping to develop that very large and powerful stomach. Why? Because the idea of the sport is to keep from being thrown out of a rather small circle while lifting your 250- to 350-pound opponent and throwing *him* out of the ring. The large abdomen also serves as a fulcrum and lever to accomplish the task. Balance, style, reflexes, and strategy are the highly tuned skills employed.

Since you're now a scholar on the backache, you know that possessing a large abdomen and lifting heavy objects out in front of your body is not good for your back. Among sumo wrestlers, there is a high incidence of spondylolysis and spondylolisthesis.

Swimming Very low risk. Swimming is excellent exercise for backache sufferers, because you work out virtually all your muscles and get cardiorespiratory conditioning as well. All this, and it doesn't put undue gravitational loads on your spine.

Sometimes, however, a patient complains that swimming irritates his/her back condition. If you have a fairly severe back problem, the breaststroke and crawl could aggravate it, perhaps because you hyperextend your back when you execute those strokes. If so, I recommend the sidestroke. There are, however, some very sensitive backs that would be uncomfortable in any swimming activity.

What about vigorous, competitive swimming? The breaststroke, particularly the dolphin breaststroke (butterfly), involves tremendous flexion and hyperextension of the spine and should be considered a risk for those with back problems. Otherwise, swimming offers good therapy and very few opportunities to hurt your back.

Tennis Low risk. Tennis gained considerable popularity in the seventies as North Americans became more fitness conscious. Not only is tennis stimulating and exciting but it's also a great equalizer. An eleven-year-old girl can have a good game with her sixty-year-old grandfather. A fifty-year-old female college professor can teach a twenty-year-old male student a few lessons. Husbands and wives, fathers and daughters, friends and lovers, can all get out on the court with reasonable chances to win or be competitive.

Two parts of tennis can cause backache, however: the serve and the backhand. Some serving styles load the lower back as you extend your back and uncoil your arm and racket to hit the ball (figure 9.8). This exerts great pressure on the spine. The follow-through is down and around to the opposite side of your body, which means a slight twist. If you have back trouble, and you're using an Australian-style or American-twist serve, try changing your serve so as to eliminate the hyperextension. If back pain occurs only occasionally with your serve, do some exercises to strengthen your back and abdominal muscles and stabilize your spine.

As for the backhand, this involves standing with your legs and lower trunk held stable while your shoulders are turned. As you swing, your shoulders, waist, and arm are uncoiled with great force, and then there's the impact of hitting the ball. This coiling and uncoiling exert twisting forces on the back.

What should you do about your backhand, which is many players' most vulnerable point anyway? Ask a pro to teach you the best technique and hope that it will let you carry out the stroke in a more relaxed way, minimizing the torsional forces. If that doesn't work, you may have to eval-

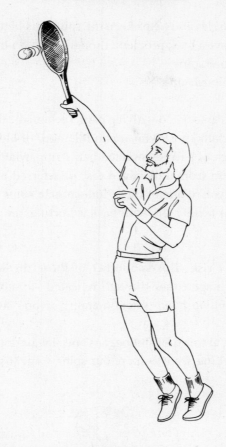

FIGURE 9.8.

It's the hyperextension arch in serving that can do it to the tennis player. Occasionally, the twist associated with the backhand will cause the tennis player to have back trouble.

uate the game's pleasure-pain ratio. Or perhaps you could go back to running around your backhand.

In general, conditioning and good technique help your back. Because tennis is a social game, most people start playing without an adequate warm-up. Try doing these warm-up exercises:

1. Stand and spread your legs to about the same width as your shoulders, then twist gently from side to side (see figure 2.8d).
2. Begin by sitting on the ground with your legs stretched out. Now come as close as you can to touching your toes. This stretches your

hamstring muscles and helps keep the spine in a better position. If you already have a back problem, though, don't do this exercise. It may irritate your spine.

3. Do at least ten push-ups.

If your backache is associated with leg pain, seek medical attention. Weekend athletes, especially those who are middle-aged or older, often attribute pain down the back of a leg to a pulled hamstring, when it may be due to nerve root irritation from a damaged disc or referred pain from another spine problem. If you're one of those unfortunate souls who plays winter tennis in an indoor facility and your back is hurting, try playing in a warm sweater.

Tobogganing Low risk. This is another of those thrilling winter sports that does back damage either through repeated vibratory loading of the spine (the *bump-bump-bump* phenomenon) or one sudden injury that fractures vertebrae.

Unfortunately, at this time, toboggans and sleighs don't come equipped with impact-absorbing seats to spare our spine some jostling. But there is

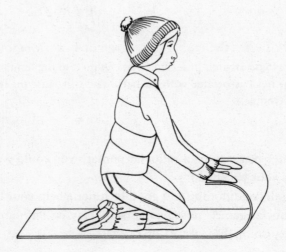

FIGURE 9.9.

By utilizing this position, actually sitting on the heels, you take advantage of the shock-absorbing capacities of your knees and ankles. This reduces the intensity of sudden impact that would otherwise be transmitted to the spine.

something you can do. Use the joints of your ankles, knees, and hips to dampen the loads that ultimately reach the lumbar spine. I advise sitting as shown in figure 9.9. As a second precaution, use common sense and don't sled or toboggan "under the influence."

Weight Lifting High risk. Weight lifting exerts immense stress on the lumbar spine. Evidence of spine damage—spondylolysis—runs as high as 40 percent among young Japanese weight lifters. However, most weight lifters are well-conditioned athletes who have carefully studied lifting techniques, and this can help reduce risks associated with the sport.

The first back-saving suggestion is to master your technique and train appropriately. Avoid jerky movements and lifting weights from the floor. Other no-no's are movements in which the spine must go from a flexed position to an erect, or hyperextended, position. If you lie flat on your back or semireclined and use your shoulder, arm, and chest muscles for lifting (bench pressing), you'll spare your back much stress. And there's an excellent theoretical and experiential basis for the use of belts in both practice and competition. By increasing intra-abdominal and thoracic pressure, belts contribute to stiffening and unweighting the spine, which diminishes the strains to it.

It has been observed that highly competitive, poorly supervised, teenage weight lifting can result in a type of fracture of the vertebral body in the region of the growth plate. If this information is relevant to you or anyone you know, use it!

Wrestling This is one of those sports with a factor X, for unknown. Although you can protect your back with careful conditioning, your opponents constitute factor X. Their moves remain a source of potential injury.

In wrestling there lurk several potential stressors to the lumbar spine. For one thing, wrestlers spend a great deal of time trying to lift each other. And each also plots to make lifting as awkward and inconvenient as possible for the opponent.

Stamina is a major factor in survival and in protection from injury. A wrestler needs superb overall conditioning, together with excellent strength and endurance in all his/her muscles. Diligent sparring and shadow practice are critical, and in sparring the use of difficult lifting moves can be controlled.

Whenever you have severe pain that lasts for several days, hold off on any training activity that aggravates the pain. This great sport has a certain baseline injury potential that is difficult to minimize.

Some Parting Shots

Of course, we haven't covered *all* sports. If your favorite has not been included, let me suggest that if it doesn't hurt your back, fine. If it does, then you should get in the best possible shape and refine your technique. Try to figure out what particular activity in the sport irritates your back. Discuss it with a fellow sportsman, coach, or pro, with the idea of altering your activity so as to maintain your competitive edge while alleviating the pain.

Since some readers are likely to be serious athletes, let me share this with you. Let's say that you're doing your sport, and you have a backache. But you want to go to the limit to gain maximum abdominal strength. Here's how to do it: Use the medicine ball. You know what I mean: the big, heavy ball (it comes in two sizes) that boxers whip into each other's abdomens to strengthen the abdominal muscles so that they can take a body punch. When you can take the medicine ball twenty-five to one hundred times in the stomach two to three times a week, you'll have an abdomen that will support any grieving back handsomely.

You may have noticed that each subheading of this chapter contains admonitions about fitness and good conditioning. Good muscle tone and endurance are of the utmost value to your health in any sport. For some sports, we've suggested that you follow the basic back-pain exercise. Properly done sit-ups should be a part of most training programs, and good abdominal tone and posture mechanics make for a healthy back.

An excellent, well-coached technique in your chosen sport improves your performance and minimizes the risk of injury. Good coaching, conscientious practice, and, in some cases, videotapes or careful reading of the right book can help sharpen your skills. Sometimes you may be able to modify your technique to spare your back. If your tennis serve, for example, causes backaches, you could work with a pro to develop one that's kinder to your spine.

Coaches can help in another way. When aware of a particular sport's risk potential, a coach can cut down on its most dangerous elements. A football team's full-blast practice scrimmage might not include a lot of kickoff plays, for instance. In this chapter, we've pinpointed some of each sport's backache-inducing activities. If these can be kept to a minimum, so much the better.

Of course, one must be circumspect about suggesting rule changes; I certainly wouldn't want anyone tampering with "my sport." But since my goal is your back's well-being, I've taken the liberty of sounding a few warnings. If this book were written by a cardiologist or an ophthalmologist, you'd be reading a different set of tips.

One more point. People often say, "Use a little common sense." My recommendation is that you use *a whole lot* of common sense, especially when engaging in recreational sports like skiing, tobogganing, snowmobiling, and diving, where you may be tempted to perform after a few drinks. Common sense is also helpful to the weekend athlete who may become overexhausted, or the football player who's trying to excite the grandstand with an overhead lifting tackle.

We've mentioned the pleasure-pain ratio. Simply put, if the pleasure derived from a sport exceeds the pain incurred, then "Batter up," "Serve 'em up," or whatever. Backache in the absence of leg pain usually has as its sole liability the misery it brings; it's not likely to result in any terrible disease or further injury. If there is associated leg pain, however, it's possible that it's early disc disease and that, if properly rested, it will have a better outcome than if it is irritated repeatedly by some athletic activity.

After following all the recommendations in this chapter, you're probably safe in regulating your sports activities on the basis of the pleasure-pain equilibrium. Good luck!

CHAPTER 10

Answers to Backache Questions Patients Frequently Ask

FOR A MOMENT, PRETEND THAT YOU ARE A STUDENT AT-tending our low back school. Now you have a chance to ask any question and to be enlightened on any point that still puzzles you. Unfortunately, books are not an interactive medium, so you'll have to hope that your questions coincide with some of those we've collected here. But since back patients tend to have similar problems, chances are that you'll get yours answered. For your convenience, we've grouped the questions by topic.

Diagnosis

Q. *When and how should I ask for a second opinion?*

A. Whenever you feel like it. Consider it seriously if (1) your doctor seems to want to rush you into surgery or gives you a heavy sales pitch, (2) you've already had one operation on your back, (3) your surgeon *promises* you an excellent result from surgery, (4) the proposed surgery and its basic techniques, risks, and benefits haven't been explained lucidly in nonmedical language, (5) there is compensation or litigation involved in your case and you don't believe you're being treated fairly, or (6) you're being treated by someone you believe is not respectful to you as a person.

The state of New Jersey has added cultural competency training as a prerequisite for medical licensure.

Q. *What should the workup consist of? Should my doctor take X-rays? Must I have an MRI?*

A. A thorough medical history and physical exam are usually enough to categorize (though maybe not diagnose) your back pain. Routine X-rays aren't essential, especially if you've had pain for less than seven weeks; but by the time you've been referred to a specialist, he'll probably ask for recent X-rays or take a new set. Some doctors routinely perform a series of lab tests, including a complete blood count, a uric acid test to rule out gout, a sedimentation rate blood test to check for an inflammatory process, and a serum test to rule out lupus erythematosus and ankylosing spondylitis.

Other physicians feel confident in diagnosing low back pain on the basis of your history and physical exam, putting the X-ray off for a while. As a matter of fact, an extensive review in 1988 of all the best clinical information on back pain led to the recommendation that no X-rays or laboratory studies are needed during the initial exam for a back problem *unless* something specific in the patient's history or physical exam so indicates.

Myelograms, CT scans, or MRIs are not ordered unless clearly indicated or surgery is proposed. (The myelogram has been virtually replaced by the MRI.) Their purpose is to confirm the diagnosis, usually of a herniated disc, and to precisely locate the abnormality. Be leery of any doctor who offers these procedures and surgery early in the nonoperative treatment process. Most people recover spontaneously after two or three months.

Q. *I feel terrible. What did my doctor mean when he said my spine was degenerating?*

A. He/she probably didn't say that the spine was *degenerating* but rather, that your spine showed *degenerative changes* or *degenerative arthritis*. What this means is simply wear and tear wrought by age.

As you get older, your spine's structures undergo inevitable changes that aren't nearly so dreadful as the word *degenerative* seems to imply (see chapter 3). These changes happen to everyone at different rates, just like gray hair and wrinkles. Some people get back pain in the process; others don't. And even though they're described as "progressive," degenerative changes don't necessarily result in worsening symptoms.

Also, don't be alarmed if you see evidence of degenerative changes on your X-rays. This doesn't mean that you can't get better. Actually, many people see extensive degenerative changes on their X-rays yet experience little or no back pain.

Q. *What causes low back pain in children?*

A. When a child who has not had a specific injury complains of persistent low back pain for one or two weeks, get him/her to a doctor. Although teenagers occasionally get low back and disc disease, it's uncommon and usually occurs as an aftereffect of a distinct injury, such as a sprain or twist. Disc disease can sometimes go undiagnosed in children for a long time, because it's rarely suspected. Most of the other, more serious diseases we worry about in adults also afflict children. Although cancer is less frequent in children, it does occur. But again, rest assured that low back pain rarely means anything dire.

Otherwise, most of what we say about back pain in adults applies to children. It is less common in children, and the psychosocial considerations are rarely factors in childhood low back pain.

Q. *Could very large breasts be the cause of my back pain? Would a breast reduction help?*

A. Mechanical and postural changes caused by excessively large breasts can provoke several clinical aches and pains. These include neck strain, headache, aching shoulders, pain and tingling in the fingers, and deep bra-strap furrows, as well as low back pain.

The added weight and the shift of the center of gravity forward can put additional strain on the muscles of the low back and more force on the upper and lower spine. Moreover, a self-conscious woman may try to minimize her prominent breasts sometimes by rolling her shoulders inward and rounding her thoracic (rib area) spine. This adds to the mechanical problem and further stresses the back muscles, joints, and nerves. Very large breasts are a mechanical liability, requiring great muscle force and stress on the lumbar spine to maintain erect posture. So it's no wonder that a large-breasted woman may fall into the posture described above, which shifts the center of gravity backward toward a more natural position. Initially voluntary, this posture can turn into a fixed deformity. Its disadvantages include lordosis of the lumbar and cervical (neck) spine, a rounding of the thoracic spine, and compromised muscle control and balance.

Would breast-reduction surgery relieve your back pain? There's no real proof, but it seems reasonable. If you're considering this operation mainly to help your back pain, you can get a better prediction from a doctor who specializes in low back problem in consultation with a plastic surgeon.

Q. *Tell me about myelograms and CT scans (CAT scan).*

A. From time to time, we run across a patient who simply says, "Do anything you wish to me, Doctor, but please don't give me a myelogram." Usually such a patient has had severe pain during a previous myelogram or an excruciating headache or backache afterward, but more likely he/she has been exposed only vicariously to the exaggerated "horrible reputation" of this procedure.

Myelograms are routinely carried out on most patients without any complication or difficulty. Since the procedure does pose certain risks, however, a myelogram probably shouldn't be done unless you and your doctor have decided to proceed with surgery if it shows an abnormality. It takes about an hour to perform.

One of two types of dye is injected into the *subarachnoid space* around the spinal cord and the nerves of the lower spine. The injected dye is called a contrast medium and shows up on X-rays as a dense white image. When it surrounds the spinal cord and nerves, anything that is pressing on them looks like an indention in the column of dye. The indention you see on the X-ray may be a disc, a tumor, an infection, or another disease process. Your doctor must interpret it.

What are myelography's risks? You may be allergic to the dye, especially if you've been found to be allergic to iodine, shellfish, or a previously administered intravenous contrast medium. Hypotension, or a drop in blood pressure, may occur during the test. The water-soluble dye can inflame brain tissue if it's allow to run too high in the neck area. Sometimes the lower back gets inflamed. The most serious complication we worry about with the water-contrast dye is *anaphylactic shock,* an acute, generalized allergic reaction that on extremely rare occasions can be fatal if not treated.

A CT scan (computed axial tomography) is a noninvasive imaging technique. It is basically a fancy X-ray machine that can generate two-dimensional or three-dimensional images by rotating the X-ray beam around an axis. The CT scan is excellent for assessing the bone architecture of the spine. It can be used in conjunction with a myelogram to better identify the neural elements as well. The MRI scan (see page 271) has virtually replaced the CT-myelogram. However, there may be times when it is still needed.

Q. *What is a discogram?*

A. In this diagnostic procedure, a needle is inserted through the lower back, flank, or midback into the intervertebral disc. A dye is then injected, and its distribution may reveal a degenerated disc. The amount absorbed by the disc can also hint that it's degenerated, as degenerated discs tend to accept more fluid. Finally, the particular location and kind of pain that you report during the test itself can help your doctor determine whether the disc space is causing your backache. Cortisone and Novocain may also be injected to reduce pain and inflammation. When the pain is eliminated in this way, it indicates that the disc receiving the injection is the one causing the problem.

While all this seems logical, a number of flaws detract from the test's accuracy. For one, most people don't remember, localize, and describe back and leg pain very precisely. Not all grossly degenerated discs are painful, either. And the injection may cause placebo pain relief.

Discograms are rather controversial. There is vigorous disagreement about this procedure among spine specialists. There are arguments about when they should be done, how they should be done, if they should be done, who should do them, where they should be done, and how they should be interpreted. A significant false-positive rate has been reported.

Okay, what is my advice, then, on discography? Maintain a significant level of skepticism, and if your doctor feels that it's really needed, he/she should explain the reason(s) satisfactorily. Despite the controversy, discography is the only available provocative test to assess a presumably painful degenerated disc. Performance of surgery may depend on the results following this test.

Q. *What is a bone scan?*

A. This X-ray technique has the advantage of little radiation exposure, but it takes four hours to complete. Because it requires you to lie face-down on a table for as long as an hour, it can make a back patient quite uncomfortable. We like to make back patients lie immobile on their stomachs as seldom as possible.

The bone scan can diagnose recent fractures as well as tumors and infections. It's half as expensive as a myelogram and is thought to expose you to less radiation. This test gives information about the possibility of tumor, fracture, infection, or arthritis in the bones and joints of the spine, whereas the myelogram tells you if there's something abnormal, such as a herniated disc, in or near the spinal canal. The study exposes patients to about one-tenth the radiation as a routine low back X-ray.

Q. *What are EMG studies?*

A. EMG stands for electromyography, a test that takes about an hour and a half and involves no radiation but can be moderately uncomfortable. The doctor, usually a neurologist, attaches little pads to the skin over your muscles; sometimes he/she will insert very fine needles into the muscles. Once the pads or needles are in place, the doctor can study the pattern of electrical recordings caused by nerve conduction. Changes in the electrical patterns and the speed of nerve conduction can help uncover various kinds of nerve pathology. Irritation of the nerve roots in the lower spine will show up as abnormal electrical responses. So the EMG can help us recognize when a disc is encroaching on the spinal canal's nerves.

Q. *What is an MRI?*

A. MRI stands for magnetic resonance imaging. This is a noninvasive system of imaging that is capable of depicting the spine from different views: front and side, as well as looking down the spinal canal to see if the disc is herniated or if something else is irritating the nerves. Various anatomic structures, such as normal and herniated discs, spinal nerves, the dura, the intervertebral joints, and tumors, can be imaged. Not only can the technology provide excellent images, it also has some capacity to characterize certain biological activities of some tissues.

This technology is an excellent tool. Unlike X-rays and the CT scan, there is no ionizing radiation associated with this imaging modality. The technology is quite complex, but in very simple terms it works in the following manner: Water molecules have magnetic properties. The many different organs and structures in our bodies have varying numbers of water molecules, based on their respective anatomies. When these water molecules are placed in a strong magnetic field, the magnetized molecules align themselves accordingly. When subjected to radio waves, the molecules in different organs will resonate at different frequencies. As the radio frequency is adjusted, this variable resonation produces small rotating magnetic signals that can be detected by the scanner and converted to an image of the area being studied. Sometimes a dye may be used to help delineate certain structures. At present, this is an appropriate test to utilize if you and your doctor think that surgery is a consideration for disc herniation or for spinal stenosis.

The test is not painful. You merely lie still on your back in a hollow tube for thirty to sixty minutes. There's also a noticeable popping sound in the machine while it works. If you're claustrophobic, let your doctor know, or just relax and keep your eyes closed. Think pleasant thoughts or, better yet, fantasize. Sometimes a sedative may be required to help you get through it.

Q. *How useful is DSSEP (dermatomal somatosensory evoked potentials) in the diagnosis of a herniated disc?*

A. This test is in its very early stages of development and has not yet been proven to be a sure and accurate method for diagnosing disc herniation. The myelogram, CT scan, and MRI are the most reliable tests. The DSSEP is an electrical test in which the skin of the foot is stimulated and the response of brain waves are recorded. An abnormal recording suggests that something, presumably a herniated disc, is interfering with the signal being transmitted from the foot to the brain. This test is often used during scoliosis surgery to monitor the spinal cord as the spine is realigned.

Self-Care

Q. *Doctor, couldn't this just be a bad muscle pull? It hurts in the muscle, and I'm getting lots of muscle spasm.*

A. If so, you're fortunate, as a muscle rupture should heal in one to two weeks. Frankly, the muscle spasm you're having is not well understood. It will gradually subside. Rest, relaxation, heat or cold, and massage are all likely to help. On rare occasions, muscle relaxants are prescribed.

Q. *Do you recommend special beds or mattresses?*

A. Chapters 5 and 6 cover this questions in some detail. If you're sleeping fine on a sofa mattress and it doesn't hurt your back, enjoy. If you want to test the idea of a harder mattress, try sleeping on the floor on a stack of blankets for a few nights. A recent study showed that a firm mattress is probably better for your back.

Q. *Someone told me that bucket seats were not good for people with backaches. What do you say about that?*

A. Certainly a number of people with or without backache find bucket seats uncomfortable. This is due to the fact that the classic bucket seats have nothing in the way of lumbar support. Based on the principle that lumbar support is desirable, the idea of a bucket seat comes up short. If you have a back problem and are considering a new car, you shouldn't buy one with bucket seats unless they have distinctly comfortable lumbar support. However, if you have been riding or driving in a bucket seat for an extended period of time and it does not interfere with your back or cause you backache, then the thing speaks for itself—but you are the exception. Many stores offer high-quality lumbar supports that are readily transferable to a variety of motor vehicles.

Q. *Does wearing high-heeled shoes hurt my back?*

A. Wearing high heels tends to shift the back into a slightly swaybacked position. Traditionally, we have thought that high heels aggravate backaches, and maybe they do. A recent study showed that high heels up to 4.5 centimeters, or 1¾ inches, do not increase or cause a swayback position. If wearing high heels definitely does not increase your backache, then go for it. If it does, I usually recommend wearing the shoes for shorter periods, which may give you a tolerable pain range.

Q. *How do I know if I'm going to have another attack of pain?*

A. Your doctor can best answer this, but, in general, there is a tendency for recurrence. Statistics show that about 60 percent of patients with acute, incapacitating low back pain are likely to have another attack within two years.

Q. *Every time I glance at a magazine or newspaper, I see an article about some new breakthrough or cure for back pain. I'm confused. How do I know what to believe? What sort of treatment should I spend my money on?*

A. Consider all advertising claims of great medical advances with the greatest skepticism. News reports of medical events merit interest and follow-up inquiries, but don't believe everything you read or hear right away. Ask your doctor about these different "cures." Don't blame him/her if he/she is prudent and doesn't immediately try out the latest vogue. The new devices and treatments you hear about are usually in the experimental stage, at best—or, at worst, aren't even solid enough to reach the experimental stage. It generally takes years for a new cure to prove itself to be better than the placebo effect and the self-limiting characteristics of the problem.

    When treatments are cheap, noninvasive, and said to be risk free, it makes sense to try some of them. But do so under your doctor's supervision.

Q. *What is your opinion about stretching exercises?*

A. Well, first of all, virtually any exercise is good for you if it doesn't hurt your back. But stretching exercises sometimes *do* hurt your back, and for patients who experience pain, they should be discontinued. These are usually patients with new, intense backache associated with severe sciatica.

    The theory of the stretching exercise is that it loosens up the ligaments in the back part of the spine, as well as tight hamstrings, making it easier to carry the spine in a straighter position, as opposed to a swayback position. This is a reasonable hypothesis and is adequate to justify the inclusion of stretching exercises in an exercise program—provided they are not irritating.

Q. *I've got sciatica, and when it's necessary to bend over to put on or tie my shoes, my leg hurts. Can I do anything about that?*

A. Ida Rolf, an organic chemist, began practicing "connective tissue therapy" in the 1940s. It's a very vigorous, even painful sort of muscular manipulation. The technique is supposed to reorder the muscles and the connecting myofascia, realigning them with gravity and thus achieving better balance. Like any other treatment, Rolfing has succeeded most with people who believe in it religiously. In my opinion, Rolfing's premise is unsound. It's an unscientific, nonmedical treatment unlikely to have any value beyond the laying-on-of-hands and placebo effect. I don't recommend it.

Q. *How would you compare the relative efficacy of transcutaneous electrical nerve stimulation (TENS) with that of acupuncture in relieving low back pain?*

A. Most likely the mechanism for the two forms of treatment is similar. That is, it works through some combination of counterstimulation, closing the "gate" for the reception of pain signals and stimulation of endorphins.

A study comparing the two methods of treatment showed a significant amount of pain reduction (about 33 percent) with both techniques. This reduction of pain was achieved in a majority of the patients (75 percent) treated with acupuncture and slightly fewer (66 percent) in those treated by electrical stimulation. Volunteers treated with acupuncture apparently enjoyed more prolonged pain relief. The average was forty hours with acupuncture and twenty-three hours with electrical stimulation. But these differences are not significant when analyzed statistically.

This particular study did not evaluate the usefulness of acupuncture supplemented by a small electrical current running through the acupuncture needle. That technique may or may not be superior.

Q. *Should I wear a lift in my shoe?*

A. Of course, if it helps—assuming that one of your legs is longer than the other. While it's controversial as to whether or not a leg-length discrepancy causes backache, it may nevertheless make you comfortable to correct it. Test the situation by having a shoe repairman do a crude adjustment on an old pair of shoes. Leg-length difference as a cause of back pain is by no means as common as some practitioners would suggest.

Q. *What do you think of DMSO for back pain?*

A. *DMSO* is an abbreviation for dimethyl sulfoxide, a substance that has been used in animal treatment for many years. More recently, it's been used to treat various human musculoskeletal disorders, especially arthritis. Athletes have used it for muscle, tendon, and joint pain. Its believers claim that it can decrease inflammation, ease pain, and speed the healing of musculoskeletal conditions. But so far, there's no proof.

When you put it on your skin, DMSO is absorbed into the bloodstream and transmitted throughout the body. This makes for some problems. Its ease of absorption raises the probability of toxicity. You can have a severe allergic reaction to it. Possible side effects include visual disturbances, headache, nausea, diarrhea, and dermatitis (pain, irritation, or itching of the skin). It has caused cancer in some animals.

In my opinion, DMSO's possible, unsubstantiated benefits for pain and arthritis don't outweigh its risks. In short, it probably shouldn't be used for backache, as there are safer methods for gaining relief.

Q. *What about gravity boots?*

A. This is a technique that involves turning the patient upside down— that is, in the vertical position, with the head down and the feet up (in boots). This has been a virtual fad among back pain sufferers. Unfortunately, the benefit is unproven; moreover, there are risks of its causing sudden increases in blood pressure as well as heart rate. The nerves in the region of your ankles can be irritated or damaged by the boots. There is also a significant risk of its causing bleeding in the back of the eye, the medical term being retinal hemorrhage.

Surgery

Q. *How do I know when I should have surgery?*

A. For the sake of this discussion, I'm assuming that you have severe low back pain with or without sciatica, and that you're considering surgery for pain relief, rather than to make a diagnosis, biopsy a tumor, or treat a tumor or infection. The recommended surgery, in your case, is probably a laminectomy with disc removal and/or fusion. Or the surgery under consideration may be a fusion needed to treat spondylolisthesis (a slipped vertebra).

First make sure that you're under the care of a spinal specialist and that you've given conservative treatment a fair try. This means two to three days' bed rest and analgesic medication and a reasonable period of some combination of physical therapy, traction, rest, and medication. A "reasonable period" means six to eight weeks for disc surgery and generally three to six months before a spinal fusion, at least. Then your doctor must have diagnosed a genuine abnormality, and you should have a positive myelogram, CT scan, or MRI before surgery if it's for disc disease, or X-ray evidence of spondylolisthesis if it's for that problem.

Anesthesia, surgery, and hospitalization carry certain inevitable risks. To justify them, your pain should be severe, incapacitating, and compromising to your quality of life (see chapter 7 for a more detailed account). Every patient is different, and there are situations in which you may elect to have surgery before two or three months are up. Ultimately the decision rests with you. If you're confused, get a second opinion.

Q. *What about my second, third, or fourth back operation?*

A. I suggest that you get a second opinion for a second operation, a third opinion for a third operation, and a fourth opinion for a fourth operation. If you get unanimity, you may be on the right track. If you don't get unanimity, you may need a tiebreaker opinion. This is a little bit facetious, but the point is, if you're having multiple back operations, you should (if you do it at all) do it with extensive consultation. The second, third, or fourth spine operation is rarely—I repeat, rarely—successful in relieving the pain and returning the patient to work.

Make sure that your doctors have made one or more specific diagnoses. X-rays and possibly EMG (electromyography) studies should probably be done. Your doctors should be able to clearly explain what is wrong and convince you it's surgically correctable.

You must accept the fact that a second operation may not help you or may even make you worse (though the odds are still slightly in your favor). Your chances of getting better with a third operation are about fifty-fifty, and they're lower with a fourth. Don't *ever* allow yourself to have multiple operations for compensation or legal reasons.

I don't mean to sound too discouraging. In some rare circumstances, a person can benefit from a second or third operation (see chapter 7). I even know a prominent orthopedic surgeon who benefited from a *fourth*. However, the message is: Be very hesitant about that second, third, or fourth operation.

Q. *Will I be completely cured by surgery?*

A. Surgical cures for back pain are generally presented in terms of success, or in terms of good and excellent results. The percentages we have discussed throughout the book are the probability of a good or an excellent result. I generally tell patients this translates into their satisfaction and their opinion that it was worth it all to go through the experience. As we discussed in chapter 7, surgery when indicated results in a more rapid recovery from disc herniation. But if you can tolerate the pain, you may do just fine without surgery.

I also like to remind patients that they won't have a new back or a perfect spine, and they may not be quite as good as they were before they had a problem.

Q. *How much of the disc do you take out?*

A. Most surgeons do not remove the entire disc, nor do they attempt it. Our practice is to remove the offending part of the disc and a margin beyond that. This usually means taking all of the extruded part of the disc and perhaps 20 percent of the remainder. This is a good compromise in terms of maintaining some mechanical integrity of the functional spine unit, avoiding any complications that could occur should one rigorously attempt to remove the entire disc, and removing enough to minimize the likelihood of material within the disc subsequently herniating. We also make a point to carefully remove all loose material inside the disc space.

Q. *Will my back collapse if you take out my disc?*

A. Sometimes with an attempt at a total discectomy, there is some collapse of the interspace. Also, disc degeneration and partial removal of the disc can sometimes result in some narrowing of the disc space. This in and of itself is not a problem.

Sometimes this question is evoked by the patient's worry that the unseparated vertebral bodies will scrape together after the disc is removed. This is not something to be concerned about. Even if there is some collapse, there is not necessarily a problem with the bones scraping together.

Sometimes, however, in association with mechanical changes, disc degeneration, and/or disc removal, changes occur in the facet joints. When this occurs, it may be arthritis, and there may be pain and difficulty.

On rare occasions, a spinal fusion is required some years after partial removal of a herniated disc. This problem can also develop without associated surgical disc removal.

Q. *Can I give my own blood before surgery?*
A. Yes. Most major hospitals do have programs that allow patients to donate their own blood for transfusion. If for any reason this does not work (the blood is not available, there are administrative problems, the timing is inappropriate, and so on), consider this: Although it is more of a risk than autotransfusion, we believe it is in your best interest to sign a release allowing your doctors to give you a transfusion from a donor if they deem it necessary. Nevertheless, it is preferable to avoid the potential exposure to diseases that can be transmitted through transfusion, even with the careful screening methods that have been in place since the 1990s.

Q. *How big will my incision be?*
A. "Just right!"

I am glad you asked that question, because I think it is an important one, and this answer should be helpful to you. The cosmetic aspect of back surgery is very important to many individuals. No one *wants* to have any scars on his/her body. Let me attempt to put this in some perspective.

The size of the incision is not a reliable measure of the seriousness, danger, extent, efficacy, or desirability of any particular operation. I believe that patients, as a result of some medical marketing, perhaps, put too much emphasis on the length of an incision. However, advancing technology and instrumentation have allowed surgery to be performed through smaller incisions. As discussed in chapters 6 and 7, there must be adequate exposure to achieve the objective of the surgery while protecting the neural elements and surrounding anatomic structures as well as controlling any bleeding.

It's quite possible to perform a huge, lousy, and ineffective operation through a rather small incision. Conversely, it is possible to do a neat, safe, and quite effective operation through a very large incision. Clearly the least amount of incision that is compatible with a safe and effective operation is desirable. However, one should never compromise an operation in any way in order to have a smaller incision.

Now let's return to the issue of cosmetics. A vertical, well-centered, midline incision in the lumbar spine is not at all cosmetically offensive. The other important issues in cosmesis of an incision are the type of suture that is used and the techniques that are used for closure. Generally, where cosmesis is of major importance, the surgeon attempts to avoid crosshatching scars from sutures. Ask your surgeon about a *subcuticular closure* (where sutures are not visable) if cosmesis is important to you.

Q. *What about this microdiscectomy procedure? The one where they claim it is possible to take out your disc through a one-inch incision?*

A. It is true that this procedure involves less surgery than the usual laminectomy for disc excision. Microdiscectomy has become the gold standard for a single disc herniation. Multiple herniations or multilevel spinal stenosis must be performed through a larger incision. Again, it must be sufficient to get the job done.

If you have a very specific kind of disc problem—that is, one where there is a clear-cut displaced fragment of disc that is lying in just the right place so that the nerves can be moved out of the way and the disc can be removed easily—then the positives of this procedure may outweigh the negatives.

On the other hand, if we have the more common situation where the offending pathology is slightly up, down, or to one side or the other, only part or none of the offending disc can be removed through this limited access. The incision would then have to be extended. This is one of the examples where a percutaneous, endoscopic, or laser procedure would not be successful.

Q. *If I have a spinal fusion, will it interfere with my lovemaking?*

A. The answer is yes and no. A mobile lumbar spine definitely contributes to the pelvic motions in sex, just as in dancing. You'll be only minimally compromised if your fusion involves just one motion segment—that is, two vertebrae fused together. Perhaps if two levels—two segments of functional spinal units—are fused, you'll experience some limitation. But we're speaking of a trade-off. The issue is not the pelvic motion of a fused back versus that of a normal back; the comparison is between a disabled, painful back and a fused back. So there's likely to be a net benefit if one is trading some loss of motion for relief from severe pain. Discuss this issue with your surgeon before your operation.

Postsurgical Care

Q. *In terms of my physical activity, will I be able to do as much—or even more—than prior to surgery?*

A. We always attempt to rehabilitate our patients back to whatever level of activity they desire. A careful rehabilitation program after successful surgery can get people to very high levels of achievement: witness Joe Montana, National Football League quarterback and Super Bowl champion, following lumbar spine disc surgery. Sometimes, though, the gradual rehabilitation process does not get patients up to the level they had hoped for. Nevertheless, the patient whose outcome is successful can do a great deal more than before the surgery and is often able to find an appropriate level of activity. Consult your physician if you have questions.

Q. *When can I take a shower after my back operation?*

A. Unless there is some complication with your incision, you may shower on the tenth postoperative day, provided that you are able to walk in the shower, balance, stand, and so forth.

Social and Psychological Issues

Q. *How do I know when to go back to work after an acute pain attack?*

A. This is a complex question, and you'll find a more detailed answer in chapter 5. The bottom line is to rely on your doctor's advice. Remember, too, that while you need to protect yourself and your earning power, you don't want to turn into a chronic "compensation-itis" sufferer. It's certainly best for your overall quality of life to prevent chronic disability and long-term pain. Let your disease process, and nothing else, dictate your work activities. However, recent programs being developed in Sweden advocate the concept that getting back to work can be therapeutic for the back pain patient.

Q. *What should I do if my doctor tells me my pain is all in my head?*

A. Psychiatrists tell us we shouldn't tell you your pain is all in your head even if we think so, since this tends to make patients angry, resentful, and uncooperative. When someone is told his pain is imaginary, he may go about consciously or unconsciously trying to prove it's real. This makes the pain more deeply ingrained and harder to dislodge. Then, of course, we may be wrong. In any case, we shouldn't operate on you when we think your pain is psychological.

There's a difference between having your pain strictly in your head and having your backache *affected* by what is going on in your head. What is occurring in your life, on the job, and in your family can certain aggravate a backache.

If your doctor says that your pain is psychological, don't feel ashamed. Realize that emotional problems, especially in our stressful society, are every bit as painful and as noble as a broken leg. There are numerous medical channels for getting emotional support. You may wish to schedule a consultation with a psychiatrist—and with another orthopedist as well. Try to avoid getting angry and to remain cooperative, as ninety-nine times out of a hundred your doctors are truly dedicated to helping you.

Q. *How do I know if the pain is in my head?*

A. Some pain is imaginary, and some pain is stimulated or made worse by tension, sleep deprivation, and morning lethargy. If pain comes on when you're frightened, guilty, angry, stressed, or tense, it may be to some extent psychological. Such pains are often subconscious, and it's difficult to recognize their pattern. Does your pain, for example, gain you more attention from your family, or let you avoid certain things like household chores, work responsibilities, sexual commitments, and so on?

Several psychological tests are designed to detect the psychological roots of a pain syndrome. The Minnesota Multiphasic Personality Inventory (MMPI) is perhaps the most common psychological screening test. A wealth of experience and data back up its accuracy. It provides a personality profile that may reveal evidence of depression, hysteria, or hypochondriasis, which is the tendency to focus on or exaggerate physical complaints. There are also many other psychological tests, such as the Mini-Mult (a short version of the MMPI), the Middlesex Hospital Questionnaire (MHQ), and the Cornell Medical Index (CMI). Much can be deciphered from the way you describe your pain, your choice of words, and the overall content.

Of course, any pain has some psychological components, and some of them are helpful. Beneficial psychological factors may include a particular philosophical outlook, religion, mysticism, autohypnosis, and the conscious utilization of the new science of endorphins, the natural painkillers produced by your central nervous system.

Undesirable psychological factors are depression, guilt, hostility, and anxiety. These are negative in themselves; moreover, they tend to aggravate and prolong back pain.

A final option is psychology or psychiatry. A skilled psychiatrist can offer an opinion about the role of psychological factors in your pain. Psychological conditions should be treated and stabilized prior to proceeding with any non-emergent surgery.

Q. *Is there too much surgery done for backache?*

A. That's a tough question. Let's examine some figures. In Canada and the United States, 760 people out of 1 million undergo disc surgery annually, compared with 125 per 1 million in Sweden and 110 per 1 million in Great Britain. In South Africa, 360 per 1 million whites have back surgery each year, but only 0.5 per 1 million blacks. These numbers raise some interesting medical, social, economic, and political speculations.

It appears that in countries with socialized medicine, perhaps too few back operations are performed, and too many in countries where there's a fee involved. Then, too, cultural demands and expectations of bodily comfort may be higher in North America than in Sweden or Britain, and U.S. and Canadian patients may demand more aggressive treatment. Medical care is more readily available in some countries than in others. There are waiting lists for elective surgery in countries with socialized medicine, such as Britain and Sweden—and South African blacks, it would appear, are virtually excluded from elective back surgery.

Since back surgery is elective and intended to improve quality of life, it's a subjective matter, making it difficult to say how much pain is enough to warrant surgery. But if you follow this book's suggestions, you needn't worry about having unnecessary surgery.

Q. *If I have a fresh, severe low back problem with or without sciatic pain (leg pain), will an orgasmic experience irritate the situation in any way or will it cause any harm or be painful?*

A. No, it will not irritate the situation. It will not cause any harm and it will not be painful. The physical activity involved in the process of achieving an orgasm may cause pain and irritate your back. But the orgasm itself is without liability. See chapter 8 for ways to avoid irritating your back while making love.

Doctors and Therapists

Q. *Can non-MD practitioners, such as osteopaths, chiropractors, acupuncturists, herbalists, or faith healers, help my back problem?*

A. Some of this is covered elsewhere in the text, but let me review some of the principles.

Now, we know that the placebo effect can crop up in connection with any treatment. And the natural course of acute back disease is such that 90 percent of patients will be better within two months. So, say that you go to an herbalist, faith healer, or some other practitioner and get well during that period. You may believe the healer performed the miracle. Maybe he or she did, but obviously you had a 90 percent chance of getting well on your own within eight weeks.

But let's not neglect psychology. Whatever his/her background, training, and tools, any practitioner can potentially use his/her personality to make you feel better. This is especially true when your major problem is pain. Anyone who exudes warmth, concern, confidence, and a positive attitude will inspire faith in the afflicted person, and this alone can ease pain.

Naturally, I can't write without bias, given my training and experience in science-based Western medicine. I think a good, well-trained MD can offer you treatment founded on solid science and adequate diagnostic and treatment procedures. This protects you from being inappropriately treated for the wrong disease while your real disease gets worse, possibly even endangering your life.

The liability of a nonmedical healer is the possibility that he or she will do more harm than good by misdiagnosis. The "quack" isn't just a figment of the American Medical Association's imagination. There are real-life con artists in the health profession, as in any other, and the stereotypical used-car dealer doesn't just turn up around defective Chevys and Cadillacs. You can waste time and money—as well as your health—on ineffective treatments.

Chiropractors come good and bad, careful and careless. Some are ethical, some aren't. However, there's no scientific basis whatsoever for the theory that all diseases emanate from *subluxations* of the vertebrae (see the next question).

Now for specifics. (See chapter 6 for more details.)

1. *Spinal manipulation,* practiced by chiropractors, is a legitimate form of symptomatic treatment for certain appropriately diagnosed spinal conditions. When done carefully, it can temporarily relieve pain, although its benefit hasn't been proven to outdo the combined benefits of the placebo effect and natural healing. Of course, the same is true of most conservative back treatments. But for some patients, chiropractic treatment is inappropriate, even dangerous. Don't stick with it for long periods if you're not getting any prolonged, objective pain relief.

2. *Acupuncture* can treat idiopathic low back pain (pain not linked to a specific disease process) without risk. Again, though, it makes no sense to continue acupuncture for long if it's not helping. A well-controlled 1983 clinical study showed the results to be the same as with a placebo. At that time there were seven high-quality studies in the medical literature. Two of the studies showed acupuncture to be superior to the placebo; in the remaining five there was no difference.

3. *Herbal therapy* raises the same points. A qualified physician should check your back first. If your herbalist is careful, your risks are very

minor. But whenever you're introducing substances into your body, you can run into complications. You should advise your doctor of any substance that is being taken. Always inform your physician of any herbal remedies or vitamin/mineral supplements that you may be taking: They can interfere with the action of prescription medications. Furthermore, none of these products are regulated by the FDA, so you don't know how much of the active substance is in each bottle.

4. *Faith healing,* again, shouldn't replace medical diagnosis. As long as you're not spending exorbitant sums, spiritual help is probably good for you.

Q. *What is subluxation? What is chiropractic adjustment?*

A. *Subluxation* can be defined as partial dislocation, a situation in which X-rays allegedly show an abnormal positioning between two adjacent vertebrae. The displacement must reach a certain point before it's called a subluxation. It may or may not cause pain. The subluxation that the chiropractor refers to cannot be seen by independent observers. This has been one of the field's major problems.

In chiropractic manipulation, the vertebrae are supposedly manipulated back into their normal position. The chiropractic hypothesis is that as a vertebra slips out again, you have pain, and it must be put back once more. This process can go on ad infinitum, and manipulations are sometimes sold in prepaid packages of a certain number.

What bothers me is this: If a vertebra is simply pushed back into place, why assume it will stay there? And why would continually pushing it back *ever* make it "stick"? It's awfully tempting to suppose that the treatment's "success" is related to the placebo effect and/or the natural course of the ailment. Although the pain probably was never related to subluxation in the first place, manipulation gets the credit for relieving it.

You may have heard the story of the man who comes in hunched over with terrible pain and muscle spasms, then has a spinal manipulation and walks away from the table standing erect and feeling wonderful. No doubt such phenomena occur, but just about any sort of practitioner using his/her favorite "treatment" can relate similar tales.

Obviously, we're looking at a complex psychophysiological problem that responds dramatically to what we dub the "placebo effect." This is the mystery and misery of low back pain.

Q. *What kind of doctor should take care of my back? When do I need a consultant or a specialist?*

A. It's a good idea to start with a general practitioner, family medicine doctor, or internist who has known you and your family for a few years. But it's not the only way to go. Group practices and health care organizations are viable alternatives.

If you have back pain associated with leg pain, go to your family, your doctor, your internist, your health care clinic, or a spine care specialty facility. They will take a medical history, examine you, and manage your ensuing workup and treatment. Most back pain is the idiopathic type, and analgesia, rest, and various forms of physical therapy are considered the best prescription.

If you haven't improved after three to six weeks of the above regimen, you may want to see a specialist. I'd recommend a board-certified orthopedic surgeon or neurosurgeon. The choice between the two is largely dictated by convenience and your own gut feelings about a particular doctor.

It's fair to say that orthopedic surgeons are generally more knowledgeable about the conservative care of spinal problems. Their training includes more attention to the mechanical, structural, architectural, and intervertebral joint factors related to the spine. However, a particular doctor's knowledge, experience, and manner are more important than his/her specialty.

Miscellaneous

Q. *Will disco, social, or ballroom dancing give me a backache?*

A. Let's start with disco, the most vigorous—and the sort most often done by untrained, occasional dancers. Twisting and jerking motions, and arching of the back, often irritate low back pain. The high heels that women often wear for ballroom dancing may also hurt the back.

If you don't have back pain while dancing, go ahead and enjoy. Nature is helpful. If you hurt a little, slow down or stop. When you feel better, gradually work back into it, staying in good condition and pacing yourself. Sometimes, though, your back won't warn you. Also, we know that a few drinks not only loosen up social inhibitions but may reduce the protective mechanisms of the muscles that support the spine. There's also a "morning-after" type of backache you can learn to avoid by pacing yourself during the midnight hours.

Q. *Can my problem recur?*

A. This patient is usually asking about a herniated disc, and the answer, of course, is that it *can* recur. It can happen at a new level or at the same level. The latter is very unlikely but nevertheless possible. Generally, when that occurs, it is managed as if it were a fresh disc herniation.

It is probably also reasonable to assume that, all other things being equal, a patient who has had one disc herniation is a little more likely than average to suffer a new or recurrent disc problem.

Q. *How much does everything you've said about backache apply to neck ache?*

A. A great deal. It's much the same, except that there are fewer visceral (internal-organ) diseases that cause neck pain, and its overall prevalence is lower. Since we know less about the biomechanics and ergonomics of neck pain, we have less advice to offer about its management.

Neck (cervical) disc surgery is similar to back disc surgery, although it's generally done from the front and more often calls for a fusion. We don't see as many totally disabled neck pain patients. For some reason, in this society, the work environment especially fosters back pain, although half of all people with work-related backache have neck pain too. Your posture while reading, writing, or working at a computer can mean a pain in the neck, as can tension and anxiety. Neck pain gained considerable attention and notoriety in the medicolegal field with the phenomenon of whiplash, which, fortunately, has been reduced by an increase in the use of car headrests.

Treatment of neck ache, like treatment of backache, should first exhaust the reasonable steps of conservative therapy. It calls for surgery only in specific correctable situations.

Q. *What does it feel like to wear a brace?*

A. Braces vary. Some immobilize and encumber the patient more than others. Some cover just the middle part of the body, from the pelvis to the rib cage. Others extend from the nipple line down one leg to the knees. Usually, a large hole is cut or it is contoured to allow your abdomen to expand.

Most patients have no problem with a cast. But some adults have trouble adjusting to its constraints. They may have anxiety or frustration or may simply be very annoyed that they must wear it. If this is the case with you, discuss it with your doctor beforehand and during the casting period. Even those who don't like casts generally manage to adapt with some support from doctors, nurses, friends, and relatives. If you're in a body cast and start vomiting repeatedly, get in touch with your doctor immediately. It may be a sign of intestinal problems caused by the cast (see chapter 6).

Q. *What is Stoshak-Mortimer syndrome? Perhaps you know of it as "jean-seam coccygodynia."*

A. This is a rather unusual medical condition in which someone, most likely a teenage girl, presents with low back pain. On careful questioning, the pain is localized mainly or in part at the coccyx, or tailbone (see figure 2.1). The patient is likely to be wearing tight-fitting jeans with a hard, reinforced midline seam and sitting in a fairly hard seat at school. The solution is not to take a vacation from school but from the jeans. The pain will disappear in two to three weeks.

Q. *Is back pain hereditary?*

A. This question usually comes from a patient with a herniated disc. There has been some recent evidence that perhaps within some families there is a higher-than-expected prevalence of disc herniation. This has not yet been precisely documented and proven, but should be considered a possibility at this point.

Q. *The doctor told me I had two or three degenerated discs. Does this mean my whole spine will degenerate?*

A. The appropriate medical term for changes within a disc is *degeneration*. Unfortunately, this carries rather threatening connotations. I like to point out to patients that as bad as the word sounds, disc degeneration is a natural process that occurs between ages thirty and fifty and is like the wrinkling of our skin and the graying of our hair.

It is the case that in this degenerative process, some discs will herniate and some others will become painful without herniating.

In answer to your question, though, having been told that you have two or three degenerating discs is no reason to be alarmed that your whole spine is going to become diseased, painful, and in need of a great deal of treatment.

CHAPTER 11

The Future of Back Care

Some Predictions, Speculations, and Hopes

IF YOU'RE BATTLING CHRONIC BACKACHE, YOU PROBABLY wonder how the future will deal with man's most important non-life-threatening ailment. Will backache one day be wiped out like smallpox or bubonic plaque? Or will we merely get more adept at diagnosing and treating it? Will our diagnostic tests and surgical procedures become less painful or risky? Will epidemiologists be able to predict—with the statistical accuracy of, say, cereal manufacturers pinpointing their markets—exactly who's at risk, and why? Will spine consultants tell us precisely how to revamp our lifestyles to spare our backs?

The predictions you'll read here are conservative, and may seem less than earthshaking to the uninitiated. On the other hand, anyone intimate with the puzzles of idiopathic back pain—and if you've read this whole book, you're included—may find the projections overly optimistic, even fantastic. Yet, I believe that most of the following forecasts will come true in your lifetime.

Epidemiology

Epidemiology is the study of the incidence of a disease in a particular population, with reference to recognizing the cause of the disease. The population is usually characterized according to age, sex, occupation, race, religion, geography, and socioeconomic standing.

- There will be more studies of the role of vibrations as a cause of disc herniation. We will learn more about why certain cars may be causing disc problems.

- One thing we have neglected up to now are studies to determine what sort of person is *unlikely* to develop serious back problems, and I think before long we'll have that demographic portrait. When we do, the rest of us may learn to imitate these backache-free types by simulating the way they live and work.
- Being in shape may prove to be one of the factors that characterize those who are unlikely to develop serious back pain.
- Evidence-based medicine will allow for a more strict definition of the type and quality of data that are being reviewed. As a result, well-designed studies in improved collaboration across international lines will allow us to address both local and global questions as we seek to develop "best practices" and treatment guidelines.

Emotions, Psychology, Socioeconomics

You've learned that your state of mind is intricately intertwined with the state of your back.

- We can look forward to more accurate psychological tests to gauge which people could benefit most from counseling or psychotherapy, and which would be better off with another form of treatment, such as medication or exercise. We'll learn even more accurately to identify patients who are likely to be helped by surgery.
- Stress, depression, and other mental states affect your body's physiology and biochemistry. As we refine our understanding of exactly how your altered biochemistry changes your spine's mechanical behavior so as to cause pain, we'll learn to protect against or even undo the damage.
- Your brain and central nervous system can produce and respond to chemicals that modify your perception of pain. Specifically, we know that our bodies produce internal opiates, called endorphins, that block pain. They aren't the only naturally produced pain-modifying "drugs" in our bodies. As we explore the biochemistry of pain, we'll be able to unlock the body's pain mechanisms. With the current knowledge explosion in the field of endorphins and related substances, we'll almost certainly develop new methods of stimulating their secretion.
- We know that psychological factors in the workplace may affect the prevalence of low back pain problems. Future studies will identify these

factors more clearly. We will discover methods and techniques for improving the psychological environment of the workplace.

- Physicians and therapists will have more psychologically based skills and methods designed to motivate, engender cooperation from, and therefore provide better results for our patients. Behavioral psychologists will help to provide the new knowledge for these skills.

- This issue may be too complex to handle succinctly here, but here is a try, as I believe that it will be useful to present it: There is considerable evidence that compensation laws—among other things, of course—play a significant role in the clinical problem of low back pain. I *am not* addressing the topic of malingering. True malingering, in my opinion, is very rare. However, there is evidence that some compensation laws and some policies and practices tend to perpetuate pain and pain behavior. These laws and practices will be revisited first in Sweden, with the goal of improving them so that they are fair to the back pain sufferer as well as just and appropriate for the overall society. At present, there is a great deal of human suffering and disability, as well as health care and administrative costs, all of which could be significantly reduced if the laws and practices could be justly improved. We may witness some serious attempts at this in the not-so-distant future.

- We are learning more about the brain. With the advent of positron emission tomography (PET), we may learn more about the psychological and psychosocial aspects of pain. A PET scan is a nuclear imaging medical modality that can provide real-time three-dimensional images of functioning organs, including the brain. It allows for an assessment of real-time functional or metabolic/chemical changes following a specific stimulus. It is also used to assess for evidence of disease such as seizure disorders, inflammatory diseases, and cancer.

Medication

- I predict we'll see safer and more effective drugs to combat stress and improve our moods. These futuristic drugs may enable us to nip many a backache in the bud.

- New drugs will fight inflammation—or the tissues' response to it—better than current anti-inflammatory drugs.

Muscles, Fascia, Discs

- Future studies and refinements of MRI techniques will help us to recognize when back pain is due to muscle and/or fascia injury or disease. The clinical science of various painful muscle fascia and tendon conditions will be discovered and described. The elusive and protean problem of muscle spasm will be analyzed.

  The clinical science of muscle development, strengthening, and conditioning, and the quantitative monitoring of muscle function, will be greatly advanced. The therapeutic benefit of muscle rehabilitation for low back pain will be more clearly delineated.

  I also look forward to being able to distinguish scientifically and clinically between actively painful discs and those that are simply wearing out.

- Not all herniated discs are painful. When we learn why some are and some aren't, we will better delineate how, when, where, and why some cause inflammation and/or pain and others do not.

Biomechanics

Biomechanics are crucial to your back. No matter what your back disease, properly controlled biomechanics can minimize pain, while improper biomechanics can aggravate it. Much future progress lies in the study of "the B and the B of the IVD"—that is, the biochemistry and biomechanics of the intervertebral disc.

- New information will permit us to improve the mechanics of work and play so as to cut down on spinal stresses and prevent injury. Back pain schools will become more numerous and effective, back care information more accurate and better disseminated.

- Disease prevention courses will enter our school systems; students will learn the rudiments of back protection. Medical students will be taught more about back pain and encouraged to do spine research.

- In industry, tests of body strength and body mechanics will match workers with appropriate jobs and protect them from spine-endangering tasks. These and other screening tests will be used to instruct employees in back-saving precautions. Employers will design workplaces to minimize back stress and injury. For example, the design and selection of seats will be based on back protection first, and only secondly on aesthetics. (These two are *not* mutually exclusive.) It has been shown that appropriate design in the workplace can prevent one-third of compensable low back injuries. Equipment in the working and/or lifting areas will be constructed to the proper height to limit bending. In my opinion, no new work environment should be built without informed and thorough consideration of the biomechanics involved in protecting the back. On-the-job information and exercise programs will emphasize general conditioning and back care.

- And what about conditions on the home front? The future will transform design there as well. We'll institute painless vacuuming methods and special exercise and back care programs for home workers. Cleaning and upkeep of floors, furniture, beds, and clothes will be revamped to minimize back strain.

- New designs in automobile seats and suspension will attenuate the *bump-bump-bump* punishment to your back. The future consumer will choose a new car as much on the basis of *vibes* per mile as on miles per gallon. New seat designs will also enhance public transportation vehicles and airplanes.

- Improvements in athletic equipment, coaching, and training techniques, and, yes, maybe even rule changes—with tradition deferring to human health—will benefit athletes' backs.

- The problem of spinal instability as we have traditionally looked at it will change radically during the next decade. One or more mechanical derangements of the spine—which can be recognized and reasonably correlated with back pain—will be discovered. Percutaneous transpedicular immobilization of the spine as a means of identifying spinal instability will be further developed and will help us to better understand this clinical problem.

- The answer to developing an effective motion-preserving device (for example, the artificial disc) lies here. The basic principle is this: Until a man-made disc is able to re-create physiologic kinematics (basically, function the way the normal spinal segment does), the implants' efficacy will be limited.

Biochemistry

The analysis of the spine's structure ultimately leads us all the way down to the chemical molecules that make up our anatomy. The intervertebral disc and cartilage, for example, are composed mainly of water, collagen, and proteoglycans (cartilage). Bone is made up of collagen and calcified hydroxyapatite crystals. The physiology and nutrition of the disc, and its water content, probably have a lot to do with backache.

- We'll learn about the normal and abnormal chemical makeup of the disc and facet joints. Circulatory, nutritional, and hormonal changes can affect the disc's biochemistry, causing pain. We know, for example, that pregnancy and menstruation often aggravate backache, probably via biochemical changes.
- Clearly, stress can provoke or worsen back pain. The following excerpt from a letter from a back patient who is also an orthopedic surgeon illustrates the delicate interplay between psychological trauma and disc disease:

> I had two episodes of moderately severe low back pain . . . and muscle spasm with no sciatica, each of which lasted about four or five days. The episodes were severe enough to make me miss work and required me to be recumbent . . . The first episode occurred about the time I was to take my Orthopaedic Boards in September of 1978. The second episode, which was practically identical to the first, occurred just over a year later at a time of major personal stress within my family . . . In the summer of 1980, I separated from the Air Force . . . and returned to my hometown of Little Rock, Arkansas, where I went into the private practice of orthopaedics. The week before I started in my new position [I developed a fresh case of severe backache].

The future will most likely *prove* that stress, such as this young doctor suffered, does indeed contribute to back pain. New medication to prevent or reverse the stress process will come to our aid.

- Smoking and prolonged riding or driving in cars, trucks, or buses, epidemiologists say, can spell backache. We have learned that nicotine or road vibrations change the spine's circulation and blood supply, hampering disc nutrition.

- Several important breakthroughs in disc biochemistry may revolutionize our understanding of disc disease. Our improved understanding of the human genome, gene expression, genetically engineered medicines, and stem cell research may bring forth the ability to repair, restore, and perhaps prevent damage to the spine. We have already begun to define the biochemical irritants in the disc that cause nerve irritation and pain. This leads us directly into the neurology of low back pain.

Nerves and Pain

The extremely complex and sophisticated science of neurophysiology has not yet told us much about backache.

- Future research is likely to identify just which nerves are transmitting pain in the back, and why. What is it that starts the chain of events that stimulates a nerve ending, and goes to the spinal cord, and the brain, to culminate in the brain's reasoning cortex saying to itself, "My back hurts"? Is it a push, a pull, a squeeze, a shear force, a chemical, an electrical charge, too little oxygen, too much acid—or what? We'll find out whether it takes place in the disc, muscle, facet joints, bone, or cartilage, or at several sites.
- We'll also learn how to better manipulate the pain-control mechanisms of the brain and spinal cord, perhaps by regulating natural painkillers like endorphins. The upshot is that you may be trained in techniques to control your own pain without drugs.

Diagnostic Tests

- The imaging capabilities and techniques based on MRI and PET scans will improve, and biochemical labeling is likely to help in clinical evaluations.
- I also envision using more dynamic imaging tests—that is, tests that image the spine in different positions with different stresses.
- Improvements in electrical diagnostic nerve and muscle testing techniques will permit them to be used more effectively.

- The idea of a "trial" of fixation of two or more vertebrae in the low back to determine whether or not pain is eliminated may prove to be a useful procedure. If so, don't be put off by the fact that there will temporarily be metal inside the vertebral bone that extends out through the skin to the outside. Sounds dramatic, and it is, but it's also quite reasonable, provided that studies show it to be useful. The idea is that this technique can thoroughly fix the vertebrae, and if this reliably eliminates the pain, then a spinal fusion may benefit the patient. Bioabsorbable implants may change the face of this approach.

Treatment

- Advances in the selection, precision, and efficacy of many surgical treatments will help back sufferers. New percutaneous discectomy techniques and instrumentation techniques will be developed and utilized. We'll have new and different surgical methods for pain arising from the facet joints. Severe arthritis will be relieved with an internally implantable spinal prosthesis.
- Better painkillers and anti-inflammatory drugs will join our arsenal.
- Exercise and ergonomic programs will improve, and we will learn precisely which exercises are best. The equipment will be developed to guide and nurture these therapeutically appropriate exercises.
- Spinal manipulation won't stay in a "Who knows?" limbo. Scientific analysis will tell us unequivocally whether it works or not.

Of course, no progress will occur through natural evolution alone. All these advances depend on extensive research in several medical and scientific fields.

What can you do about it? You can, of course, contribute to a university, medical school, hospital, or researcher of your choice. Or you can use your influence in a corporation, insurance company, foundation, or labor union. *Advocate preventive programs in your sphere of influence.*

It's estimated that two billion people will have backache this year and that two million doctors will treat them. But only a small number of people on earth will be carefully researching back disease. We have a long way to go.

So ends the proselytizing part of this book. I hope you won't think a couple of brief paragraphs in support of your local back pain researcher too much of an imposition.

The Compensation Issue

There is a very serious, expensive, and complex game that's played in our society. The players are the patient (worker or professional), lawyer, doctor, employer, union, insurance company, and society. In any given game, there may be any combination of winners and losers. Unfortunately, the patient and society are often the losers. Our compensation laws, labor practices, employee policies, and insurance and legal systems all somehow work in such a way as to potentiate, foster, and perpetuate pain behavior and disability. In the future, our society will improve this current counterproductive situation in the following manner: A multidisciplinary panel of experts—economists, lawyers, clinicians, psychologists, psychiatrists, ethicists, labor leaders, and insurance and corporate leaders—will convene. The purpose will be to study the problem with the goal of rewriting the compensation laws so that justice is ensured to the individual back pain sufferer and to our society. It is possible to devise fair, humanitarian laws and practices that do not perpetuate illness or engender a great deal of nonproductive expenditure of time and money on the parts of doctors, lawyers, judges, therapists, insurance personnel, employers, and on and on.

Conclusion

If you have journeyed through this book from start to finish, thanks for staying with me. I sincerely hope that the information here has diminished your pain, frustration, and confusion, and enhanced your strength, optimism, determination, and ability to beat the backache and get on with your life!

Glossary*

AEROBIC EXERCISE: Any of a variety of sustained exercises, such as jogging or rowing, that stimulate and strengthen the heart and lungs, thereby improving the body's utilization of oxygen.

AIDS: Acquired immunodeficiency syndrome. A fatal viral infection in which the body's ability to combat infection and certain cancers is reduced to the point that the patient succumbs to one or both.

ANALGESIC: Pain-controlling medications such as Tylenol, aspirin, Darvon, Darvocet, Demerol, and codeine.

ANKYLOSING SPONDYLITIS: An inflammatory disease of the spine that causes pain and leads to bony ankylosis of the vertebral articulations.

ANNULUS: The tough outer fibrous portion of the intervertebral disc. (See figures 2.3 and 2.6b.)

ANTI-INFLAMMATORY: Drugs such as Feldene (piroxicam), Motrin (ibuprofen), Naprosyn (naproxen), and Voltaren (diclofenac sodium), to name a few, that tend to reduce swelling, inflammation, and pain.

ARACHNOIDITIS: Inflammatory disease leading to fibrosis that binds the roots of the cauda equina.

ARTHRITIS: Inflammation and irritation of the joints. It is associated with swelling, secretion of fluid, and usually pain. It may be degenerative (osteoarthritis) or autoimmune (rheumatoid) in nature.

ARTHRODESIS: A synonym for spinal fusion. (See "Fusion.")

AXIAL ROTATION: Twisting of the spine about the long axis of the body. (See figure 2.8.)

BEHAVIOR MODIFICATION: The utilization of one or more of a number of techniques based on learning theory and the principles of

---

* This glossary was prepared with the help of *Dorland's Medical Dictionary* and the American Academy of Orthopaedic Surgeons' *Glossary of Spinal Terminology*.

learning to effect specific changes in behavior. In this context, we want the patient's behavior (hurting and suffering) to change.

BENDING MOMENT: When a load is applied to a long structure that is not directly supported at the point of application of the load, the structure deforms, and this deformation is called bending. The bending moment is a product of the force applied times the distance between the point of application and the point of attachment of the long structure.

BIOFEEDBACK: A process whereby one or more physiological systems is monitored, usually electronically, and the information is fed back to the individual in a usable form so that he/she can learn to exercise voluntary control over the physiological system. The aim is to reduce or remove unpleasant experiences associated with bodily functions.

BONE SCAN: A scan in which an image of the bone is produced after the patient is given a radioactive material. The material then collects in the bone, with an increased concentration in areas where there is an increased blood supply to the bone. This is done by moving a detector with a sweeping beam across the area of interest. The image of the bone produced by a bone scan is an area of concentrated activity that can be developed and interpreted.

CAT SCAN (CT SCAN): A computerized tomography (an X-ray image) that can be reconstituted by a computer to depict bone and soft tissues in several planes. It provides visual slices of the material from several perspectives. One important point for readers here is that a CT scan allows a view of the spinal canal and evidence of soft-tissue encroachment by, say, a herniated disc.

CENTER OF GRAVITY: The point in a body where the body mass is centered.

CHEMONUCLEOLYSIS: A process through which biological or biochemical substances (enzymes) are placed in the intervertebral disc in order to break down the chemical substances within the disc. The enzymes chymopapain and collagenase are commonly used for this purpose.

CLIMAX: A synonym for orgasm.

CLINICAL STABILITY: The ability of the spine under physiological loads to limit patterns of displacement so as not to damage or irritate the spinal cord or nerve root and, in addition, to prevent incapacitating deformity or pain due to structural changes. This is commonly measured as excessive motion on X-rays with the patient in full flexion and full extension.

COCCYX: The structure at the very tip of the spine; the tailbone. This structure is connected to the bottom of the sacrum.

COMPENSATION-ITIS: Medical jargon for pain behavior that may be subconsciously influenced by issues of compensation and/or litigation.

COMPRESSION: The normal force that tends to push together material fibers. The unit of force is measured in newtons (N).

CONSCIOUS: That part of a person's psychological functioning of which he/she is generally aware.

DAMPING: A material property that constitutes resistance to speed.

DEGENERATION: A change of tissue from one form and function to another. Commonly used to describe changes in the intervertebral disc, which is transformed over many years from an elastic, resilient, strong structure with a jellylike center and firm periphery to a dried-out structure with a relatively inelastic, fragmented periphery. Usually in this process the disc loses some of its height. (See figures 3.1a and 3.1b.)

DEGENERATIVE DISC DISEASE: A situation in which disc degeneration produces clinical symptoms and signs.

DEGENERATIVE JOINT DISEASE OF THE ZYGAPOPHYSEAL (FACET) JOINT: Degenerative changes in the facet joints characterized by cartilage thinning and osteophyte formation. (See figure 3.6.)

DENIAL: A defense mechanism whereby the individual rejects certain aspects or interpretations of external reality. They may be replaced by unrealistic or wish-fulfilling ideation.

DEPRESSIVE NEUROSIS: An excessive reaction of depression due to an internal conflict or an identifiable event, such as the loss of a loved one or a cherished possession.

DISC DEGENERATION: The loss of the structural and functional integrity of the disc. This may or may not be a cause of pain. (See figure 3.1a.)

DISCECTOMY: The removal of all or part of the intervertebral disc.

DISC NARROWING: A situation in which a disc is degenerating. It loses its height, and the two vertebral bodies come closer together as a result of the narrowing of the disc. (See figure 3.1b.)

DISCOGRAPHY: The introduction of radiopaque fluid into the nucleus pulposus for purposes of identifying disc configuration. This may include evaluation of the amount of fluid injected or the resistance to fluid injected. Some clinicians also assess the pain response to injection of radiopaque media and/or other substances designed to either stimulate or relieve pain.

DISC SCARRING: Medical jargon for soft tissue that is sometimes seen on an X-ray to surround a nerve root in the region or at the level of a previously operated-on herniated disc.

DISPLACED DISC: A situation in which fragments of a disc move away from their normal positions. (See figure 2.6b.)

DRUG DEPENDENCE: This category is for patients who are addicted or dependent on drugs other than alcohol, tobacco, and ordinary caffeine-containing beverages. Dependence on medically prescribed drugs is also excluded, so long as the drug is medically indicated and the intake is proportionate to the medical need. This diagnosis requires evidence of habitual use or a clear sense of need for the drug.

DURA: The strongest and outermost of three membranes that protect the brain, spinal cord, and nerves of the cauda equina. (See figure 2.6b.)

ELASTICITY: The ability of a material or a structure to return to its original form following the removal of the deforming load.

ENERGY-ABSORPTION CAPACITY: The mechanical energy absorbed by a structure when loaded (pressed, bent, or twisted) to failure. The unit of measure is newton meters (foot poundforce).

EPIDEMIOLOGY: The science that concerns itself with the study of factors that influence the frequency and distribution of various human diseases within a defined community.

EQUILIBRIUM: The body is said to be in a state of equilibrium if it is at rest or in uniform motion under a given set of forces.

ERGONOMICS: The scientific and clinical study of the most healthy use of the body in a work, sports, or recreational setting.

EXERCISE, LOW-IMPACT AEROBIC: Aerobic exercise in which at least one foot must be kept on the floor at all times.

EXTENSION: Backward bending of the spine. (See figure 2.8.)

FACETECTOMY: Excision of the articular process that contains the facets of a zygapophyseal joint.

FACET JOINTS: Located behind the vertebral body, these paired joints connect the posterior elements of the vertebra. They have a slick surface and a lubricating substance, and are covered by a capsule of sinewy tissue. (See figure 2.2.)

FACET RHIZOTOMY: Denervation of a zygapophyseal joint by destruction of capsular and pericapsular tissue.

FASCIA: A sheet or band of fibrous tissue that separates various muscles and organs within the body. Analogous to files in a file cabinet, where our body is the file cabinet, the various organs and muscle groups are the individual files, and the fasciae the manila folders separating each of these files.

FATIGUE (MECHANICAL): A process of birth and growth of cracks in structures subjected to repetitive load cycles. The load is generally below the failure load of the structure.

FLEXION: Forward bending of the spine. (See figure 2.8.)

FORCE: Any action that tends to change the state of rest or motion of a body to which it is applied. The unit of measure for the magnitude of force is newtons (N).

FRACTURE: A break in the continuity of bone; a failure of the bone. There are two types of fracture. A regular fracture occurs with one particular episode of force, loading, or energy input. A fatigue fracture occurs as a result of repeated loading at a level that does not cause fracture in a single episode, but rather after repeated episodes finally cause the bone to fail.

FUNCTIONAL SPINAL UNIT: Also referred to as the motion segment. This biomechanical term is defined as two adjacent vertebrae and their intervening soft tissue.

FUSION: A process in which a bone graft either from the patient or from another human being, or from an animal, is selected, processed, and preserved, and then placed in and about the bone of a patient. The goal is to achieve a solid union between the bone graft and the bone to which it is attached. Through that coupling, the two bones are united ("welded together," like grafting a limb onto a tree). As a consequence, the region is considerably immobilized. A spinal fusion is the process by which two or more vertebrae are connected with a bone graft to reduce motion and eliminate pain. (See figure 7.11.)

HEMILAMINECTOMY: Removal of a vertebral laminae on one side only. (See figure 7.2.)

HEPATITIS: An infection and inflammation of the liver that prevents the organ from performing many of its important functions.

HERNIATED DISC: Displacement of nuclear material and other disc components beyond the normal confines of the annulus. Four degrees of displacement are recognized:

1. Intraspongy nuclear herniation.
2. Protrusion: The displaced material causes a discrete bulge in the annulus but remains connected to material persisting within the disc.
3. Extrusion: The displaced material is present in the spinal canal through disrupted fibers of the annulus but remains connected to material persisting within the disc.
4. Sequestration: Nuclear material escapes into the spinal canal as free fragments that may migrate to other locations.

HYPOCHONDRIACAL NEUROSIS: A condition dominated by preoccupation with the body and with fear of presumed diseases of various organs. Those fears are not delusional, as in psychotic depressions; they persist despite reassurance. The condition differs from hysterical neurosis in that there are no actual losses or distortions of function.

HYSTERIA: An abnormal psychological condition in which symptoms observed in the patient are due more to the dynamics of the emotions than to identifiable changes in organs or tissues.

HYSTERICAL NEUROSIS: A neurosis characterized by an involuntary psychogenic loss or disorder of function. Symptoms characteristically begin and end suddenly in emotionally charged situations and are symbolic of the underlying conflict. Often they can be modified by suggestion alone. The disorder is limited to the voluntary musculature or the organs of special sense.

HYSTERICAL NEUROSIS, CONVERSION TYPE: In the conversion type, the special senses or voluntary nervous system are affected, causing such symptoms as blindness, deafness, anosmia, anesthesia, paresthesias, paralysis, ataxias, akinesias, and dyskinesias. Often the patient shows an inappropriate lack of concern or indifference about these symptoms that may actually provide secondary gains by winning him/her sympathy or relieving him/her of unpleasant

Types of Intervertebral Disc Displacements

TERMS	DEFINITION	EXAMPLE
Bulging annulus fibrosus Intraspongy nuclear herniation Bulging disc	General extension of disc beyond boundary of adjacent vertebral body end plates	Figure 7.5
Protrusion Prolapsed disc	Distinct bulge in annulus, created by dispaced material beyond the margin of the vertebral end plate. Nuclear material may or may not have extended through the annulus. But, though herniated, it remains in continuity with the more central nuclear material.	Figure 7.5
Extrusion Extruded disc	Large displacement of a portion of the disc material into the spinal canal, with persistent connection of extruded material with the more central nucleus of the disc.	Figures 2.6a, 2.6b, 3.3, 7.2
Sequestration Free fragment	Complete displacement of nuclear material into the spinal canal with no connection to remaining disc. This sequestrated fragment may migrate to locations away from the level of the disc.	Figure 7.3 (but with fragment completely separated)

Comments: Clearly this is a spectrum of severity as one moves from the top of this chart to the bottom, there is some clinical relevance to this grouping of degrees of disc herniation. This is more cogent now that MRI technology makes it possible to identify the various types of disc displacement. Generally, the more severe the type of herniation bulge, protrusion, extrusion, or sequestration, the more severe the symptoms. All should be initially treated conservatively. Surgery will work for any of the four but should not be done for a mere bulging disc. The selection of treatment is not based on the imaging studies of the type of disc displacement but on the patient's entire clinical picture.

responsibilities. This type of hysterical neurosis must be distinguished from psychophysiologic disorders, which are mediated by the autonomic nervous system; from malingering, which is done consciously; and from neurological lesions, which cause anatomically circumscribed symptoms.

IMPOTENCE: Loss of the ability of the male to attain and maintain an erection up until the point of ejaculation.

INFERIOR ARTICULAR PROCESS: Part of the back of the vertebra, this projection articulates with a similar structure on the vertebra below. The structure also forms part of the bony spinal canal. The bony projection is partially covered with cartilage that forms part of the small paired facet joints in the back of the spine. (See figure 2.2.)

INTERNAL FIXATION: The binding together of two or more vertebrae with implants of metal and other material.

INTERVERTEBRAL DISC: An energy-absorbent structure that lies between the cylinderlike vertebral bodies in the spine. It is made up of a jellylike center and a sinewy arrangement of crossing tissues. (See figure 2.3.)

JOINT REACTION FORCE: If a joint in the body is subjected to external forces in the form of external loads and/or muscle forces, the internal reaction forces acting at the contact surfaces are called the joint reaction forces. The unit of measure is newtons (poundforce).

KINEMATICS: That division of mechanics (dynamics) that deals with the geometry of the motion of bodies—displacement, velocity, and acceleration—without taking into account the forces that produce the motion.

LAMINECTOMY: A surgical procedure in which a portion of the lamina (the platelike configuration of bone that lies posterior to the vertebral canal) is removed. (See figure 7.2.)

LAMINOTOMY: Creating an opening in one or more lamina. (See figure 7.2.)

LATERAL BENDING: Bending of the spine to either side. (See figure 2.8.)

LEVEL: This is often seen as *spinal level,* and for the purposes of this book, it would be *lumbar spinal level.* It relates to the number of the vertebra to which one is referring. There are fiver lumbar vertebra; the fifth sits on top of the sacral vertebra that is the next level down, the fourth sits on top of the fifth, the third sits on the fourth, and so on, up to the first. When people describe a herniated disc that is between the L4 and L5 level, they say it is located at the L4–L5 level. (See figure 3.4a.) Similarly, a herniated disc between L5 and S1 is said to be located at the L5–S1 level. (See figure 8.1.)

LIGAMENT: Fibrous collagenous connective tissue that connects bones to other bones.

LOAD: A general term describing the application of a force and/or moment (torque) to a structure. The units of measure are newtons (poundforce) for the force and newton meters (foot poundforce) for the moment.

LUMBAR LORDOSIS: The position of the vertebra of the lumbar spine in which the convexity of the curve as we look from the side is anterior. (See figure 8.1.)

LUMBOSACRAL SPRAIN: A ligamentous injury of the lumbosacral region. This term is imprecise but frequently used when localized pain follows a specific moderately traumatic injury.

LUMBOSACRAL STRAIN: A musculature injury of the lumbosacral region. Like the preceding term, this is imprecise and used in a similar fashion.

MALINGERING: Consciously feigning illness or pain.

MASOCHISM: A state in which pleasure is derived from suffering physiological or psychological pain. The reason is usually unconscious and has some sexual basis, either apparent or concealed.

MASS: The quantitative measure of inertia for linear motion. The unit of measure is kilograms or pounds.

MOTION: The relative displacement with time of a body to space with respect to other bodies or some reference system.

MOTION SEGMENT: A unit of the spine representing inherent biomechanical characteristics of the ligamentous spine. Two vertebrae, the intervertebral disc, and all the connecting ligaments are included in the motion segment. (See also "Functional Spinal Unit.")

MUSCLE SPASMS: Involuntarily contracted, intensely painful muscles.

MYELOGRAM: A radiologic test in which X-rays are taken after a radiopaque medium has been placed into the dural sheath with the cauda equina. This allows visualization of the spinal cord, cauda equina, and nerve roots. A water-soluble myelogram is done with a contrast medium that is absorbed by the body. A fat-soluble myelogram involves a contrast medium that is not absorbed by the body and must be removed.

NARCOTIC: A drug that tends to put one in a state of narcosis—that is, a stupor or sense of insensibility. Narcotics tend to combat pain more by causing the patient to become indifferent to it than by actually reducing the sensation of pain. Unfortunately, these drugs are clinically addictive.

NERVE ROOT: The portion of the nerve as it leaves the dural sheath goes through the foramen and out just beyond the vertebra. (See figure

2.6.) It combines with other nerve roots to form a larger nerve, such as the sciatic nerve.

NEUROLOGIC DEFICIT: Loss of a reflex, such as a knee-jerk reflex (the patella tendon in front of the knee is hit with a hammer, and the patient involuntarily kicks the leg). Loss of normal motor strength, or loss of ability to feel light touch or pain, would also be a neurological deficit.

NEUROLOGIC PROBLEM: A situation in which the patient and/or physician is aware of an abnormality due to some malfunction of the nerves. Obvious examples would be weakness, numbness, and loss of reflexes.

NUCLEUS PULPOSUS: The central gelatinlike component of the intervertebral disc. (See figure 3.4.)

OCCULT DISC: A small, sometimes overlooked, discrete disc herniation that may be difficult to diagnose and may require several different imaging studies to characterize it.

ORGANIC: Used in medical jargon to describe disease or pain that can be recognized as related to some physical abnormality in the body. This is in contradistinction to *psychosomatic,* a term that is used to describe disease or pain for which there is unlikely to be any physical explanation; the implication is that the disease or pain could have a psychological or emotional component. Such disease or pain is no less "worthy" and no less "real," however.

ORGASM: A peak of sexual excitement and/or culmination of an episode of sexual excitement.

OSTEOMALACIA: Reduction in the physical strength of bone due to its decreased mineralization.

OSTEOPENIA: Any state in which bone mass is reduced below normal.

OSTEOPOROSIS: Diminution in both the mineral and matrix components of bone. A condition in which the bone loses it strength and the various materials of which it is composed.

PARS INTERARTICULARIS: The part of the neural arch between the superior and inferior articular processes. (See figure 2.2.)

PEDICLE: A tubular bony structure that connects the vertebral body to the posterior elements. (See figure 3.5a.)

PLACEBO: A substance or procedure that is given as treatment but has no known or recognizable therapeutic effect. This is sometimes used to satisfy a patient's psychological need for medicine or treatment. More often it is used in controlled experimental studies as a standard of comparison to measure the efficacy of some drug treatment modality that is thought to be specifically useful in combating a disease or condition.

PREMATURE EJACULATION: Ejaculation that occurs prior to the time that the sexual partner has achieved satisfaction.

PSEUDOARTHROSIS: A situation in which there has been an attempt to create an arthrodesis of the spine (i.e., healing of a spinal fusion), but this has not healed in such a way that there is bone formation across the region in which the bone graft was applied. A defect in bone secondary to failure of healing of a bone.

PSYCHOLOGICAL TESTING: The employment of various standardized techniques in which an individual responds either verbally or behaviorally to various commands. The manner in which he/she responds tends to reveal significant information about him/her that is not obtained through physical examination or interview.

PSYCHOTHERAPY: The use of learning, conditioning methods, and emotional reactions in a professional relationship to assist persons to modify feelings, attitudes, and behaviors that are intellectually, socially, or emotionally maladjustive or ineffectual.

RADICULITIS: Inflammation of a spinal nerve in the spinal or neural canal.

RANGE OF MOTION: Quantities that indicate the extremes of the physiological range of translation and rotation of a joint. The units of measure are meters and degrees, respectively.

RETROLISTHESIS: Posterior displacement of a vertebra in relation to the one below.

RUPTURED DISC: See "Herniated Disc."

SACROILIAC JOINT: The connection of the sacrum to the pelvis on each side. (See figure 3.8.)

SCIATICA: The name given to a situation in which a patient complains of pain in the region of the body that is supplied by the sciatic nerve. This pain is usually in the buttock, posterior thigh, and lateral aspect of the leg and/or the foot. The most likely cause of sciatica, though certainly not the only cause, is a herniated disc. (See figures 2.6a and 2.6b.)

SCOLIOSIS: An abnormal curvature of the spine. (See figures 3.8 and 3.9.)

SECONDARY GAIN: An external situational gain derived from any illness.

SPINAL NERVE ROOT: Those neural structures (motor nerve and sensory root) that combine to form a single entity that begins at the emergence from the dura and extends to the level of the sensory ganglion, and are invested by an extension of the common dural sac. (See figure 2.6b.)

SPINAL STENOSIS: Reduction in the size of the spinal canal or regions thereof to a pathological degree. (See figure 3.3.) The classifications:

1. Congenital stenosis: malformation present at birth.
2. Developmental stenosis: malformation of genetic origin.
3. Acquired stenosis: malformation developed after birth; a lateral stenosis of the nerve canal (lateral recess entrapment).

SPINE: The midline and posteriormost portion of the vertebra, the tips of which can be felt as the line of bones just beneath the skin going down the middle of your back. Also, the entire group of articulated bones that connect to the skull and end with the coccyx. (See figure 2.1.)

SPONDYLOLYSIS: A defect in the pars interarticularis. (See figure 3.5a.)

SPONDYLOLISTHESIS: Anterior displacement of a vertebra on the adjacent vertebra below, which occurs in one of several ways. (See figure 3.5a.) The ones that are most important are described here:

1. Isthmic: Fibrous defects are present in the pars interarticularis, permitting forward displacement of the upper vertebra and separation of the anterior aspects of that vertebra from its neural arch. We think this one occurs as a birth defect.
2. Degenerative: Anterior displacement of the upper vertebra and separation of the anterior aspects of that vertebra from its neural arch. We think this one also occurs as a birth defect.
3. Traumatic: Anterior displacement of a vertebra due to traumatic injury to its restraining structures. This is what we see in a gymnast, weight lifter, or sumo wrestler.

SPONDYLOSIS: Degenerative disease of both the disc and the facet joints.

STRESS: The force per unit area of a structure and a measurement of the intensity of the force.

SUBLUXATIONS AND DISLOCATIONS: A subluxation may be defined as a partial dislocation. It is any pathological situation in which there is not a normal physiological juxtaposition of the articular surfaces of a joint. Such situations should be reliably demonstrable on an X-ray.

SUPERIOR ARTICULAR PROCESS OR SUPERIOR ARTICULAR FACET: This forms part of the facet joint, which connects it to the posterior parts of the vertebra above. (See also figure 2.2; see also "Inferior Articular Process.")

SYMPTOMS: A complaint from a patient regarding something that is wrong as perceived by the patient. This could be pain, as it commonly is, or some other bodily function that the patient perceives as abnormal, such as weakness, burning, or numbness.

TENDON: A fibrous cord that attaches a muscle to a particular bony structure or joint.

TENSION: A normal force that tends to elongate the fiber of a material. The unit of measurement is newtons (N).

TORQUE: When we twist something with a force, we apply a torque. We apply a torque when we use our steering wheel to turn a corner. When we wring out our T-shirt (after our vigorous trunk-strengthening exercises), we apply a torque.

TORSION: Same as a torque. A type of load that is applied by a couple of forces (parallel and directed opposite each other) about the long axis of a structure.

TRANSVERSE PROCESS: Winglike projection at the side of the vertebra. (See figure 2.6b.)

TRIGGER POINT: A localized area of pain or tenderness that reproduces pain symptoms on application of mechanical pressure, and that results from referred pain.

TRUNK MUSCLES: The abdominal and back muscles, including the iliopsoas. (See figure 2.4.)

UNCONSCIOUS: That part of an individual's psychological functioning of which he/she is not aware.

VERTEBRAL BODY: A large cylindrical portion of vertebra attached to the disc above and below. (See figure 2.1.)

VERTEBRAL CANAL: Sometimes called spinal canal. The tunnel that runs down the spine just behind the vertebral bodies and just in front of the vertebral arch (base of the spinous process and lamina). Above the lumbar spine (low back), the spinal cord lies in this tunnel and ends at the level of the first lumbar vertebra (L1). Below that zone in the low back, the spinal nerves run in that tunnel, and we call them the cauda equina. (See figures 2.6a and 2.6b.)

VERTEBRAL OSTEOMYELITIS: Infection in the bony structures of the spine.

X-RAY: Electromagnetic radiation that has a wavelength capable of penetrating, among other things, the human body, and providing a differential simulation on a photographic plate, giving a picture of bone and other structures within the body.

Bibliography

CHAPTER 1

General Epidemiology

Hult, L. "Cervical Dorsal and Lumbar Spine Syndromes." *Acta Orthopaedica Scandinavica* 17, supplement (1954): 1–102. (This publication provides reliable information about the natural course of the disease.)

Kelsey, J. L., and A. M. Ostfeld. "Demographic Characteristics of Persons with Acute Herniated Lumbar Intervertebral Disc." *Journal of Chronic Diseases* 28, no. 1 (1975), 37–50. (A high-quality epidemiological study done in Connecticut.)

Kelsey, J. L., and A. A. White. "Epidemiology and Impact of Low Back Pain." *Spine* 5, no. 2 (1980): 133–42. (This publication summarizes the effects of back pain on society through a review of most of the cogent epidemiological studies.)

White, A. A., and S. L. Gordon, eds. *Symposium on Idiopathic Low Back Pain.* St. Louis: C. V. Mosby Company, 1982. (This book includes several publications by world authorities on the epidemiology of back pain.)

White, A. A., and M. M. Panjabi. "The Clinical Biomechanics of Spine Pain." Chap. 6 in *Clinical Biomechanics of the Spine.* 2nd ed. Philadelphia: J. B. Lippincott, 1990. (This chapter provides an illustrated overview of the epidemiology and treatment of spine pain.)

Occupational Factors

Magora, A. "Investigation of the Relationship Between Low Back Pain and Occupation. IV. Physical Requirements: Bending, Rotation, Reaching, and Sudden Maximal Effort." *Scandinavian Journal of Rehabilitation Medicine* 5, no. 4 (1973): 186–90. (This important study showed that, among other things, back pain may be caused by a sudden unexpected exertion while carrying a heavy object.)

Rowe, M. L. "Low Back Pain in Industry: A Position Paper." *Journal of Occupa-*

tional Medicine 11, no. 4 (April 1969): 161–69. (One of the first industrial epidemiological surveys of back problems. This was a long-range study of Kodak employees in Rochester, New York, with back disability.)

———. "Low Back Pain in Industry: Updated Position." *Journal of Occupational Medicine* 13, no. 10 (October 1971): 476–78.

Westrin, C. G. "Low Back Pain Sick Listing: A Nosological and Medical Insurance Investigation." *Scandinavian Journal of Social Medicine* 7, supplement (1973): 1–116. (An enlightening and important study. For the laborer, the supervisor, and the high-level executive.)

Driving and Back Pain

Frymoyer, J. W., M. H. Pope, M. C. Costanza, M. C. Rosen, J. E. Goggin, and D. G. Wilder. "Epidemiological Studies of Low Back Pain." *Spine* 5 (1980): 419–23. (This study shows the association of back pain with driving and also with smoking.)

Kelsey, J. L., and R. J. Hardy. "Driving of Motor Vehicles as a Risk Factor for Acute Herniated Lumbar Disc." *American Journal of Epidemiology* 102 (1975): 63–73. (This was probably the first study to show the relationship between driving and back problems.)

Pope, M. H., D. G. Wilder, and J. W. Frymoyer: "Vibration as an Etiologic Factor in Low Back Pain: Engineering Aspects of the Spine." Proceedings of conference. Joint meeting of the British Orthopaedic Association and the Institute of Medical Engineering. Westminster, May 7–9, 1980.

Pregnancy

Kelsey, J. L., R. A. Greenberg, R. J. Hardy, and M. F. Johnson. "Pregnancy and the Syndrome of Herniated Lumbar Intervertebral Disc." *Yale Journal of Biology and Medicine* 48, no. 5 (November 1975): 361–68. (This is a report on part of a very large yet well-conceived epidemiological study done in Connecticut.)

CHAPTER 2

Anderson, G. B. J. "Measurements of Loads on the Lumbar Spine." *Symposium on Idiopathic Low Back Pain,* A. A. White and S. L. Gordon, eds. St. Louis: C. V. Mosby Company, 1982. (A thorough review of the forces exerted on the spine with various activities.)

Keim, H. A., and W. H. Kirkaldy. "Low Back Pain." *CIBA Clinical Symposia* 32, no. 6 (1980). Summit, NJ: Willis, 1980. (Beautifully illustrated and well-labeled color drawing by the great medical illustrator Dr. Frank Netter.)

White, A. A., and M. M. Panjabi. "Physical Properties and Functional Biomechanics of the Spine." Chap. 1 in *Clinical Biomechanics of the Spine*. 2nd ed. Philadelphia: J. B. Lippincott, 1990. (This is advanced reading for those seeking detailed data and theory, as well as in-depth knowledge of the biomechanics of the spine as it relates to back pain.)

CHAPTER 3

Aloia, J. F., S. H. Cohn, J. A. Ostuni, R. Cane, and K. Ellis. "Prevention of Involuntary Bone Loss by Exercise." *Annals of Internal Medicine* 89, no. 3 (September 1, 1978): 356–58.

Arnoldi, C. C., A. E. Brodsky, J. Cauchoix, H. V. Crock, G. F. Dommisse, M. A. Edgar, F. P. Gargano, R. E. Jacobson, W. H. Kirkaldi-Willis, A. Kurihara, et al. "Lumbar Spinal Stenosis and Nerve Root Entrapment Syndromes: Definition and Classification." *Clinical Orthopaedics and Related Research* 115 (March–April 1976): 4–5. (A clear description of the disease and all the situations that can cause it.)

Dillane, J. B., J. Fry, and G. Kalton. "Acute Low Back Syndrome: A Study from General Practice." *British Medical Journal* 2, no. 5505 (July 9, 1966): 82–84. (This study showed that a large majority of patients who presented with backache could not be diagnosed.)

Farfan, H. F., and J. D. Sullivan. "The Relation of Facet Orientation to Intervertebral Disc Failure." *Canadian Journal of Surgery* 10, no. 2 (April 1967): 179–85. (A good discussion of the associations of facet joint position and disc herniation.)

Frymoyer, J. W. "Back Pain and Sciatica." *New England Journal of Medicine* 318, no. 5 (February 4, 1988): 291–300.

Frymoyer, J. W., and S. L. Gordon. "New Perspectives on Low Back Pain." *American Academy of Orthopaedic Surgeons*, 1989. (The latest "state-of-the-art" scientific document on low back pain. A must for the reader who wants experimentally documented facts and references.)

Mankin, J. J., and R. D. Adams. "Pain in the Back and the Neck." Chap. 7 in *Harrison's Principles of Internal Medicine*. K. J. Isselbacher, R. D. Adams, E. Braunwald, R. G. Petersdorf, and J. D. Wilson, eds. New York: McGraw-Hill Book Company, 1980. (The textbook of medicine.)

Menard, D., W. D. Stanish. "The Aging Athlete." *American Journal of Sports Medicine* 17, no. 2 (March–April 1989): 187–96.

Mixter, W. J., and J. S. Barr. "Ruptures of the Intervertebral Disc with Involvement of the Spinal Canal." *New England Journal of Medicine* 211 (1934): 210–15. (This is the article that put the focus of the medical world and its surgeons on the disc as a cause of back pain.)

O'Connor, B. L. "The Vertebral Columns of Monkeys, Apes, and Men." *Symposium on Low Back Pain.* A. A. White and S. L. Gordon, eds. St. Louis: C. V. Mosby Company, 1982. (An expert on comparative anatomy reviews the problem and lays to rest the hypothesis that our backs hurt because we don't walk on all fours.)

Rockwood, C. A., and R. E. Eilert. "Camptocormia." *Journal of Bone and Joint Surgery* 51, no. 3 (April 1969): 553–56. (A good synopsis and a clear description of a very interesting hysterical disease process.)

Stadnik, T. W., R. R. Lee, H. L. Coen, E. C. Neiryuck, T. S. Buisseret, M. J. C. Osteaux. "Annular Tears and Disk Herniation: Prevalence and Contrast Enhancement on MR Images in the Absence of Low Back Pain or Sciatica." *Radiology.* 206 (1998): 49–56

Wiesel, S. W., N. Tsourmas, H. L. Feffer. "A Study of Computer Assisted Tomography. I. Incidence of Positive CAT Scans in an Asymptomatic Group of Patients." *Spine* 9 (1984): 549–51.

Wiltse, L. L. "The Etiology of Spondylolisthesis." *Journal of Bone and Joint Surgery* 57A:17, 1975. (A thorough review of most aspects of this disease.)

CHAPTER 4

Anderson, B. J. G. "A Quantitative Study of Back Loads in Lifting." *Spine* 1 (1976): 178–85. (This shows in the real world the importance of lifting objects close to the body.)

Bartelink, D. L. "The Role of Abdominal Pressure in Relieving the Pressure on the Lumbar Intervertebral Disc." *Journal of Bone and Joint Surgery.* 39-B, no. 4 (November 1957): 718–25. (Discussion of the mechanism of the protection of the spine by the abdominal muscles.)

Beals, R. K., and N. W. Hickman. "Industrial Injuries of the Back and the Extremities: Comprehensive Evaluation." *Journal of Bone and Joint Surgery* 54, no. 8 (December 1972): 1593–1611. (This gives some concrete information showing the effect of compensation factors on the problem of back pain.)

Benson, Herbert, with Miriam Z. Klipper: *The Relaxation Response.* New York: Avon Books, 1975. (A neatly and interestingly written exposition of a skill that may help not only your backache but other aspects of your life as well.)

Bergquist-Ullman, M., and U. Larsson. "Acute Back Pain in Industry: A Controlled Prospective Study with Special Reference to Therapy and Confounding Factors." *Acta Orthopaedica Scandinavica* 170, supplement (1977): 1–117. (This study demonstrates the effectiveness of the low back school.)

Bigos S., O. Bowyer, G. Braen, K. Brown, R. Deyo, S. Haldeman, J. L. Hart, E. W. Johnson, R. Keller, D. Kido, M. H. Liang, R. M. Nelson, M. Nordin, B. D. Owen, M. H. Pope. "Acute Low Back Problems in Adults." *Clinical Practice Guideline,* no. 14, AHCPR. (1994): 95–0643.

Blummer, D. "Psychiatric Considerations in Pain." Chap. 6 in *The Spine.* Vol. 2. R. H. Rothmann and F. A. Simeone, eds. Philadelphia: W. B. Saunders, 1975. (One of the most comprehensive works on the psychopathophysiological aspects of spine pain.)

Caddy, L. D., D. P. Bischoff, E. R. O'Connell, P. C. Thomas, and J. H. Allan. "Strength and Fitness and Subsequent Back Injuries in Firefighters." *Journal of Occupational Medicine* 21, no. 4 (April 1979): 269–72. (This is a well-done study showing that physical fitness helped prevent back injuries in these workers.)

Chaffin, D. B. "Human Strength Capacity and Low Back Pain." *Journal of Occupational Medicine* 16 (1974): 248–54. (This shows the possible benefits of strength testing for selection for certain jobs.)

———. "An Occupational Biomechanics of Low Back Injury." *Symposium on Idiopathic Low Back Pain.* A. A. White and S. L. Gordon, eds. St. Louis: C. V. Mosby Company, 1982. (An excellent summary of all the practical considerations of back mechanics as it relates to the worker.)

Deyo R. A. "Acute low back pain: a new paradigm for management." *BMJ* (1996): 313:1343.

Epps, Charles H. "Secondary Gain as a Factor in Results of Treatment." Chap. 8 in *Complications in Orthopaedic Surgery.* Vol. 1. Charles H. Epps, ed. Philadelphia: J. B. Lippincott, 1978. (Here we have a frank discussion of how patients, therapists, doctors, and lawyers can consciously conspire to profit from someone's back.)

Holmes, T. H., and N. Masuda. *Life Changes and Illness Susceptibility Separation and Depression.* American Association Advancement of Science publication no. 14 (1973): 161–86. (A fascinating and thoroughly documented demonstration of the relationship between the onset of life crises and disease.)

Kendall, P. H., and J. M. Jenkins. "Exercise for Backache: A Double Blind Controlled Trial." *Physiotherapy* 54 (1968): 154–57. (This study shows the value of isometric abdominal exercises.)

Melzack, R., and P. D. Wall. "Pain Mechanisms: A New Theory." *Science* 150, no. 699 (November 19, 1965): 971–79. (This, dear readers, is the classic exposition on the important gate-control theory of pain. Highly recommended for those who wish to study it in detail. Moreover, this article contains an excellent review of the literature on the pathophysiological aspects of pain.)

Mossfledt, Folke, and Mary Susan Miller. *SAS In-the-Chair Exercise Book.* New York: Bantam Books Inc., 1979. (Recommended for the frequent sitter or traveler.)

Poussaint, A. F. "Psychological/Psychiatric Factors in the Low Back Patient." *Symposium on Idiopathic Low Back Pain.* A. A. White and S. L. Gordon, eds. St. Louis: C. V. Mosby Company, 1982. (This publication gives a thorough review of the important emotional aspects of low back pain.)

Singleton, W. T. *Introduction to Ergonomics.* Geneva, Switzerland: World Health Organization, 1972. (A good synopsis and thorough explanation of ergonomics.)

Swedlow A, Johnson G, Smithline N, Milstein A. "Increased Costs and Rates of Use in the California Workers' Compensation System as a Result of Self-Referral by Physicians." *New England Journal of Medicine* 207 (1992): 1502–6.

Troup, J. D. "Relation of Lumbar Spine Disorders to Heavy Manual Work and Lifting." *Lancet* 1, no. 7390 (April 17, 1965): 857–61. (A good synopsis and excellent review of the biomechanics of lifting.)

Volinn E. "Between the Idea and the Reality: Research on Bed Rest for Uncomplicated Acute Low Back Pain and Implications for Clinical Practice Patterns." *Clinical Journal of Pain* 12 (1996): 166–70.

Waddell G., G. Feder, M. Lewis. "Systematic Reviews of Bed Rest and Advice to Stay Active for Acute Low Back Pain." *British Journal of General Practice,* no. 47 (1997): 647–52.

Zborowski, M. "Cultural Components in Responses to Pain." *Journal of Social Issues* 8, no. 4 (1952): 16–30. (This interesting work studies pain responses among patients of Jewish, Italian, and "Old American" [Anglo-Saxon] cultural origins.)

Zborowski, Mark. *People in Pain.* San Francisco: Jossey-Bass Inc., 1969. (Several intergroup statistical comparisons among individuals from Jewish, Italian, Anglo-Saxon, and Irish cultures in their responses to pain.)

CHAPTER 5

Berwick, D. M. "Continuous Improvement as an Ideal in Health Care." *New England Journal of Medicine* 320 (1989): 53–6.

Berwick, D. M. and T. W. Nolan. "Physicians as Leaders in Improving Health Care: A New Series in Annals of Internal Medicine." *Annals of Internal Medicine.* 128 (1998): 289–92.

Cherkin, D. C., R. A. Deyo, A. O. Berg. "Evaluation of a Physician Education Intervention to Improve Primary Care for Low-Back Pain. II. Impact on Patients." *Spine* 16 (1991): 1173–8.

Cherkin, D. C., R. A. Deyo, A. O. Berg, J. J. Bergman, D. M. Lishner. "Evaluation of a Physician Education Intervention to Improve Primary Care for Low-Back Pain. I. Impact on Physicians." *Spine* 16 (1991): 1168–72.

Cherkin, D. C., R. A. Deyo, J. H. Street, M. Hunt, W. Barlow. "Pitfalls of Patient Education. Limited Success of a Program for Back Pain in Primary Care." *Spine* 21 (1996): 345–55.

Cherkin, D. C., R. A. Deyo, K. Wheeler, M. A. Ciol. "Physician Views about Treating Low Back Pain. The Results of a National Survey." *Spine* 20 (1995): 1–9.

Daltroy, L. H., W. L. Cats-Baril, J. N. Katz, A. H. Fossel, M. H. Liang. "The North American Spine Society Lumbar Spine Outcome Assessment Instrument: Reliability and Validity Tests." *Spine* 21 (1996): 741–9.

Deyo, R. A, M. Battie, AJHM Beurskens, et al. "Outcome Measures for Low Back Pain Research: a Proposal for Standardized Use." *Spine* 23 (1998): 2003–13.

Deyo, R. A., A. K. Diehl, and M. Rosenthal. "How Many Days of Bed Rest for Acute Low Back Pain? A Randomized Clinical Trial." *New England Journal of Medicine* 315, no. 17 (October 23, 1986): 1064–70.

Garfin, S. R., and S. A. Pye: "Bed Design and Its Effect on Chronic Low Back Pain." *Pain* 10, no. 1 (February 1981): 87–91. (A neat, very much needed study on an immensely important topic. Probably the first and only research on an environment in which we spend approximately one-third of our time.)

Kilo, C. M. "A Framework for Collaborative Improvement: Lessons from the Institute for Healthcare Improvement's Breakthrough Series." *Quality Management in Health Care* 6 (1998): 1–13.

Kilo, C. M. "Improving Care Through Collaboration." *Pediatric* 103 (suppl) (1999): 384–93.

Langley, G. J., K. M. Nolan, T. W. Nolan, C. L. Norman, L. P. Provost. "The Improvement Guide: A Practical Approach to Enhancing Organizational Performance." San Francisco, California: Jossey-Bass Publishers; 1996.

Schroth, W. S., J. M. Schectman, E. G. Elinsky, J. C. Panagides. "Utilization of Medical Services for the Treatment of Acute Low Back Pain: Conformance with Clinical Guidelines." *Journal of General Internal Medicine* 7 (1992): 486–91.

Waddell, G. "A New Clinical Model for the Treatment of Low-Back Pain." *Spine* 12 (1987): 632–44.

Ware, J. E., C. Sherbourne. "The MOS 36-Item Short-Form Survey (SF-36). I. Conceptual Framework and Item Selection." *Medical Care* 30 (1992): 473–83.

CHAPTER 6

Bergquist-Ullman, M., and U. Larsson. "Acute Back Pain in Industry: A Controlled Prospective Study with Special Reference to Therapy and Confounding Factors." *Acta Orthopaedica Scandinavica* 170, supplement (1977): 1–117. (This justifies the back school.)

Chrisman, O. D., A. Mittnacht, and G. A. Snook. "A Study of the Results Following Rotatory Manipulation in the Lumbar Intervertebral Disc Syndrome." *Journal of Bone and Joint Surgery* 46-A, no. 3 (April 1964): 517–24. (An informative clinical study of spinal manipulative therapy.)

Crelin, E. S. "A Scientific Test of Chiropractic Theory." *American Scientist* 61, no. 5 (September–October 1973): 574–90. (Professor Crelin of Yale Medical School has been an outspoken opponent of chiropractic theory for many years. Some of his views are expressed in this publication.)

Deyo, R. "Conservative Therapy for Low Back Pain: Distinguishing Useful from Useless Therapy." *Journal of the American Medical Association (JAMA)* 250, no. 8 (August 26, 1983): 1057–62. (A milestone publication.)

Dimaggio, A., and V. Mooney: "The McKenzie Program: Exercise Effective Against Low Back Pain." *Journal of Musculoskeletal Medicine* (December 1987). (A preliminary study.)

Dimond, E. G., C. F. Kittle, and J. E. Crockett. "Comparison of Internal Mammary Artery Ligation and Sham Operation for Angina Pectoris." *American Journal of Cardiology* 5, no. 4 (April 1960): 483–86. (A fascinating and classical ethical study demonstrating some powerful placebo effects from surgery.)

Doran, D. M., and D. J. Newell. "Manipulation in Treatment of Low Back Pain: A Multicentre Study." *British Medical Journal* 2, no. 5964 (April 26, 1975): 161–64. (This is one of the studies that show quick but rapidly fading pain with manipulation.)

Fisher, E. D. "Report of a Case of Ruptured Intervertebral Disc Following Chiropractic Manipulation." *Kentucky Medical Journal* 41 (1943): 14. (This is why we discourage manipulations when you haven't had an adequate medical diagnostic evaluation.)

Glover, J. R., J. G. Morris, and T. Khosla. "Back Pain: A Randomized Clinical

Trial of Rotational Manipulation of the Trunk." *British Journal of Industrial Medicine* 31, no. 1 (January 1974): 59–64. (An important, informative, well-designed, and well-executed study.)

Goldstein, M., ed. *The Research Status of Spinal Manipulative Therapy.* HEW publication no. 76: U.S. Department of Health, Education, and Welfare, 1975. Bethesda, MD, 1975. (This publication does an excellent job of presenting a large amount of information on this topic, including several points of view. The document does not answer the question of effectiveness of spinal-manipulative therapy, nor does it resolve controversy.)

Green, D., and R. J. Joynt. "Vascular Accidents to the Brain Stem Associated with Neck Manipulation." *Journal of the American Medical Association (JAMA)* 170, no. 5 (May 30, 1959): 522–24. (This time the complication was death when an undiagnosed disease was manipulated.)

Jackson, C. P. "Physical Therapy for Lumbar Disc Disease." *Seminars in Spine Surgery* 1, no. 1 (1989): 28–34. (A cogent, concise, well-referenced, useful review.)

Judovich, B. D. "Lumbar Traction Theory: Elimination of Physical Factors That Prevent Lumbar Stretch." *Journal of the American Medical Association (JAMA)* 159, no. 6 (October 8, 1955): 549–50.

Kane, R. L., D. Olsen, C. Leymaster, F. R. Woolley, and F. D. Fisher. "Manipulating the Patient: A Comparison of the Effectiveness of Physician and Chiropractor Care." *Lancet* 1, no. 7870 (June 29, 1974): 1333–36. (This is the study demonstrating that patients responded favorably to certain personality characteristics in their therapists.)

Larsson, U., U. Choler, A. Lidstrom, G. Lind, A. Nachemson, B. Nilsson, and J. Roslund. "Auto-traction for Treatment of Lumbago-Sciatica: A Multicentre Controlled Investigation." *Acta Orthopaedica Scandinavica* 51, no. 5 (October 1980): 791–98. (This study shows the value of auto-traction treatment over that of a corset and bed rest alone.)

Maitland, G. D. *Vertebral Manipulation.* 3rd ed. London: Butterworth, 1973. (Spinal manipulation is viewed differently in various countries. This is the way the English see it.)

Mayer, T. G., R. J. Gatchel, M. Kishino, J. Keeley, P. Capra, H. Mayer, J. Barnett, and V. Mooney. "Objective Assessment of Spine Functioning Following Industrial Injury: A Prospective Study with Comparison Group and a One-Year Follow-up." *Spine* 10, no. 6 (July–August 1985): 482–93. (A milestone study in the science of low back pain rehabilitation.)

McCullough, J. A. "Chemonucleolysis: Experience with 2000 Cases." *Clinical Orthopaedics and Related Research* 146 (January–February 1980): 128–35.

(A comprehensive report of one surgeon's experience. This explains indications for and complications of the procedure.)

Nachemson, A. L. "The Natural Course of Low Back Pain." *Symposium on Idiopathic Low Back Pain*. A. A. White and S. L. Gordon, eds. St. Louis: C. V. Mosby Company, 1982. (This gives a detailed statistical account of what you can expect to happen to your back pain in a variety of different circumstances.)

Nordby, E. J., and G. L. Lucas. "A Comparative Analysis of Lumbar Disc Disease Treated by Laminectomy or Chemonucleolysis." *Clinical Orthopaedics and Related Research* 90 (January–February 1973): 119–29.

Norton, P. L., and T. Brown: "The Immobilizing Efficiency of Back Braces: Their Effect on the Posture and Motion of the Lumbosacral Spine." *Journal of Bone and Joint Surgery* 39A (January 1957): 111–39. (A good study of the assets and limitations of braces.)

Poppen, J. L. "The Herniated Intervertebral Disc: An Analysis of 400 Verified Cases." *New England Journal of Medicine* 232 (1945): 211–15. (This shows the serious complications of spinal manipulation in the patient with a herniated disc.)

Sampson, P. "Chymopapain: A Case Study in Federal Drug Regulations." *Journal of the American Medical Association (JAMA)* 240, no. 3 (July 21, 1978): 195–205. (A superb review of the question, with good illustrations.)

Stambough, J. L., R. E. Booth, and R. H. Rothman. "Transient Hypercorticism After Epidural Steroid Injection: A Case Report." *Journal of Bone and Joint Surgery* 66, no. 7 (September 1984): 1115–16. (This case is accompanied by a superb preview and summary of the complications associated with the use of epidural steroids.)

Stern, M. B., ed. "Symposium: Percutaneous Nucleotomy." *Clinical Orthopaedics and Related Research* (1989): 1–106. (This is the best synopsis of our current knowledge of this important development.)

White, A. A., and M. M. Panjabi. "The Clinical Biomechanics of Spine Pain." Chap. 6 in *Clinical Biomechanics of the Spine*. 2nd ed. Philadelphia: J. B. Lippincott, 1990. (This contains a detailed review of the various studies of spinal-manipulative therapy.)

———. "Spinal Braces: Functional Analysis and Clinical Application." Chap. 7 in *Clinical Biomechanics of the Spine*. Philadelphia: J. B. Lippincott, 1990, 2nd ed. (There's probably as much here as anyone would like to know about bracing.)

Williams, P. C. "Lesions of the Lumbosacral Spine. Part II. Chronic Traumatic

(Postural) Destruction of the Lumbosacral Intervertebral Disc." *Journal of Bone and Joint Surgery* 19 (1937): 690–703.

Position Paper on Chiropractic. The National Council Against Health Fraud, Inc.: Box 1276, Loma Linda, CA 92354 (1985).

CHAPTER 7

"End-Result Study of the Treatment of Herniated Nucleus Pulposus by Excision with Fusion and Without Fusion." *Journal of Bone and Joint Surgery* 34A, no. 4 (1952): 981–98. (Some evidence to suggest that routine fusion is not necessary with a routine disc operation.)

Finnegan, W. J., J. M. Fenlin, J. P. Marvel, R. J. Nardini, and R. H. Rothman: "Results of Surgical Intervention in the Symptomatic Multiply Operated Back Patient: Analysis of Sixty-seven Cases Followed for Three to Seven Years." *Journal of Bone and Joint Surgery* 61, no. 7 (October 1979): 1077–82. (This article demonstrates the complexity of evaluating a patient with back pain after several operations have been done.)

Flynn, J. C., and C. T. Price. "Sexual Complications of Anterior Fusion of the Lumbar Spine." *Spine* 9, no. 5 (July–August 1984): 489–92. (This study suggests that the complications of fusions from the front for low back pain, though quite rare, can be serious for the male.)

Hakelius, A. "A Prognosis in Sciatica: A Clinical Follow-up of Surgical and Nonsurgical Treatment." *Acta Orthopaedica Scandinavica* 129, supplement (1970): 1–76. (This gives some idea of outcomes in disc disease patients with and without surgery. The study is difficult to interpret, especially when one tries to apply it to an individual patient. Discuss it with your surgeon.)

McCullough, J. A. "Percutaneous Radiofrequency Lumbar Rhizolysis (Rhizotomy)." *Applied Neurophysiology* 39, no. 2 (1976–77): 87–96. (A very good explanation of the procedure and its rationale. The procedure, however, has not yet distinguished itself.)

Nachemson, A. L. "The Lumbar Spine, an Orthopaedic Challenge." *Spine* 1 (1976): 59. (Some good guidelines for expected results of disc surgery with various preoperative findings.)

Selecki, B. R., T. D. Ness, P. Limbers, P. Blum, and W. R. Stening. "Low Back Pain: A Joint Neurosurgical and Orthopaedic Project." *Medical Journal of Australia* 2, no. 19 (November 10, 1973): 889–93. (A detailed study comparing the results and frequency of surgery done by a group of orthopedic surgeons and neurosurgeons in Australia.)

Spangfort, E. V. "The Lumbar Disc Herniation: A Computer-Aided Analysis of 2,504 Operations." *Acta Orthopaedica Scandinavica* 142, supplement (1972): 1–95. (This shows how the results of disc surgery are very much related to the findings of abnormality at the time of surgery.)

Surin, V. V. "Duration of Disability Following Lumbar Disc Surgery." *Acta Orthopaedica Scandinavica* 48, no. 5 (1977): 466–71. (Some good data to help in the decision "to operate or not to operate, and when."

Weber, H. "The Effects of Delayed Disc Surgery on Muscular Paresis." *Acta Orthopaedica Scandinavica* 46 (1975): 631. (This study tells what happens to moderate leg weakness without surgery. Answer: You can get over it even without surgery.)

White, A. A., and M. M. Panjabi. "Biomechanical Consideration in the Surgical Management of the Spine." Chap. 8 in *Clinical Biomechanics of the Spine.* 2nd ed. Philadelphia: J. B. Lippincott, 1990. (This chapter includes a brief description and illustrations of virtually all the operations done on the lumbar spine.)

White, A. A., R. Voy, E. Ryan, and R. Beeten. "A Program for the Evaluation and Management of the High-Performance Athlete with Acute Low Back Pain." *Athletic Training* 23, no. 3 (Fall 1990): 228–32.

CHAPTER 8

Comfort, Alex, ed. *The Joy of Sex: A Gourmet Guide to Love Making.* New York: Crown Publishers Inc., 1972. (This book should help you to establish communication with your lover about lovemaking. There are enough options on the menu to suit the taste of just about all you good readers.)

———. *Sexual Consequences of Disability.* Philadelphia: G. F. Stickley Co., 1978. (This is a description of severe sexual disabilities. Several chapters are potentially relevant, however.)

Edwards, A., and R. E. L. Masters. *The Cradle of Erotica.* New York: The Julian Press, 1963. (A marvelous study of Afro-Asian sexual expression, certain to stimulate your imagination and feed your ingenuity.)

Frank, E., C. Anderson, and D. Rubenstein. "Frequency of Sexual Dysfunction in 'Normal' Couples." *New England Journal of Medicine* 299, no. 3 (July 20, 1978): 111–15. (This study showed that roughly half of all men and women had some problem.)

Moore, J. T., and Y. Goldstein. "Sexual Problems Among Family Medicine Patients." *Journal of Family Practice* 10, no. 2 (February 1980): 243–47. (This piece shows that even without backache, sexual problems are present in over 50 percent of couples.)

Osborne, D., and T. Maruta. "Sexual Adjustment and Chronic Back Pain." *Medi-*

cal Aspects of Human Sexuality 14 (1980): 94–113. (A good discussion of some of the problems that may relate to medications you may be taking and long-standing disability.)

CHAPTER 9

Aggragal, N. D., R. Kaur, S. Kumar, and D. N. Nathur. "A Study of Changes in the Spine in Weight Lifters and Other Athletes." *British Journal of Sports Medicine* 13, no. 2 (June 1979): 58–61. (Shows frequency of backache and describes some of the associated X-ray irregularities in the spine.)

Blyth, C. S., and F. O. Mueller. "Injury Rates Vary with Coaching: Football Injury Survey." *Physician and Sports Medicine* 2, no. 11 (1974): 45–50. (This shows that coaching can make a difference.)

Canale, S. T., E. D. Cantler, T. D. Sisk, and B. L. Freeman "A Chronicle of Injuries of an American Intercollegiate Football Team." *American Journal of Sports Medicine* 9, no. 6 (November–December 1981): 384–89. (This publication and its references give a good idea of the various injuries sustained by players on a college football team.)

DiLibero, R. J., and A. Pilmanis. "Spinal Cord Injury Resulting from Scuba Diving." *American Journal of Sports Medicine* 11, no. 1 (January–February 1983): 29–33. (This describes an unusual yet serious mechanism of back pain from scuba diving.)

Eie, N., and P. Wehn. "Measurement of the Intra-Abdominal Pressure in Relation to Weight Bearing of the Lumbar Spine." *Journal of Oslo City Hospital* 12 (1962): 205–17. (This is an interesting, informative study that would be particularly useful for the weight lifter.)

Farfan, H. F., J. W. Cossette, G. H. Robertson, R. V. Wells, and H. Kraus. "The Effects of Torsion on the Lumbar Intervertebral Joint: The Role of Torsion in the Production of Disc Degeneration." *Journal of Bone and Joint Surgery* 52, no. 3 (April 1970): 468–97. (This explains in biomechanical terms why there's so much talk about twisting.)

Harman, Bob, and Keith Monroe. *Use Your Head in Tennis.* Revised edition. New York: Thomas Y. Crowell Company, 1974. (This book will help you to enjoy your tennis so much more that you will forget your backache.)

Jackson, D. W., L. L. Wiltse, and R. J. Cirincione. "Spondylolysis in the Female Gymnast." *Clinical Orthopaedics and Related Research* 117 (June 1976): 68–73. (An excellent review of the cause and treatment of this problem.)

Lawrence, J. P., H. S. Greene, J. N. Grauer. "Back Pain in Athletes." *Journal of the American Academy of Orthopaedic Surgeons* 14, no. 13 (December 2006): 726–35.

Miller, E. H., H. J. Schneider, J. L. Bronson, and D. McLain. "A New Consideration in Athletic Injuries: The Classical Ballet Dancer." *Clinical Orthopaedics and Related Research* 111 (September 1975): 181–91. (This shows the importance to the dancer as well as the athlete of special attention in matters of backache and other clinical problems.)

Stallard, M. C. "Backache in Oarsmen." *British Journal of Sports Medicine* 14, nos. 2–3 (July 1980: 105–8. (An excellent exposition on this subject.)

White, A. A., and M. M. Panjabi. "Physical Properties and Functional Biomechanics of the Spine." Chap. 1 in *Clinical Biomechanics of the Spine*. 2nd ed. Philadelphia: J. B. Lippincott, 1990. (This contains some detailed analyses of the mechanics that cause damage to the spine.)

CHAPTER 10

Letterman, G., and M. Schurter. "The Effects of Mammary Hypertrophy [large breasts] on the Skeletal System." *Annals of Plastic Surgery* 5, no. 6 (December 1980): 425–31.

Mendelson, G., T. S. Selwood, H. Kranz, T. S. Loh, M. A. Kidson, and D. S. Scott. "Acupuncture Treatment of Chronic Back Pain: A Double-Blind Placebo-Controlled Trial." *American Journal of Medicine* 74, no. 1 (January 1983): 49–55.

Spitzer, W. O., F. E. LeBlanc, and M. Dupuis, et al. "Scientific Approach to the Assessment and Management of Activity-Related Spinal Disorders." *Spine* 12, supplement (September 1987): S1–S9. (A milestone publication on the clinical care of spine problems. Cuts through all the bs [bold speculation].)

CHAPTER 11

Basbaum A. I., and H. L. Fields. "Endogenous Pain Control Systems: Brainstem Spinal Pathways and Endorphin Circuitry." *Annual Review of Neuroscience,* vol. 7 (March 1984): 309–338.

Boden, S. D., D. O. Davis, T. S. Dina, N. J. Patronas, and S. W. Wiesel. "Abnormal Magnetic-Resonance Scans of the Lumbar Spine in Asymptomatic Subjects: a Prospective Investigation." *Journal of Bone and Joint Surgery,* 72A: 403–8, 1990.

Casey, K. L. "The Imaging of Pain: Background and Rationale, in Pain Imaging: Progress in Pain Research and Management." *IASP Press,* no.18 (2000): 1–29.

Chaffin, D. B., and J. A. Ashton-Miller. "Biomechanical Aspects of Low Back Pain in the Older Worker." *Experimental Aging Research,* 17(3) (1991): 177–188.

Chaffin, D. B., G. B. J. Andersson and B. J. Martin. "Occupational Biomechanics" (4th Edition) New York: J. Wiley & Sons; 2006.

Eisenberg, R. L., M. W. Hedgcock, E. A. Williams, et al. "Optimum Radiographic Examination for Consideration of Compensation Awards: II. Cervical and Lumbar Spines." *American Journal of Radiology* 135 (1980): 1071–4.

Eisenberg, R. L., J. R. Akin, M. W. Hedgcock. "Single, Well-centered Lateral View of Lumbosacral Spine: Is Coned View Necessary?" *American Journal of Radiology* 133 (1979): 711–3.

Frymoyer, J. W., and Gordon S. L., eds. "New Perspectives on Low Back Pain" *American Academy of Orthopaedic Surgeons"* (1989): 1–406.

Gehweiler J. A., and R. H. Daffner. "Low Back Pain: The Controversy of Radiologic Evaluation." *American Journal Radiology* 140 (1983): 109–12.

Rhea, J. T., S. A. DeLuca, H. J. Llewellyn, R. J. Boyd. "The Oblique View: An Unnecessary Component of the Initial Adult Lumbar Spine Examination" *Radiology* 134 (1980): 45–7.

Scavone, J. G., R. F. Latshaw, W. A. Weidner. "Anteroposterior and Lateral Radiographs: An Adequate Lumbar Spine Examination." *American Journal Radiology* 136 (1981): 715–7.

Snook, S. H. "The Costs of Back Pain in Industry." *Occupational Medicine* (Jan.-March 1988) 3(1):1–5.

White, Augustus A. III DrMedSci, Stephen L. Gordon Phd. "Synopsis: Workshop on Idiopathic Low-Back Pain Spine." (March/April 1982), volume 7, issue 2: 141–149.

GLOSSARY

Dorland's Illustrated Medical Dictionary. 25th ed. Philadelphia: W. B. Saunders Company, 1974.

Glossary of Spinal Terminology. Park Ridge, IL: American Academy of Orthopaedic Surgeons, 1985

Masayk, T. J., J. S. Ross, M. T. Modic, F. Boumphrey, H. Bohlman, and G. Wilber. "High-Resolution MR Imaging of Sequestrated Lumbar Intervertebral Discs." *American Journal of Neuroradiology* 9 (1988): 351.

Standard for Surgical Bone Banking. Arlington, VA: American Association of Tissue Banks, 1987. (Revision to standards, effective January 15, 1988, section C1.330.)

Arden, N. K., C. Price, I. Reading, J. Stubbing, J. Hazelgrove, C. Dunne, M. Michel, P. Rogers, and C. Cooper. "A Multicentre Randomized Controlled Trial of Epidural Corticosteroid Injections for Sciatica: The WEST Study." *Rheumatology* 44, no. 11 (November 2005): 1399–1406.

Biyani A, and G. B. Andersson. "Low Back Pain: Pathophysiology and Management." *Journal of the American Academy of Orthopaedic Surgeons* 12, no. 2 (March–April 2004): 106–15.

Blau, L. A., and J. D. Hoehns. "Analgesic Efficacy of Calcitonin for Vertebral Fracture Pain." *Annals of Pharmacotherapy* 37, no. 4 (April 2003): 564–70.

Brown, M. D., and A. D. Levi. "Surgery for Lumbar Disc Herniation During Pregnancy." *Spine* 26, no. 4 (February 15, 2001): 440–43.

Carey, T. S., J. Garrett, A. Jackman, C. McLaughlin, J. Fryer, and D. R. Smucker. "The Outcomes and Costs of Care for Acute Low Back Pain Among Patients Seen by Primary Care Practitioners, Chiropractors, and Orthopedic Surgeons: The North Carolina Back Pain Project." *New England Journal of Medicine* 333, no. 14 (October 5, 1995): 913–17.

Cherkin, D. C., Y. A. Dayo, M. Battié, J. Street, W. Barlow. "A Comparison of Physical Therapy, Chiropractic Manipulation, and Provision of an Educational Booklet for the Treatment of Patients with Low Back Pain." *New England Journal of Medicine* 339, no. 15 (October 8, 1998): 1021–29.

Chou, R., and L. H. Huffman. "Nonpharmacologic Therapies for Acute and Chronic Low Back Pain: A Review of the Evidence for an American Pain Society/American College of Physicians Clinical Practice Guideline." *Annals of Internal Medicine* 147, no. 7 (October 2, 2007): 492–504.

Chou, R., A. Qaseem, V. Snow, D. Casey, J. T. Cross Jr., P. Shekelle, and D. K. Owens. "Diagnosis and Treatment of Low Back Pain: A Joint Clinical Practice Guideline from the American College of Physicians and the American Pain Society." *Annals of Internal Medicine* 147, no. 7 (October 2, 2007): 478–91.

Cooney III, William P. "Evidence-Based Medicine." *Journal of the American Academy of Orthopaedic Surgeons* 13, no. 4 (July–August 2005): 219.

Davidson, Dan. "Commitment to Injury Reduction Programs Paying Off for USPS." FederalTimes.com, September 7, 2006.

Deyo, R. A., D. C. Cherkin, J. Weinstein, J. Howe, M. Ciol, and A. G. Mulley Jr. "Involving Patients in Clinical Decisions: Impact of an Interactive Video Program on Use of Back Surgery." *Medical Care* 38, no. 9 (September 2000): 959–69.

Deyo, R. A., J. Rainville, and D. L. Kent. "What Can the History and Physical Exam Tell Us About Low Back Pain?" *Journal of the American Medical Association (JAMA)* 268, no. 6 (August 12, 1992): 760–65.

Einhorn, T. A., and C. A. Lee. "Bone Regeneration: New Findings and Potential Clinical Applications." *Journal of the American Academy of Orthopaedic Surgeons* 9, no. 3 (May–June 2001): 157–65.

French, S. D., M. Cameron, B. F. Walker, J. W. Reggars, and A. J. Esterman. "A Cochrane Review of Superficial Heat or Cold for Low Back Pain." *Spine* 31, no. 9 (April 20, 2006): 998–1006.

Furlan, A. D., L. Brosseau, M. Imamura, and E. Irvin. "Massage for Low-Back Pain: A Systematic Review Within the Framework of the Cochrane Collaboration Review Group." *Spine* 27, no. 17 (September 1, 2002): 1896–1910.

Furlan, A. D., M. van Tulder, D. Cherkin, H. Tsukayama, L. Lao, B. Koes, and B. Beman. "Acupuncture and Dry-Needling for Low Back Pain: An Updated Systematic Review Within the Framework of the Cochrane Collaboration." *Spine* 30, no. 8 (April 15, 2005): 944–63.

Gitelis, S., R. M. Wilkins, and A. W. Yasko. "BMPs and Cancer: Is the Risk Real?" *AAOS Now* 2, no. 5 (May 2008): www.aaos.org/news/aaosnow/may08/research7.asp.

Gordon, G. A. "Molecular Basis for Low Back Pain in Western Industrialized Cultures." *Medical Hypotheses* 33, no. 4 (December 1990): 251–56.

Greenhalgh, Trisha. *How to Read a Paper: The Basis of Evidence-Based Medicine.* 2nd ed. London: BMJ Publishing Group, 2001.

Grundy, P. F., and C. J. Roberts. "Does Unequal Leg Length Cause Back Pain? A Case-Control Study." *Lancet* 2, no. 8397 (August 4, 1984): 256–58.

Guidelines: Occupational Health Physical Therapy: Work Conditioning and Work Hardening Programs BOD G03-01-17-58 (Program 32). Alexandria, VA: American Physical Therapy Association.

Guyer, R. D., M. Patterson, and D. D. Ohnmeiss. "Failed Back Surgery Syndrome: Diagnostic Evaluation." *Journal of the American Academy of Orthopaedic Surgeons* 14, no. 9 (September 2006): 534–43.

Hagen, K. B., G. Hilde, G. Jamtvedt, and M. Winnem. "The Cochrane Review of Advice to Stay Active as a Single Treatment for Low Back Pain." *Spine* 27, no. 16 (August 15, 2002): 1736–41.

Hagen, K. B., G. Jamtvedt, G. Hilde, and M. Winnem. "The Updated Cochrane Review of Bedrest for Low Back Pain and Sciatica." *Spine* 30, no. 5 (March 1, 2005): 542–46.

Heymans, M. W., M. W. van Tulder, R. Esmail, C. Bombardier, and B. W. Koes. "Back Schools for Nonspecific Low Back Pain: A Systematic Review Within the Framework of the Cochrane Collaboration Back Review Group." *Spine* 30, no. 19 (October 1, 2005): 2153–63.

Hodges, S. D., J. C. Eck, and S. C. Humphreys. "Use of Electrical Bone Stimulation in Spinal Fusion." *Journal of the American Academy of Orthopaedic Surgeons* 11, no. 2 (March–April 2003): 81–88.

Hoikka, V., M. Ylikoski, and K. Tallroth. "Leg-Length Inequality Has Poor Correlation with Lumbar Scoliosis: A Radiological Study of 100 Patients with Chronic Low Back Pain." *Archives of Orthopaedic and Trauma Surgery* 108, no. 3 (1989): 173–79.

Hubert, M. G., G. Vadala, G. Sowa, R. K. Studer, and J. D. Kang. "Gene Therapy for the Treatment of Degenerative Disk Disease." *Journal of the American Academy of Orthopaedic Surgeons* 16, no. 6 (June 2008): 312–19.

Kim, D. H., and T. J. Albert. "Interspinous Process Spacers." *Journal of the American Academy of Orthopaedic Surgeons* 15, no. 4 (April 2007): 200–7.

Jellema, P., M. W. van Tulder, M. N. van Poppel, A. L. Nachemson, and L. M. Bouter. "Lumbar Supports for Prevention and Treatment of Low Back Pain: A Systematic Review Within the Framework of the Cochrane Back Review Group." *Spine* 26, no. 4 (February 15, 2001): 337–86.

Lagarrigue, J., and P. Chaynes. "Comparative Study of Disc Surgery With or Without Microsurgery: A Prospective Study of 80 Cases." *Neurochirurgie* 40, no. 2 (1994): 116–20.

Laurencin C. T., and S. F. El-Amin. "Xenotransplantation in Orthopaedic Surgery." *Journal of the American Academy of Orthopaedic Surgeons* 16, no. 1 (January 2008): 4–8.

Lin, E. L, and J. C. Wang. "Total Disk Arthroplasty." *Journal of the American Academy of Orthopaedic Surgeons* 14, no. 13 (December 2006): 705–17.

Mackowiak, Philip A. *Post Mortem: Solving History's Great Medical Mysteries.* Philadelphia: American College of Physicians (ACP) Press, 2007, and American Medical News, *Post Mortem* 50, no. 30 (August 13, 2007).

Majid, K., and J. S. Fischgrund. "Degenerative Lumbar Spondylolisthesis: Trends in Management." *Journal of the American Academy of Orthopaedic Surgeons* 16, no. 4 (April 2008): 208–15.

Mathews, H. H., and B. H. Long. "Minimally Invasive Techniques for the Treatment of Intervertebral Disk Herniation." *Journal of the American Academy of Orthopaedic Surgeons* 10, no. 2 (March–April 2002): 80–85.

Mauritis W., M. W. van Tulder, Raymond Ostelo, Johan Vlaeyen, Steven J. Linton, Stephen J. Morely, and Willem Assendelft. *Spine* 26, no. 3 (2000): 270–81.

Nachemson, Alf, and Egon Jonsson. *Neck and Back Pain: The Scientific Evidence of Causes, Diagnosis, and Treatment.* Philadelphia: Lippincott Williams & Wilkins, 2000.

Niemistö, L., E. Kalso, A. Malmivaara, S. Seitsalo, and H. Hurri. "Radiofrequency Denervation for Neck and Back Pain: A Systematic Review Within the Framework of the Cochrane Collaboration Back Review Group." *Spine* 28, no. 16 (August 15, 2003): 1877–88.

Norris, M. "Study: Surgery Just One Option for Herniated Disk. *All Things Considered,* NPR, November 21, 2006.

Phillips, W. J., and B. L. Currier. "Analgesic Pharmacology I: Neurophysiology." *Journal of the American Academy of Orthopaedic Surgeons* 12, no. 4 (July–August 2004): 213–20.

Pneumaticos, S. G., C. A. Reitman, and R. W. Lindsey. "Discography in the Evaluation of Low Back Pain." *Journal of the American Academy of Orthopaedic Surgeons* 14, no. 1 (January 2006): 46–55.

"Public Health Advisory: Update on Magnetic Resonance Imaging (MRI) Contrast Agents Containing Gadolinium and Nephrogenic Fibrosing Dermopathy." U.S. Food and Drug Administration, 2006. www.fda.gov/CDER/drug/advisory/gadolinium_agents_20061222.htm.

Roelofs, P. D., R. A. Deyo, B. W. Koes, R. J. Scholten, and M. W. van Tulder. "Nonsteroidal Anti-inflammatory Drugs for Low Back Pain." *Spine* 33, no. 16 (July 15, 2008): 1766–74.

Sackett, D. L., W. M. Rosenberg, J. A. Gray, R. B. Haynes, and W. S. Richardson. "Evidence-Based Medicine: What It Is and What It Isn't." *BMJ* 312, no. 7032 (January 13, 1996): 71–72.

Sapico, F. L., and J. Z. Montgomerie. "Vertebral Osteomyelitis." *Infectious Disease Clinics of North America* 4, no. 3 (September 1990): 539–50.

Shen, F. S., D. Samartzis, and G. B. Andersson. "Nonsurgical Management of Acute and Chronic Low Back Pain." *Journal of the American Academy of Orthopaedic Surgeons* 14, no. 8 (August 2006): 477–87.

Smedley, Brian D., Adrienne Y. Stith, and Alan R. Nelson, eds. *Unequal Treatment: Confronting Racial and Ethnic Disparities in Healthcare.* Washington, DC: National Academies Press, 2003.

Sneag, D. B., and J. A. Bendo. "Pregnancy-Related Low Back Pain." *Orthopedics* 30, no. 10 (October 2007): 839–45.

Soehle, M., and T. Wallenfang. "Spinal Epidural Abscesses: Clinical Manifestations, Prognostic Factors, and Outcomes." *Neurosurgery* 51, no. 1 (July 2002): 79–85.

Spindler, K. P., J. E. Kuhn, W. Dunn, C. E. Matthews, F. E. Harrell Jr., and R. S. Dittus. "Reading and Reviewing the Orthopaedic Literature: A Systematic, Evidence-Based Medicine Approach." *Journal of the American Academy of Orthopaedic Surgeons* 13, no. 4 (July–August 2005): 220–29.

Spivak, J. M., and M. G. Johnson. "Percutaneous Treatment of Vertebral Body Pathology." *Journal of the American Academy of Orthopaedic Surgeons* 13, no. 1 (January–February 2005): 6–17.

Swenson, R., and S. Haldeman. "Spinal Manipulative Therapy for Low Back Pain." *Journal of the American Academy of Orthopaedic Surgeons* 11, no. 4 (July–August 2003): 228–37.

Tullberg, T., J. Isaacson, and L. Weidenhielm. "Does Microscopic Removal of Disc Herniation Lead to Better Results Than the Standard Procedure? Results of a One-Year Randomized Study." *Spine* 18, no. 1 (September 1, 1993): 24–27.

Van Tulder, M. W., T. Touray, A. D. Furlan, S. Solway, and L. M. Bouter. "Muscle Relaxants for Nonspecific Low Back Pain: A Systematic Review Within the Framework of the Cochrane Collaboration." *Spine* 29, no. 17 (September 1, 2003): 1978–92.

Vogt, M. T., D. A. Rubin, L. Palermo, L. Christianson, J. D. Kang, M. C. Nevitt, and J. A. Cauley. "Lumbar Spine Listhesis in Older African American Women. *Spine Journal* 3, no. 4 (July 2003): 255–61.

Weber, H. "Disc Herniation: A Controlled, Prospective Study with Ten Years of Observation." *Lumbar Spine* 8, no. 2 (March 1983): 131–40.

Weinstein, J. N., T. D. Tosteson, J. D. Lurie, A. N. Tosteson, B. Hanscom, J. S. Skinner, W. A. Abdu, A. S. Hilibrand, S. D. Boden, and R. A. Deyo. "Surgical vs. Nonoperative Treatment for Lumbar Disk Herniation: The Spine Patient Outcomes Research Trial (SPORT): Randomized Trial." *Journal of the American Medical Association (JAMA)* 296, no. 20 (November 22/29, 2006): 2441–50.

Wetzel, F. T., and T. A. McNally. "Treatment of Chronic Low Back Pain with Intradiskal Electrothermal Therapy." *Journal of the American Academy of Orthopaedic Surgeons* 11, no. 1 (January–February 2003): 6–11.

Wilson J. D., C. P. Dougherty, M. L. Ireland, and I. M. Davis. "Core Stability and Its Relationship to Lower Extremity Function and Injury." *Journal of the American Academy of Orthopaedic Surgeons* 13, no. 5 (September 2005): 315–25.

Young, I. A., G. S. Hyman, L. N. Packia-Raj, and A. J. Cole. "The Use of Lumbar Epidural/Transforaminal Steroids for Managing Spinal Disease. *Journal of the American Academy of Orthopaedic Surgeons* 15, no. 4 (April 2007): 228–38.

Zlotolow, D. A., A. R. Vaccaro, M. L. Salamon, and T. J. Albert. "The Role of Human Bone Morphogenetic Proteins in Spinal Fusion." *Journal of the American Academy of Orthopaedic Surgeons* 8, no. 1 (January–February 2000): 3–9.

Rheumatoid Arthritis. The Johns Hopkins Arthritis Center. www.hopkins-arthritis.org.

Index

Note: Page numbers in *italics* refer to illustrations.